...with liberty and sickness for all.

The toxins in our food, our environment, and our minds...

An in-depth look at toxic food additives and GMOs, and their
contribution to cancer and other diseases and disorders

JOHN Y. KAMIN

...with liberty and sickness for all.
The toxins in our food, our environment, and our minds...
An in-depth look at toxic food additives and GMOs, and their contribution to cancer and other diseases and disorders

Copyright © 2017 by John Y. Kamin

DISCLAIMERS: The author of this book is not a medical professional. This book is not intended as a substitute for the medical advice of physicians. The reader should regularly consult a physician in matters relating to his/her health and particularly with respect to any symptoms that may require diagnosis or medical attention.

Whenever possible, when a reference is made to an external source, several methods are provided for finding the source, such as the name of the author(s), the name of the article or study, a digital object identifier (doi) or PubMed ID (PMID) number. In most cases, an internet address will also be provided when one is available. Neither the author nor the publisher assume responsibility for errors in internet addresses or for changes in the addresses, nor are they responsible for the contents of websites they do not own.

Trademark Acknowledgements:
Roundup® and Roundup Ready® are registered trademarks of Monsanto Company.
Flavr Savr™ is a registered trademark of Calgene and Monsanto Company.
Arctic® apples is a registered trademark of Okanagan Specifalty Fruits Inc.

Cover illustration by Anton Rosovsky

DEDICATION

This book is dedicated to my beautiful wife Naya, for without her, I would have not been on the path of learning about this subject matter, and would have not written this book.

"One cannot resist an idea whose time has come"

Victor Hugo

CONTENTS

FOREWORD

STEPHANIE SENEFF

America faces a crisis today with a looming healthcare burden that will bankrupt the country if the escalating costs continue unabated. Nobody in the media seems to be willing to ask the obvious question: why is healthcare so much more expensive in America than everywhere else in the world? To me, the answer is obvious: toxic food and toxic drugs. In short, we in the United States are, collectively, much sicker than everybody else, and the reason is that our processed food industry has played a leadership role in promoting the development of essentially synthetic foods with severe nutritional deficiencies assembled with a multitude of toxic chemicals, added either intentionally or unintentionally. Food dyes, artificial sweeteners, processed sugars, preservatives, taste enhancers, synthetic flavors, emulsifiers, the list goes on and on. And, in my opinion, the worst offenders, the most damaging disruptors of body chemistry, are the pesticides that are routinely used in agriculture to enable the production of massive amounts of core food crops efficiently and cheaply on huge agricultural fields, with very little labor. Herbicides, insecticides, and fungicides are all "biocides," as indicated by the suffix "cide." They kill life.

I have heard that, in terms of percent of income spent on food, the United States spends less than any other nation. This is not a bargain, because I suspect that we spend far more treating illness than we gain by eating cheap food. And being sick is not fun! Especially neurologically debilitating diseases like Alzheimer's and autism. We are losing the "war on cancer" initiated by Richard Nixon in 1971. As each country, one by one, starts to adopt a Western diet, their population begins to grow fat and diabetes becomes an epidemic. Today, over half of children in the United States suffer from one or more debilitating autoimmune or neurological disease, such as type I diabetes, gastroesophageal reflux disease (GERD), inflammatory bowel disease, fatty liver, obesity, eczema, asthma, seizures, attention deficit hyperactivity disorder (ADHD), autism, depression, Tourette syndrome, etc. Formerly rare illnesses like chronic fatigue syndrome, fibromyalgia, eosinophilic esophagitis, Lyme disease, Celiac disease, lupus, Morgellons and antiphospholipid syndrome are now becoming household words. We face a crisis from an opioid overdose epidemic that is probably due in large part to the fact that so many people need opioid drugs just to be able to endure the pain and suffering of chronic inflammatory diseases.

There is a way out of this mess, and the very good news is that this book provides answers. John Kamin and his wife had a wake-up call when his wife was diagnosed with cancer, and a visit to the shiny new oncology center revealed a sinister backdrop of a medical system gone awry. The doctor offered a depressing surgical option, involving the removal of multiple organs. Courageously, they opted out of everything the oncologist recommended, and they chose a natural treatment protocol that led eventually to a resolution of the cancer with welcomed beneficial side effects that improved her quality of life.

This book describes their personal story in lively and entertaining prose, and then provides a wealth of information on the dangers of all the additives in our processed foods, a historical perspective on the development of genetically modified foods and the associated pesticides, and, most importantly, the new methods that are being developed to restore the soil to good health and to find ways to grow foods economically without the use of chemicals. Furthermore, the book details the multitude of nasty side effects associated with traditional cancer treatment methods, and provides priceless information about natural ways to treat cancer, by taking advantage of the healing properties of medicinal foods, herbs and spices such as reishi mushrooms, ginger, turmeric, cardamom, dandelions, milk thistle, artichokes, and cannabis.

I was pleased to see that glyphosate, the active ingredient in the pervasive herbicide, Roundup, was recognized by John Kamin as one of the significant toxic chemicals in food. I believe that glyphosate is the most egregious example of what is wrong with our food supply. Because we have been led to believe that it is essentially harmless to humans, we make little effort even to monitor how much is in our food. The approval process that took place back in the 1970's was fraught with fraud, and only now are we being made aware of its carcinogenic potential. As I write this, there is hope that Europe might phase out glyphosate usage in agriculture, finally wising up to its true colors. The development of GMOs that are resistant to glyphosate led to exponential growth in the use of Roundup on crops, because glyphosate-resistant weeds began to appear among the glyphosate-resistant crops. Today, the industry faces a crisis as Roundup no longer controls the weeds. They are now forced to introduce new GMOs that are resistant to other toxic herbicides such as 2,4-D, a component of agent orange, and dicamba, which has caused numerous lawsuits among farmers in the Midwest due to its tendency to drift into the neighbor's crop that is not genetically engineered to resist it. At the same time that chemical-based agriculture is crumbling, consumer demand for sustainable organic food production is growing exponentially, and this gives us hope that we all will eventually recognize that consuming wholesome organic food is the most important formula for a long and healthy life.

By buying off the regulators, the industry has kept us in the dark on the degree to which we are being poisoned every day, by our food, our pharmaceutical drugs and our vaccines. This book offers practical solutions through wholesome food and Eastern medicine, and a way forward that can give us hope for a future time when humans are stewards of the earth.

> — *Dr. Stephanie Seneff, PhD, Senior Research Scientist*
> *MIT Computer Science and Artificial Intelligence*
> *Laboratory*

PREFACE

The day was Thursday; May 23, 2013. It started like any other day, but soon, everything changed. That day my wife was diagnosed with cancer. However, having grown up exposed to knowledge of alternative medicine, and having been let down again and again by western medicine, we had already at that point in our lives known the limitation and prejudices of modern medicine, and were aware of the amazing wealth of knowledge that was passed down through the ages for curing all sorts of ailments, including ones that modern medicine had determined to be incurable. By the time we were scheduled for a consultation with the oncologist, we had already done extensive research, zeroed in on a plan for natural treatment, and had already begun treatment. During the visit to the oncologist, even though the cancer was detected fairly early, the oncologist was pushing my wife to have surgery to remove several of her organs. Of course, no surprise, both my wife and I said hell no and told the doctor that we will be continuing with the natural path that we were on, which angered him quite a bit, I might add. "Well, I cannot condone that" he said angrily.

Just to paint a pretty picture in your mind, the oncology center that we had visited was not like any other healthcare facility. It was large, with lots of wide open spaces, quite beautiful and lavish, with hardwood and marble all over the place. It was immediately obvious what cancer pays for and why there is no will by the cancer industry to find a cure (as opposed to perpetual treatments) for cancer or admit that there are already cures for most, if not all the types of cancer out there. After all, if they did, they would all be out of a job overnight. According to the National Cancer Institute, cancer research has been going on for 250 years. Isn't it interesting that in that time frame cancer has exploded in numbers, rather than decline? Is that simply a case of incompetence, or is it by design?

My wife continued with her course of natural treatment, and today she is cancer free. She did not have to go through nauseating, toxic chemotherapy treatments, or devastating radiation therapy. She did not have a single incision made to her body and she did not lose a single hair (with the exception of normal hair shedding of course). She did however have several side effects as a result of her treatment. Not the conventional type of side effects that you might expect from taking conventional medications, such as constipation, incontinence, nose bleeds, stroke, coma, or death, etc., etc., but rather, her side effects were inadvertently curing other life-long conditions that she had. Not only was the cancer gone, but for the first time in her life, she was also free of other conditions that had plagued her for decades.

We had learned so much as a result of this event that you might say it was a blessing. We are both now the healthiest we have been since childhood.

It is not my intent for this book to sound like an attack on modern medicine or any particular industry. It is meant to bring to light the wrongs that are being done by those systems and hopefully change the status quo. It is also meant to open the reader's eyes and to hopefully encourage people to do their own research and explore alternatives; to seek out the truth and true causes of things rather than focusing on symptoms and "killing the messenger over the message". The mission statement of the medical industry is to control and dominate, rather than to promote health. The mission statement of the medical and food industries alike <u>should be</u> to understand the natural functioning of the body and allow it to heal itself through proper nutrition, both for the body and mind. Because the body cannot function properly with a sick mind, and the mind cannot function properly with a sick body. In today's day and age, with the internet at your fingertips, there is no excuse for not knowing. All it takes is the will to look, and a little bit of knowledge of how and where to look, and more importantly, where not to look.

In some cases when I present references in this book, I will provide several or many studies as supporting evidence. But in some cases, the evidence is scant, but nevertheless sufficiently alarming to justify precaution. Replication studies - those attempting to replicate the results of a prior study, are critical for determining a scientific truth. Unfortunately, in today's age of grabbing headlines, and the fact that replication studies will not get you a Nobel Prize or grant money; replication studies are rarely performed. The problem is, replication is the hallmark of scientific truth, and without replication, nothing can be known with a high degree of certainty.

To compound the issue, in many fields, such as toxicology, holistic cancer research, and other fields affecting mega-industries, when a researcher comes out with results that are seen as threatening to the industry, whether they are true or not, the industry immediately sets out to discredit, defame, and destroy the scientists involved[1,2,3,4,5,6,7]. The result is that scientists are afraid to perform research in certain areas, or they design their studies to make their results look favorable for the industry in order to gain financially. Consequently, the public is left with one simple principle to rely on, and that is the precautionary principle. That is to say, if a study shows adverse effects to health from a certain substance, whether or not it was replicated, precaution should be taken on the part of the consumer, to reduce or eliminate exposure to said substance. It is a small sacrifice for me to not eat, or greatly reduce my consumption of processed foods that contain chemicals which have been shown in one or a few studies to be toxic, in exchange for a greatly reduced risk of being chronically ill later in life. For example, many studies have shown that vegetarian and vegans have a lower incidence of cancers, by a wide margin, and lower incidences of other diseases than non-vegetarians/vegans[8,9,10]. Many studies over several decades have linked many food colorings to cancers and other disorders, but nevertheless those colorings are still approved by the FDA and are still being used. So I don't eat foods containing dies, and I limit my intake of animal products as much as possible. Keep in mind that being vegan does not only mean not eating animal products, but it also means not being exposed to chemicals and hormones that are used in farming, processing, preservation, and preparation of animal products, which is a very long list of substances, of which many have been proven to be carcinogenic, and otherwise toxic.

Additionally, many studies are performed on rats and other animals, or human cells in petri dishes. In some instances, there is no direct correlation between humans and animals, or the effects on individual cells and the effects of ingesting a certain substance, however, those results are nevertheless relevant for the stage of testing at which they are performed. Furthermore, some studies cannot be performed on human beings for ethical reasons, such as studies testing for carcinogenicity, genotoxicity, mutagenicity and others. In those instances, lab tests on animals or human cells are the only lab tests that can be had, and outside of that, epidemiological studies are the only studies that are specifically relevant to human beings, but are not always feasible, such as in the case of newly created or newly discovered substances of which not much is known.

It is also worth mentioning that while correlation is not causation, there can be no causation without correlation, and when a correlation is claimed that seems plausible, the first response should not be dismissal, but investigation – especially when health and safety is involved.

Buckminster Fuller said "You never change things by fighting the existing reality. To change something, build a new model that makes the existing model obsolete."

It is my goal to raise enough funds from sales of this book to start organic neighborhood farms all over the United States that will offer people an alternative to the status quo, create good jobs and raise awareness of the importance of healthy, toxin-free whole foods.

ABOUT THE TITLE

The title of the book – "…with liberty and sickness for all" is a twist on the ending of The Pledge of Allegiance – "…with liberty and justice for all".

The reason that I picked this title is because it illustrates precisely the state of affairs in the United States today. As citizens, we have a choice about what we eat, when we eat it, how much of it we eat and so on. Corporations as well have significant liberties over what chemicals they put in our foods, and even in determining whether or not those chemicals are safe (whether or not they are telling the truth).

Additionally, I had replaced "and justice for all" with "and sickness for all" for two very specific reasons. The first reason is, our justice system has been hijacked by multinational corporations in favor of unhindered economic wealth. The second reason is, their economic wealth is usually at the expense of human and environmental health.

In such a system, liberty and justice are neither of those things at all – it is only the illusion of liberty and justice. When nearly the entire food supply is full of toxins, having a choice to pick what we buy is akin to a prisoner on death row having a choice as to the method of execution. No matter what he chooses, the end result will be the same. In many cases we don't have a choice at all, such as with the roll-out of the smart grid, which according to large scale, long-term studies performed by both the U.S. National Institutes of Health and the World Health Organization, is already exposing hundreds of millions of people to dangerous levels of harmful radiation, yet the government and utility companies lie to the public about the system's supposed safety. As a matter of fact – take a look at your electric meter and you will notice that unlike every other device that is plugged into the electric grid, it is neither UL nor CSA certified. That is because it is neither safe for humans, nor the electric grid itself.

Chapter 1

THE STATE OF OUR FOOD
A TOXIC SOUP

1.1   PROBLEM STATEMENT

It is no secret that the state of health around the world, and especially in the United States is on a downward spiral. You cannot turn on your television without being bombarded by dozens of medication commercials, or listening to the radio and hearing commercials for class-action lawsuits against pharmaceutical companies for horrible side effects or deaths caused by their products. It both amuses and horrifies me to listen to those commercials, because while I know that most of the conditions they claim to treat are bogus, as in they are not actual conditions, but rather a sign of another problem in the body – in other words, they are symptoms, not root causes; it horrifies me because I realize that while they are rattling off those long lists of side effects, people seem to completely ignore them. Why else would people take those medications?

The rates of cancer, diabetes, heart disease, obesity and many other ailments are out of control and no one seems to be talking about what is really causing it. Over the past 100 years, according to the U.S. census, The New England Medical Gazette, and American Cancer Society data, deaths from cancer have gone up from 79.4 people per 100,000 population in 1914[11,12] to 183.7 per 100,000 in 2014[13]. In other words, based on U.S. population then and now, 52,420 people died from cancer in 1914 and 585,720 died in 2014. The total number of new cancer cases in the U.S. in 2014 was 1,665,540, and an estimated 13.7 million Americans (4.4% of the population) with a history of cancer were alive on January 1, 2012, of which some still had evidence of cancer.

According to the American Association for Cancer Research 2015 Cancer Progress Report[14], 1 out of 4 deaths in the U.S. is due to cancer. It is also worth mentioning that the medical industry defines "cure" as 5-year survival, so although they claim to have cured a certain percentage of cancer patients, that percentage is actually a lot smaller, because more of those "survivors" don't live much past 5 years, mostly due to the toxic treatments themselves.

In patents filed by the U.S. government[15] for a cancer treatment stolen from Dr. Stanislaw Burzynski by Dvorit Samid on behalf of the government, and assigned to the U.S. Department of Health and Human Services (HSS), they admit that "Current approaches to combat cancer rely primarily on the use of chemicals and radiation, which are themselves carcinogenic and may promote recurrences and the development of metastatic disease." Although Dr. Burzynski has received FDA approval for using his medicine on his patients, and has had tremendous success in truly curing cancer patients (not just for 5 years) of cancers that the industry claims to be incurable, and has done so for decades, they have tried and failed for decades to put him out of business, jail him, discredit him, and finally, even though he has already patented his cure, the U.S. government had stolen that cure from him and filed numerous patents of their own, and directed the patent office to fraudulently approve those patents. I highly recommend watching the Burzynski movie, which can be found in its entirety on YouTube, with more information available at burzynskimovie.com

There is a lot of misinformation being spread by the "healthcare" industry and the FDA about what causes disease and how to prevent or treat it. At the same time that the FDA legalizes all sorts of toxins to be used in food production or medications they illegalize natural, health-promoting products, such as Vitamin B17[16] or cannabis, which has wide-ranging health benefits as will be discussed in detail later on in the book. Likewise, did you know that you cannot buy raw almonds in the U.S.? The FDA and USDA had mandated that from 2007 and on, almonds must be pasteurized. Their reasoning is salmonella contamination. However, salmonella comes from one place and one place only - from feces - feces from animals or water contaminated with feces. However, if you use that argument you would have to also pasteurize lettuce, tomatoes, spinach, and every other fruit, vegetable, nut, grain and legume. The pasteurization process not only eliminates some health-promoting compounds in almonds, but studies have also shown that pasteurizing almonds creates potentially harmful levels of acrylamide (as does roasting of various nuts), which is a byproduct of the amino acid asparagine that results from heating up almonds. According to the National Cancer Institute Acrylamide has been found in certain foods, with especially high levels in potato chips, French fries, and other food products produced by high-temperature cooking[17]. What is more disturbing is that the FDA and USDA allow labeling pasteurized almonds as raw, fooling consumers who might not read the fine print or understand its implications.

In addition, non-organic almonds could be pasteurized using Propylene Oxide (PPO) in a process called Propylene Oxide Fumigation. PPO has been classified by the EPA as a possible human carcinogen[18].

Modern medicine has compartmentalized the human body into its constituents, and as a result, doctors don't look at the body as a system. Cardiologist, pulmonologist, gastroenterologist, etc., etc., etc., and they all live in their own bubble and don't look at the system as a whole. You have acid reflux? Let's put it out with antacids… But what is causing the acid reflux in the first place? Who cares!!! But what are the antacids doing to my liver? Don't worry about it!!! Acid reflux, headaches, stomach aches, oily skin, acne, rashes, and so on are signals from your body telling you that something is wrong or out of balance. So rather than fix the problem, modern medicine seeks to cover it up; eliminate the symptom rather than the root cause. Because eliminating the symptom will keep you a paying customer.

In addition, doctors have become little more than glorified drug dealers. It is common practice in the pharmaceutical industry to bribe doctors for prescribing their medications and encouraging them to "go off label", which means to prescribe medications for non-FDA-approved purposes, and since pharmacies sell prescription sales data back to the pharmaceutical companies, they immediately know which doctor prescribed what, using that information to intimidate doctors if they don't prescribe as promised. The pharmaceutical companies even pay doctors to casually speak with other doctors about specific medications, or to give scripted lectures, as if they are speaking from personal experience with the product being peddled.

According to a Mayo Clinic study, 70% of Americans take at least 1 prescription drug, and more than 50% take at least 2. In 2011, 4.02 Billion prescriptions were written and in 2013 U.S. spending on prescription drugs reached $329.2 Billion. A review of the efficacy of pharmaceutical medications found that since the mid-1990's "85 to 90 percent of new drugs don't offer any clinical advantages for users"[19].

In contrast, eastern medicine (Chinese medicine, Ayurveda, etc.) seeks to find the cause of the problem and correct it, and the cause is not always a single thing, and therefore neither is the course of treatment. But more importantly, they recognize that a healthy lifestyle, a healthy diet, and a healthy mind, are critical for good overall health. You might say, "So why aren't all Chinese and Indian people healthy and vibrant?" Well... Having the knowledge and using the knowledge are two separate things. Theodore Roosevelt said "Knowing what's right doesn't mean much unless you do what's right". Many people in those regions don't have the means to eat healthy. Many people who have the means would rather indulge on rich foods that give them pleasure in the moment, but ravage their body in the long run. And yet others simply are not aware of this knowledge. Of course, there are many other reasons, such as pollution, access to a diverse diet, and other factors.

Some studies show that we live longer than past generations. What is true is that the rate of infant and child mortality has gone down, not due to advancement in medicine so much, but mostly because of hygiene - both personal and in the medical industry. Although, according to a 2014 National Vital Statistics Report[20] the U.S. has the highest pre-term births and highest rates of infant mortality in the developed world.

Adulthood diseases, such as diabetes, are becoming commonplace in young children. Certainly, something has gone awry.

But let's assume for a moment that we are living longer... Would you want to live to 120 or 200 years of age, but be in pain and discomfort every day? Having surgery every year to fix or replace your organs or joints? Taking pills every day to supposedly keep you healthy? Or would you rather live to be

75 years old but live pain free and in excellent health every moment of your life?

1.2   WHERE DID WE GO WRONG?

It's hard to know where to start...   There are many areas that we can do better in, but perhaps the biggest problem facing us today, when it comes to our health, as well as the health of our domesticated animals is the food supply. What is passed for food nowadays is disturbing. Some "food" products on the supermarket shelves nowadays have nearly no natural ingredients in them – they are comprised almost exclusively of synthetic chemicals, of which many are known carcinogens, immunosuppressants, genotixins and mutagens. Let's look at some of those chemicals and their health effects:

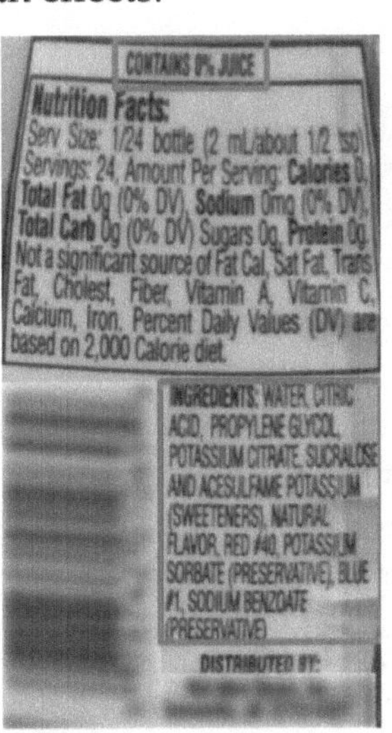

Nutritional information and ingredients of a common "liquid water enhancer". Looking through this list, you can see that it is full of toxic chemicals that cause cancer, suppression of the immune system, and damage to and mutation of DNA.

1.2.1   <u>Acesulfame Potassium (Artificial Sweetener)</u>

Acesulfame Potassium, also known as Acesulfame K and Ace-K, is an artificial sweetener that is up to 200 times sweeter than table sugar. However, because it has a bitter after-taste, it is usually combined with other sweeteners such as Aspartame and sucralose. Although Ace-K is approved by the FDA, it's approval was based on sub-standard and insufficient testing that nevertheless showed evidence of carcinogenicity[21]. To date there has not been sufficient testing done to determine if Acesulfame Potassium is safe for human consumption.

1.2.2 <u>Sucralose (Artificial Sweetener)</u>

Sucralose, best known by its brand name Splenda, is an artificial sweetener that is 320 to 1,000 times as sweet as table sugar. Like Ace-K, there is limited data on its safety, and some data suggests changes to CYP enzymes responsible for detoxification, among other functions, suppression and elimination of beneficial gastrointestinal bacteria, increase in fecal pH and abnormal changes to the intestinal lining and DNA damage in the gastrointestinal tract[22]. When combined with Ace-K, it has been shown to increase the secretion of regulatory hormones.

1.2.3 <u>Aspartame (Artificial Sweetener)</u>

Aspartame, also known as NutraSweet, AminoSweet, Equal, Canderel, E951, Naturnaste, Benevia, Spoonful and a new, more concentrated and heat-resistant version called Neotame (aspartame + 3-di-methylbutyl, which can be found on the EPA's list of most hazardous chemicals) is one of the most prolific and toxic chemicals in the food supply. Along with many side effects and debilitating conditions reported to the FDA over the years, it has been shown to cause tumors[25,26], lymphoma/leukemia[25,26], transitional cell carcinomas[26], malignant schwannomas of the peripheral nerves[26], hepatocellular carcinoma and alveolar/bronchiolar carcinoma[27], mammary cancer[25], and various other cancers in rats and mice in testing by the original manufacturer G.D. Searle & Company[28] and the FDA before its forced approval, as well as after its approval, by numerous independent labs in studies on mice, rats and humans[28,29]. It has also been shown to cause leukemia[29], non-Hodgkin lymphoma[29] and multiple myeloma[29] and other cancers of the central nervous system in humans. As evidenced in the studies cited above, Aspartame is a "multipotential carcinogenic agent"[26].

It is interesting to note that all publicized industry-funded studies found aspartame to be safe even though their own data showed many cancers and organ damage, while 92% of independent studies identified one or more problems with its safety[25-31]. Also, by 1998, 80% of complaints to the FDA about food additives were about aspartame products[32]. This goes back to my statement in the preface about where not to look for information. Industry funded studies should never be accepted by the FDA or any public safety authority, or the public, and although I use Wikipedia extensively – since it can be edited by anyone, and it is edited extensively by special interests, it needs to be backed up by independent, non-industry funded research.

The history of Aspartame's development and approval for use in foods and drugs sounds more like a soap opera or a gangster movie than reality. I will go into it in more detail later on in the book.

1.2.4   <u>Sodium Benzoate (Preservative)</u>

Sodium Benzoate (E211), which is used in countless food products as a preservative has been shown in tests on rats to induce anxiety and motor impairment[33], and in cultured human peripheral lymphocytes (white blood cells) to cause significant DNA damage[34]. In the latter reference study, the authors concluded that "The present results indicate that SB [Sodium Benzoate] and PB [Potassium Benzoate] are clastogenic, mutagenic and cytotoxic to human lymphocytes in vitro"[34].

In a randomized, double-blinded, placebo controlled trial on children, published in the world's most prestigious journal - the Lancet, Sodium Benzoate and food colorings had been shown to cause hyperactivity and decreased intelligence[35]. In a preceding randomized, double blind, placebo controlled study on artificial colors and sodium benzoate, the authors found that not only did artificial colors and sodium benzoate increase hyperactivity in children, but removing those chemicals from the diet led to a reduction in hyperactive behavior[36].

Randomized, double-blinded, placebo controlled clinical trials are the gold standard of research.

1.2.5   <u>Genetically Modified Organisms (GMOs)</u>

GMOs or Genetically Modified Organisms, also referred to as GE (Genetically Engineered) crops are one of the most controversial food additives/modifications. The awareness of the existence of GMOs is (relatively) widespread, but the GMO seed manufacturers have done a great job of purposely misinforming the public, authorities, and the scientific community, spreading rumors, discrediting good science and manipulating politics and the justice system, all the way to the supreme court of the United States to get their way. There have been countless independent studies that repeatedly demonstrated that GMOs and the herbicides that are used along with GMO crops have caused cancers, immune disorders, and other toxic effects to humans, animals, and the environment. Remember that earlier I said that replications studies are critical to scientific truth? Since this is such a hot-button topic, I will go into more detail about GMOs later in the book, where you will discover how many studies have been performed by scientists all over the world, and they all say the same thing.

You must be asking yourself at this point, "Why would food companies knowingly and willingly poison entire populations?" Usually, the motive is very simple… Money! If they can simulate a taste with a chemical less expensively than by using real ingredients, they will do so. If they could make a product last on the shelf for 10 years so that they can produce in enormous quantities, or keep it on the shelf rather than in the more expensive refrigerated section, they will do so. If they could spray produce with toxic chemicals to keep them looking fresh and blemish-free, or fumigate meat to make it look fresh, even though it's not, why not? Never mind that those chemicals are absorbed into the produce and meat and cannot be washed away. But money alone does not make people willingly do harm onto others, it takes a certain mindset; a certain immorality. If you think that people are not capable of such callousness, there are many examples in world history that would make you think twice.

It is important that I set a tone for the rest of the book by providing the following examples of government and corporate atrocities, because they demonstrate a phenomenon that many people would not believe is possible. It demonstrates that governments and corporations care more about power and money than about human life, or even inflicting pain and suffering on their own citizens and fellow countrymen, and when given the opportunity, they would not think twice about inflicting harm on the masses.

1.3   THE ATROCITIES OF OUR FELLOW COUNTRYMEN - A LESSON IN HISTORY

1.3.1   <u>The Tuskegee Syphilis Experiment</u>[37]

The Tuskegee Syphilis Experiment, where between 1932 and 1972 the U.S. Public Health Service studied the natural progression of untreated syphilis in 600 rural African American men who thought they were receiving free health care from the U.S. government. 399 of those men had contracted syphilis before the study began, and 201 of the men were infected with the disease by the clinicians. The men were not told that they had syphilis, nor were they ever treated for it even though a cure was discovered in the 1940's in the form of penicillin. Instead, the men were told that they were being treated for "bad blood". By the end of the study in 1972, only 74 of the test subjects were alive. Of the original 399 men, 28 had died of syphilis, 100 died of related complications, 40 of their wives had been infected, and 19 of their children were born with congenital syphilis.

1.3.2   <u>The St. Louis Radiation Experiment</u>[38,39]

The St. Louis Radiation Experiment involved the spraying of radioactive Zinc Cadmium Sulfide by the U.S. Army on impoverished, predominantly black St. Louis neighborhoods. Local authorities at the time were told that the government were testing a smoke screen that could shield St. Louis from aerial observations in case of a Russian attack. In 1994 the government had confessed to the experiment and stated that the tests were part of a biological weapons program. They said that St. Louis was chosen because it bore some resemblance to Russian cities that the U.S. would potentially attack.

1.3.3   H.I.V. & Hepatitis C Tainted Hemophilia Product[40-43]

In the 1980's, a subsidiary of Bayer was producing a hemophilia blood product when they had discovered that their product had infected thousands of people in the United States with H.I.V. and around 60,000 people with Hepatitis C. Rather than destroy the tainted product, internal memos obtained in court cases show that the company, with the cooperation of the FDA, had decided to sell those products overseas.

"'Can we in good faith continue to ship nonheat-treated coagulation products to Japan?'" a company task force asked in February 1985, fearing that some of its plasma donors might be H.I.V. positive. The decision, records show, was yes. [40]

An estimated 6,000 to 10,000 people were infected with H.I.V. in the united states, and thousands more in nearly a dozen countries, of which most were children [41,42]. In the U.S. alone, more than 4,000 died of AIDS. [43].

1.3.4   DuPont Poisons the World with PFOA[44]

You've most likely heard of PFOA in the context of PFOA-Free cookware, but you most likely have not heard about why cookware manufacturers make such a big deal about placing that statement on their product labeling.

PFOA was developed by 3M in 1947. Four years later, in 1951, DuPont started purchasing PFOA from 3M. "3M sent DuPont recommendations on how to dispose of it. It was to be incinerated or sent to chemical-waste facilities."[44]   Even though DuPont's own instructions specified that the chemical is not to be disposed of in surface water or sewers, for decades they proceeded to dump hundreds of thousands of pounds of it into the Ohio river, and thousands of tons into open, unlined pits where the chemical could seep into the ground, and into the water table.

For more than four decades, both 3M and DuPont had been conducting medical studies on PFOA in secret. They had found that PFOA binds to plasma proteins in the blood, and that it circulated in the bloodstream through every organ in the body, causing liver damage, birth defects, DNA damage, and multiple types of cancer in lab animals and in DuPont's own workers, their spouses, and their children. DuPont had also discovered that PFOA dust from their factory had settled beyond their property and had entered the local water supply. All those findings were kept from authorities and the public.

"In 1991, DuPont scientists determined an internal safety limit for PFOA concentration in drinking water: one part per billion [ppb]. The same year, DuPont found that water in one local district contained PFOA levels at three times that figure." [44] Subsequently, after a comprehensive review of previous health studies, Philippe Grandjean of the Harvard School of Public Health and Richard Clapp of the University of Massachusetts-Lowell named an "approximate" safe level of 0.001ppb (or one part per trillion). To put that in perspective, 1 part per trillion is equivalent to 1 drop of water divided into 20 Olympic-sized swimming pools.

In 1993, internal memos show that for the first time, DuPont scientists had found an alternative to PFOA which was less toxic and stays in the body for a shorter period of time.

"Discussions were held at DuPont's corporate headquarters to discuss switching to the new compound. DuPont decided against it. The risk was too great: Products manufactured with

PFOA were an important part of DuPont's business, worth $1 billion in annual profit." [44]

Although the new alternative was "safer" according to DuPont's scientists, "200 scientists from a variety of disciplines signed the Madrid Statement, which expresses concern about the production of all fluorochemicals"[44], which the alternative is.

In 2002, the E.P.A. had released initial findings from a toxicity study it has been conducting on PFOA. In their report, they stated that "PFOA might pose human health risks not only to those drinking tainted water, but also to the general public — anyone, for instance, who cooked with Teflon pans ... By 2003 the average concentration of PFOA in the blood of an adult American was four to five parts per billion." [44] That is 4,000 to 5,000 times the limit set for drinking water by Philippe Grandjean and Richard Clapp. Both 3M and DuPont were aware of the presence of PFOA in the blood of the population as early as 1976.

To date, wherever scientists have tested for the presence of PFOA, they have found it. It is present in the blood and vital organs of every living creature on earth, from major population centers, to the most remote places on earth.

This short blurb cannot do justice to the scope of this story. I highly recommend that you read The New York Times article "The Lawyer Who Became DuPont's Worst Nightmare"[44] by Nathaniel Rich.

Those were but a few examples from recent U.S. history. Many other examples exist, in the U.S. and globally.

Today, more than ever, it is critical to be aware and educate yourself. It is also important to not be gullible. For example; in articles where I've written about the dangers of GMOs, and in response to the numerous studies that I've quoted, I've had people refer me to articles from the GMO manufacturers' websites claiming that GMOs are perfectly safe. What I am getting to is, if you want unbiased information; never ask the person who stands to gain the most from it, such as the case with DuPont as outlined above. Second, you always have to be true to yourself, so if you read conflicting information and don't know if something is safe to consume, ask yourself what is right for you. Your decision may differ depending on your personal preferences – if you believe that your body is your temple, you may not compromise and not take a chance. If you believe that a little bit of toxins here and there will most likely be okay, as long as you eat mostly wholesome foods, then that is the right decision for you, although, especially with endocrine disruptors, even parts per trillion are toxic. On the other hand, you may live in a small town where the only option is deep fried, processed, GMO, chemical-ladened food (to be dramatic). In that case, you have only three options; eat what you've got, starve, or move to another city, state, or country.

Another big threat to our health is the industry that is claiming to be our guardians in health; the pharmaceutical industry, who's only goal is to make more and more money, regardless of the consequences. So as a result, they have invented medical conditions to explain everyday events, they have created vaccines to lower our immune system and make us sick, and they have created an atmosphere of misinformation to keep people (and doctors) ignorant in order to further their mission. They have stolen trillions of dollars in donations over the years to develop "cures" for diseases that they then turn around and charge the same people who paid for their development handsomely. And, of course, they never really cure anything. They only suppress. Because when you suppress something, it will come back, and so will you when you need your next fix. That is the business model of the pharmaceutical industry - "A patient cured is a customer lost".

The following statement from the Susan G. Komen website should tell you something about where their true allegiances lie:

"...consumption of organic food is a controversial issue and high quality human research is lacking in this area. Specifically, claims of higher nutritional value and lower toxic contaminants in organic foods currently have little scientific evidence supporting pronounced benefits. Some studies have shown that organic food has a lower amount of pesticides, but research has not confirmed that lower amounts of pesticides are causally related to preventing certain diseases or conditions."

Not only does this statement ignore countless scientific studies which have shown that pesticides and herbicides cause all sorts of physical illnesses and conditions, and cause soil microbiota and nutrient depletion through chemicals which compete with those nutrients, which then lowers the nutrient value of the crops, but even a minimally intelligent person should be offended by it.

An ancient Greek physician by the name of Hippocrates, who is considered to be the father of modern medicine, said nearly two and a half millennia ago, "Let food be thy medicine". Nature has given us all of the tools we need to lead a healthy life, if we only open our eyes to see it. Not to say that there is no place for modern medicine – modern medicine has saved countless lives, but for the most part, it has been at the expense of a lot of misery, through horrible side effects and debilitation, of which most is by design.

T. Colin Campbell, PhD, a world-renowned biochemist and researcher at the forefront of nutritional science who was one of the directors of the China Project - acclaimed as being the most comprehensive study of health and nutrition ever conducted had this to say about modern medicine:

"I know that there are some few drugs that can be life-saving and may be useful if used judiciously. But our dependence on drugs and our addiction to the marketplace and its claims about nutrition supplements, drugs and other medical paraphernalia is sickening–literally so."[45]

Additionally, a 2013 report in the Journal of Patient Safety[46] revealed that about 400,000 people in the United States die each year due to preventable medical harm, and an additional 4 to 8 million incur serious harm due to medical malpractice.

Ultimately, the individual is responsible for what food or drugs they put into their body, and what environment they choose to remain in.

The importance of eating natural, clean, whole foods cannot be overstated. Here are a couple of interesting, recent scientific studies into natural foods and their health effects:

Coconut oil is about 50% Lauric Acid, which has been shown in published studies to kill colon cancer cells[47].

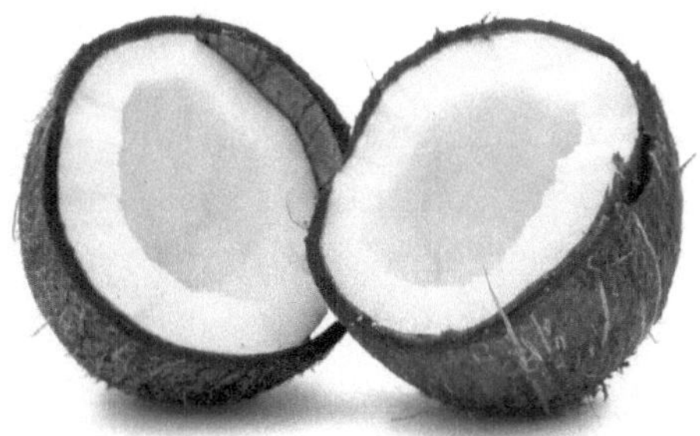

Oleocanthal, a phenolic compound present in extra-virgin olive oil kills cancer cells in 30 to 60 minutes. As a bonus, it also has positive effects on inflammation, Osteoporosis, and age-related diseases [48,49,50].

1.4   HOW DO TOXINS AFFECT OUR BIOLOGY?

Obviously, different toxins affect our biology in different ways, but let's focus on toxins that don't kill us immediately, but rather cause a cumulative and chronic effect on our bodies that leads to disorder and disease.

When you ingest food, your digestive system breaks the food down to its constituents; sodium, magnesium, glucose, etc. Those constituents go into your bloodstream and are distributed throughout your body as nourishment for your cells and for other biological activities. The cells of the body have hundreds of thousands of little sensors on their surface called Integral Membrane Proteins (IMP), with each IMP recognizing a specific mineral or compound, or hormone, etc., collectively called signals. If the IMP recognizes a signal in the environment surrounding it, it will couple with the signal and initiate a cellular function within the cell. If it does not recognize the signal it will not couple with it. If a toxin is present in the environment surrounding the cell, the IMP's will recognize it as a toxin and actually move away from the toxin. If it cannot distance itself from the toxin, the cell will shut itself down until the toxin is no longer in the environment. If the toxin remains in the environment, the cell will remain inactive and will eventually starve of nutrition. When the cell weakens, opportunistic organisms, such as Candida will proliferate and take over the cells, and eventually cause disease, dysfunction and even cancer. So, eradicating the cancer or Candida for example without eliminating the toxins, and eliminating the continual intake of toxins will only serve to delay the disease and not eradicate it. That is why it is so important to take a holistic approach by not only treating the effect, but also eliminating the cause. Dr. Bruce H. Lipton, Ph.D., a cellular biologist and one of the pioneers of epigenetics calls those IMP's "Perception Switches" for the reason that they perceive the conditions of the environment around them and react accordingly. If you would like more in-depth information about cellular biology and how cells and DNA, and therefore the human, is affected by the environment, I would highly recommend reading Dr. Lipton's book "The Biology of Belief". In it, Dr. Lipton does a fantastic job of explaining complex concepts in a very simple and easy to understand way.

However, the word "toxin" is a little lacking in the context of food safety/health. When talking about health, something like water, which is healthy in the proper quantity, could become toxic to the body if taken in excess. Of course, water would not be thought of as toxic, but other chemicals which are used in foods, and which are known to cause cancer and be destructive to DNA for example, have been argued in favor of by food manufacturers and the FDA to not be toxic in the quantities which they are used. However, how do you determine how many pickles any particular person eats in an average day? How do you quantify how many different products that contain the same chemical are consumed by a single individual in the course of a day? In that case, it is easy to see how a person may ingest more than the safe limit. And ethically, if you demonstrate that 90% of the population does not consume those ingredients in sufficient quantities to be harmful, do you damn the 10% that do?

Furthermore, there are many links to disease and disorders that have not been made (or acknowledged) by food manufacturers for the obvious reason that why would they search for something if they are not required to? And with all of the medical conditions that are plaguing the public, which are growing by the day, at the same time that the number of chemicals in our foods have gone up, the correlation can no longer be denied. For instance, it has been clearly demonstrated that the rate of increase of food allergies, toxic levels of Glyphosate in the blood of humans, and rates of certain cancers and other conditions correspond directly with the introduction of GMOs into the food supply, and the increased use of GMOs over the years[51,52,53].

A study published in the journal Food and Chemical Toxicology (FCT) in September 2012 reported that a GM corn and Roundup caused organ damage and increased rates of tumors and premature death in rats.

Just months after the study was published showing that the two Monsanto products damaged the health of rats, the journal that published the study appointed a former Monsanto scientist – Richard E. Goodman to the upper editorial board of FCT, to decide which papers on GM foods and crops should be published and which should not.

According to Dr. Jonathan Latham, executive director of the nonprofit Bioscience Resource Project, "Unfortunately, the public and the scientific community can no longer trust that peer-reviewed journals reflect the true state of scientific knowledge. Some journals have become a vehicle for a narrow interest group – biotechnology corporations – to control scientific discourse."

1.4.1   pH BALANCE

One of the most critical aspects to the health of any organism; whether it be humans, animals, plants, bacteria or any other living organism, is a proper pH. pH, which stands for potential of hydrogen, is the measure of acidity or basicity (alkalinity) and is measured on a logarithmic scale. This means that a pH of 6 is ten times more acidic that a pH of 7, and a pH of 9 is ten times more alkaline than a pH of 8. Every organism has its own range of pH where it can live in balance.

If you're growing tomatoes in your garden, you want the soil pH to be between 5.5 and 7.5. If you're growing blueberries on the other hand, your soil needs to be more acidic – in the range of 4.0 to 5.0. If the soil is higher or lower than the range necessary for the particular plant, the plant will suffer, get diseased, die, or not sprout at all. It is no different for humans. A pH that is too low (acidic), which is very common in humans nowadays, leads to an entire host of diseases and disorders. A pH that is too high (alkaline), which is not very common, can likewise lead to other disorders.

"Dietary lifestyles can alter systemic acid-base balance over time. Acidogenic diets, which are typically high in animal protein and salt and low in fruits and vegetables, can lead to a sub-clinical or low-grade state of metabolic acidosis."[54]

You can check your urine pH on a regular basis to determine if your eating habits are generally acidifying or alkalizing by using litmus paper, by checking preferably the second elimination of the day. The ideal urine pH range for humans is 6.5 to 7.5, however, you want to be on the high end of that range more often than not. pH will fluctuate somewhat throughout the day, and day to day, depending on what you eat and drink, but if you are usually within that range, you should be doing well. If you are out of that range on a regular basis, you should bring your pH back into balance. Depending on your needs, eating more alkalizing foods or more acidifying foods will change your pH in that direction. The more alkalizing or more acidifying the food item is, the faster and more drastic impact it will have on your body pH.

Acidic foods are not necessarily bad. The problem occurs when your net dietary intake is more acidifying than alkalizing over a long period of time, which the standard American diet is. If your battling cancer however, you might want to forego acidifying foods altogether until you have brought your body back to health.

Blood pH however is more tightly regulated and needs to be in the range of 7.35 to 7.45.

Although the kidneys and lungs typically keep the blood pH at this tight range, what people who claim that it is impossible to sufficiently alter blood pH with food fail to understand is that when you keep on flooding your body with acidifying foods and substances, your lungs and kidneys will struggle to keep up, and eventually will lag behind, which leads to low-grade systemic metabolic acidosis, which can go unnoticed for years while doing serious harm to organs and tissues, the immune system, causing inflammation, and even cancer.

Additionally, as a result of the acid load, the renal system will compensate by pulling calcium carbonate and calcium phosphate from your bones, and wasting away your bones and muscles to keep the blood at its optimal range[55].   In additional to many other disorders, a reduction in the absorption of vitamin D results from an acidic diet[55]. Nearly all Americans are deficient in vitamin D. Low vitamin D is likewise associated with cancer development.

Much misinformation has been presented to the public by so-called health authorities in regards to which foods promote health and which do not. On the one hand, they claim no benefit from an alkaline diet, stating that there is no connection between acidic diets and the formation of cancer, while on the other hand claiming that incorporating more alkaline foods and reducing or eliminating acidic foods tilts the scale towards health and the prevention of cancer[56]. It has now been demonstrated beyond a shadow of a doubt that a diet high in alkalizing foods, such as fruits and vegetables, and low in acidifying foods, such as meat, dairy, sugars, processed foods and refined grains leads to a reduction in all diseases, including incidences of all forms of cancer. The China Project, has done more than any other scientific study to unravel the link between animal products – meat and milk proteins, and nearly every chronic disease – the so-called diseases of affluence. The book "The China Study" outlines all of the findings of the China Project, as well as those of many high-quality studies prior to, and following the China Project. This book should be required reading for every man, woman, and child.

"Most fruits and vegetables are net-base producing foods since the metabolized products are organic anion precursors such as citrate, succinate, and conjugate bases of carboxylic acids. The final metabolite of these precursors is bicarbonate anion. Sulfur containing amino acids, methionine and cysteine, typically found in meats, eggs and dairy products, are oxidized into sulfuric acid which is ultimately net-acid producing ... Sodium chloride [table salt] is reported to be an independent and causal factor for inducing metabolic acidosis in a dose-dependent manner. Conversely, potassium salts, and to a lesser degree magnesium, serve as a countervailing effect on net acid excretion and help to promote alkaline balance."[54]

1.4.2 <u>ASPARTAME</u>

<u>THE LEGALIZATION OF ASPARTAME</u>

In 1965 James M. Schlatter, a chemist working for G.D. Searle & Company was working on an anti-ulcer drug, when he accidentally discovered that one of the compounds that he created had a sweet taste, when some of it spilled on his finger and he licked it. G.D. Searle proceeded to test this compound on lab animals in efforts to turn this sweet compound into a marketable sweetener as an alternative to sugar, but they quickly discovered that it had some very serious effects on the test animals. In a very short period of time the test animals developed large tumors and a host of other conditions, and died very quickly. G.D. Searle wasn't interested however in those results, so they directed their scientists to alter the tests in such a way that the results will either be benign or show only favorable results. And so, they took the tumor riddled animals, cut out their tumors and presented the rest of the animal as a healthy specimen. In other tests, rather than perform autopsies on the animals immediately after death, they left the dead animals for many months, and in some cases over a year to decompose so that any testing on the decomposed tissue would not show any abnormalities.

They then took their "findings" to the FDA in an attempt to get this chemical approved as a sweetener for human consumption. The FDA looked at the information and immediately noticed problems with the data and requested that additional testing be performed. G.D. Searle continued trying to swindle the FDA, but the FDA were not going to be fooled. After four times that G.D. Searle tried to get this chemical approved by the FDA and were rejected, the FDA and the CDC filed a lawsuit against G.D. Searle for intentionally altering test results and reports to remove damaging information in an attempt to fool the FDA.

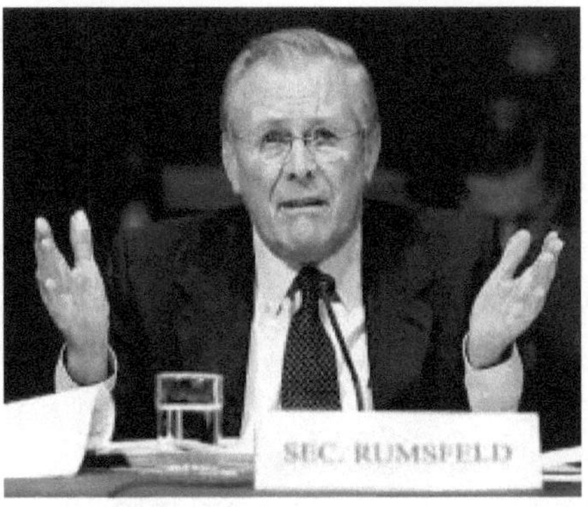

In 1977 Donald Rumsfeld was hired by G.D. Searle as their CEO. By that time Rumsfeld was already a Washington veteran. Rumsfeld vowed that he will get this chemical approved for human consumption by the FDA. On January 21, 1981, the day after Ronald Reagan's inauguration, G.D. Searle reapplied to the FDA to use this chemical as a food sweetener. Reagan's new FDA commissioner, Arthur Hayes Hull, Jr. appointed a 5-person scientific commission to review the board of inquiry's decision to ban this chemical.

The commission reviewed the board's finding and rules 3 to 2 to uphold the ban. Hull then installed a sixth commission member, which tied the vote, and then used his position as the FDA commissioner to break the tie to approve this chemical. Hull later left the FDA under allegations of impropriety, and later on went to work for Burston-Marsteller, the chief public relations firm for both G.D. Searle and Monsanto.

Donald Rumsfeld subsequently used his power within the government to get the FDA and CDC lawsuits dropped, and so, they were.

Since the approval of aspartame, it has been adopted in all sorts of diet soft drinks and snacks, and at the same time, incidents of cancer, diabetes, and a host of brain disorders drastically shot up.

Rumsfeld then used his political influence again to get Aspartame approved in the U.K., and once it was approved in both the U.S. and the U.K., Europe and other countries automatically approved it for use in their countries without further review.

Aspartame has also found its way into the pharmaceutical industry and is used to induce cancerous tumors in rats and mice so that anti-cancer drugs can be tested on them.

Since then, G.D. Searle had been purchased by none other than Monsanto – one of the most evil corporations of all time.   It was later purchased by Pfizer (which is the current owner), however, because the name G.D. Searle was so damaged over the years, Pfizer has dropped it.

In 1995 the FDA, under the Freedom of Information Act, were forced to release a list of Aspartame symptoms that was compiled from 10,000 consumer complaints. The list outlines 92 symptoms, including death.

<u>THE CHEMISTRY OF ASPARTAME</u>

Aspartame is comprised of aspartic acid, phenylalanine, and methanol.

Aspartic acid (40% of aspartame) is a naturally occurring amino acid which is a component of all proteins.   It is classified as a "non-essential" amino acid, which means that humans do not need to get it from their diets since they can make it from other things in the diet. However, when unbound to proteins, as in aspartame, aspartic acid leads to a variety of harmful effects.

"Dr. Russell L. Blaylock, a professor of neurosurgery at the Medical University of Mississippi, recently published a book thoroughly detailing the damage that is caused by the ingestion of excessive aspartic acid from Aspartame. Blaylock makes use of almost 500 scientific references to show how excess free excitatory amino acids such as aspartic acid and glutamic acid (such as in MSG) in our food supply are causing serious chronic neurological disorders and a myriad of other acute symptoms.

Aspartic acid (also called aspartate) and glutamate act as neurotransmitters in the brain by facilitating the transmission of information from neuron to neuron. Too much aspartate or glutamate in the brain kills certain neurons by allowing the influx of too much calcium into the cells. This influx triggers excessive amounts of free radicals, which kill the cells. The neural cell damage that can be caused by excessive aspartate and glutamate is why they are referred to as 'excitotoxins.' They 'excite' or stimulate the neural cells to death.

Aspartic acid is an amino acid. Taken in its free form (unbound to proteins), it significantly raises the blood plasma level of aspartate and glutamate. The excess aspartate and glutamate in the blood plasma shortly after ingesting aspartame or products with free glutamic acid (glutamate precursor) leads to a high level of those neurotransmitters in certain areas of the brain.
The blood brain barrier (BBB), which normally protects the brain from excess glutamate and aspartate as well as toxins, 1)

is not fully developed during childhood, 2) does not fully protect all areas of the brain, 3) is damaged by numerous chronic and acute conditions, and 4) allows seepage of excess glutamate and aspartate into the brain even when intact.

The excess glutamate and aspartate slowly begin to destroy neurons. The large majority (75 percent or more) of neural cells in a particular area of the brain are killed before any clinical symptoms of a chronic illness are noticed.

The risk to infants, children, pregnant women, the elderly and persons with certain chronic health problems from excitotoxins are great. Even the Federation of American Societies for Experimental Biology (FASEB), which usually understates problems and mimics the FDA party-line, recently stated in a review that glutamic acid should be avoided by women of childbearing age.

Aspartic acid from aspartame has the same harmful effects on the body as glutamic acid isolated from its naturally protein-bound state, causing it to become a neurotoxin instead of a non-essential amino acid.

Aspartame in diet sodas or in other liquid forms are absorbed more quickly and have been shown to spike plasma levels of aspartic acid.

One common complaint of persons suffering from the effect of aspartame is memory loss. Ironically, in 1987, G.D. Searle, the original manufacturer of aspartame, undertook a search for a drug to combat memory loss caused by excitatory amino acid damage.

Blaylock is one of many scientists and physicians who are concerned about excitatory amino acid damage caused by ingestion of aspartame and MSG.

A few of the many experts who have spoken out against the damage being caused by aspartate and glutamate include Adrienne Samuels, Ph.D., an experimental psychologist specializing in research design. Another is Dr. John Olney, a professor in the department of psychiatry, School of Medicine, Washington University, a neuroscientist and researcher, and one of the world's foremost authorities on excitotoxins. (He informed Searle in 1971 that aspartic acid caused holes in the brains of mice.)

Phenylalanine (50% of aspartame) is an amino acid normally found in the brain. Persons with the genetic disorder phenylketonuria (PKU) cannot metabolize phenylalanine. This leads to dangerously high levels of phenylalanine in the brain (sometimes lethal). It has been shown that ingesting aspartame, especially along with carbohydrates, can lead to excess levels of phenylalanine in the brain even in persons who do not have PKU.

This is not just a theory, as many people who have eaten large amounts of aspartame over a long period of time and do not have PKU have been shown to have excessive levels of phenylalanine in the blood. Excessive levels of phenylalanine in the brain can cause the levels of serotonin in the brain to decrease, leading to emotional disorders such as depression. It was shown in human testing that phenylalanine levels of the blood were increased significantly in human subjects who chronically used aspartame. Even a single use of aspartame raised the blood phenylalanine levels.

In his testimony before the U.S. Congress, Dr. Louis J. Elsas showed that high blood phenylalanine can be concentrated in parts of the brain and is especially dangerous for infants and fetuses. He also showed that phenylalanine is metabolized much more efficiently by rodents than by humans.

As Blaylock points out in his book, early studies measuring phenylalanine buildup in the brain were flawed. Investigators who measured specific brain regions and not the average throughout the brain notice significant rises in phenylalanine levels. Specifically, the hypothalamus, medulla oblongata, and corpus striatum areas of the brain had the largest increases in phenylalanine. Blaylock goes on to point out that excessive buildup of phenylalanine in the brain can cause schizophrenia or make one more susceptible to seizures.

Therefore, long-term, excessive use of aspartame may provide a boost to sales of serotonin reuptake inhibitors such as Prozac and drugs to control schizophrenia and seizures.

Methanol (10% of aspartame), also called wood alcohol is a deadly poison. Some people may remember methanol as the poison that has caused some 'skid row' alcoholics to end up blind or dead. Methanol is gradually released in the small intestine when the methyl group of aspartame encounters the enzyme chymotrypsin.

The absorption of methanol into the body is sped up considerably when free methanol is ingested. Free methanol is created from aspartame when it is heated to above 86°F (30°C). This would occur when aspartame-containing product is improperly stored or when it is heated (e.g. as part of a 'food' product such as Jello) [and when ingested - normal body temperature is 98.6°F (37°C)].

Methanol breaks down into formaldehyde in the body. Formaldehyde is a deadly neurotoxin. An EPA assessment of methanol states that methanol 'is considered a cumulative poison due to the low rate of excretion once it is absorbed. In the body, methanol is oxidized to formaldehyde.' They recommend a limit of consumption of 7.8mg/day. A one-liter (approx. 1 quart) aspartame-sweetened beverage contains about 56mg of methanol. [A 16 ounce beverage would have about 28mg of methanol]. Heavy users of aspartame-containing products consume as much as 250mg of methanol daily or 32 times the EPA limit.

Symptoms from methanol poisoning include headaches, ear buzzing, dizziness, nausea, gastrointestinal disturbances, weakness, vertigo, chills, memory lapses, numbness and shooting pains in the extremities, behavioral disturbances, and neuritis. The most well-known problems from methanol poisoning are vision problems including misty vision, progressive contraction of visual fields, blurring of vision, obscuration of vision, retinal damage, and blindness. Formaldehyde is a known carcinogen, causes retinal damage, interferes with DNA replication and causes birth defects.

Due to the lack of a couple of key enzymes, humans are many times more sensitive to the toxic effects of methanol than animals. Therefore, tests of aspartame or methanol on animals do not accurately reflect the danger for humans.

As pointed out by Dr. Woodrow C. Monte, director of the food science and nutrition laboratory at Arizona State University: 'There are no human or mammalian studies to evaluate the possible mutagenic, teratogenic or carcinogenic effects of chronic administration of methyl alcohol. [57]'

He was so concerned about the unresolved safety issues that he filed suit with the FDA requesting a hearing to address these issues. He asked the FDA to:

'...Slow down on this soft drink issue long enough to answer some of the important questions. It's not fair that you are leaving the full burden of proof on the few of us who are concerned and have such limited resources. You must remember that you are the American public's last defense. Once you allow usage (of aspartame) there is literally nothing I or my colleagues can do to reverse the course. Aspartame will then join saccharin, the sulfiting agents, and God knows how many other questionable compounds enjoined to insult the human constitution with governmental approval.'

Shortly thereafter, the Commissioner of the FDA, Arthur Hull Hayes, Jr., approved the use of aspartame in carbonated beverage. He then left for a position with G.D. Searle's public relations firm.

It has been pointed out that some fruit juices and alcoholic beverages contain small amounts of methanol. It is important to remember, however, that [in nature] methanol never appears alone. In every case, ethanol is present, usually in much higher amounts. Ethanol is an antidote for methanol toxicity in humans. The troops of Desert Storm were 'treated' to large amounts of aspartame-sweetened beverages, which had been heated to over 86°F in the Saudi Arabian sun. Many of them returned home with numerous disorders similar to what has been seen in persons who have been chemically poisoned by formaldehyde. The free methanol in the beverages may have been a contributing factor in these illnesses. Other breakdown products of aspartame such as DKP also have been a factor.

In a 1993 act that can only be described as 'unconscionable', the FDA approved aspartame as an ingredient in numerous food items that would always be heated to above 86°F (30°C)."[58]

Chapter 2

GMOs
A COUNTDOWN TO EXTINCTION

"Recombinant DNA technology faces our society with problems unprecedented not only in the history of science, but of life on the Earth. It places in human hands the capacity to redesign living organisms… Such intervention must not be confused with previous intrusions upon the natural order of living organisms… [it is] the biggest break in nature that has occurred in human history."

George Wald, Nobel Laureate; Professor of Biology Emeritus, Harvard University

---

"The genetic modification of food is intrinsically dangerous. It involves making irreversible changes in a random manner to a complex level of life about which little is known. It is inevitable that this hit-and-miss approach will lead to disasters. It must disrupt the natural intelligence of the plant or animal to which it is applied, and lead to health-damaging side-effects."

Dr. Geoffrey Clements, leader of the Natural Law Party, UK.

2.1   WHAT ARE GMOs?

GMO stands for "Genetically Modified Organisms" and is sometimes abbreviated as GM (Genetically modified), GE (Genetically Engineered), as well as Transgenic, gene splicing, and recombinant DNA technology. More specifically, the uproar recently has been over genetically modified crops, although those are not the only GMOs that present an imminent danger to the health of every living organism on this planet.   GMOs include genetically engineered bacteria, genetically engineered mosquitos (which have already been released in several U.S. cities), genetically modified animals, and other forms of genetically modified living organisms.

The genetic engineering process introduces foreign genetic material into a host plant / plant cells. The reason for the modification is to introduce a desirable trait to the organism (corn, soy, etc.) that they do not naturally possess, or that they only possess in small amounts, in order to allegedly increase crop yields and for other reasons. Some of those claimed traits are drought resistance, which doesn't sound so bad, and traits that will allow farmers to grow their crops closer together to maximize the yield of their land – again, doesn't sound so bad… But then, here are some traits that raise a few eyebrows - the seed is genetically modified to enable the plant to produce its own insecticide within each and every cell, and genetically modified to resist enormous amounts of herbicides that are sprayed onto the crops regularly, such as Monsanto's Roundup and Dow Chemical's 2,4-D, among others.

There are two processes by which the foreign genetic code is introduced into the plant. One way involves what's called a gene gun. Essentially the desired genetic material, as well as a genetic code for antibiotic resistance or pesticide resistance (marker gene), along with a viral promoter and a terminator sequence are coated onto gold or tungsten nanoparticles. These DNA-coated particles are inserted into the gene gun. This genetic material is then shot into a petri dish containing plant cells in a process called particle bombardment, or biolistics. A very small portion of the DNA-coated particles enters the nucleus of some of the cells in the dish, and an even smaller number actually get incorporated into the genetic makeup (through unknown mechanisms). The process relies entirely on luck, because it is entirely random. You will hear GMO proponents talk about how precise the genetic engineering process is, and while the selection and isolation processes of the desired DNA from the parent organism is precise science, the insertion of that DNA into the host organism is entirely random and success rates are extremely low. Saying that particle bombardment is a precise process is tantamount to saying that one could paint a Mona Lisa with a pipe bomb.

In addition, the foreign DNA that does make its way into the nucleus of the host cell and gets incorporated into its DNA does so in a completely random order. In other words, the location along the strand of DNA where the foreign gene inserts itself is random. This has enormous implications for the ability to even test for safety, since genes are not isolated units of information and therefore products that are derived from those genes are derived from either those genes on their own, or a combination with adjoining genes. Since there is no control or uniformity to the exact location of the inserted gene from plant to plant, or even within the same plant, the expressions of those genes will also be random and unpredictable. So, even if health safety testing is performed on one batch, it does not mean that the next batch will have the same protein expressions, which may include allergens, toxins, and/or an altered nutritional profile.

The next step of the genetic engineering process is to put antibiotics or pesticides into the petri dish to separate the cells which have been successfully modified from those which were not. The cells that have been modified resist the antibiotics or pesticides and stay alive, and the cells which were not modified die off. The genetic engineers then add a growth medium into the dish to make the cells multiply and grow into a plant that can be transplanted into the soil. From there, more plants get rejected for defects caused by genetic mutations, abnormalities, or other undesired protein expressions which may or may not be detected by the genetic engineers. This is done mostly by visual inspection.

Another genetic engineering method is using a bacterium which is normally found in the soil, called Agrobacterium tumefaciens (or A. tumefaciens for short). *Tumefacient means "tumor inducing"*. This bacterium has the natural ability to insert small segments of its DNA, called T-DNA (Transfer DNA) into a plant host. It does this in order to make the host plant produce nutrients that it likes. Genetic engineers use this to their advantage, for example to insert genetic material from the bacterium Bacillus thuringiensis into a host plant, so it produces a toxin called Bt toxin. They do this by first linking the gene for Bt toxin production, along with the antibiotic or herbicide resistance gene, the viral promoter and the terminator sequence to the T-DNA and introducing it back into the A. tumefaciens bacterium, which then introduces it into the host plant DNA. Bt toxin is an extremely potent toxin which causes the stomachs of insects to literally burst. B. thuringiensis is in the same family of such bacteria as B. anthracis, which causes anthrax, and B. cereus, which causes food poisoning. Crops that contain this Bt toxin are called "Bt" crops, as in Bt Corn, Bt Soy and Bt Canola for instance. When A. tumefaciens inserts its genes in nature, or the targeted GE genes in a lab, it does it randomly, as is the case with the gene gun method. In nature however, the infection occurs when the plant is already mature, and it is localized at the base of the stalk, forming a tumor called a Crow Gall which does not infect the remaining plant cells or the fruit of the plant, and does not propagate to future generations. In the lab on the other hand, with either method, the infection is made to single cells, and the infected cells get propagated to form a complete plant, and therefore the inserted DNA, which has caused a modification in the genetic code is present in all cells of the plant, and therefore every cell of that plant has an altered genetic expression.

As stated above, with both methods, in addition to the gene or genes responsible for the trait(s) that the genetic engineer wants to introduce to the plant, an antibiotic marker gene is introduced, as well as a viral promoter, such as the 35S enhanced cauliflower mosaic virus promoter, and a terminator sequence. This combination of genetic information and promoters is called the gene cassette.

The antibiotic resistance gene (marker gene) is inserted so that when the plant cell is infected with the gene cassette in the petri dish, antibiotics is introduced into the culture to kill off all unmodified cells. This is a way of separating modified cells from unmodified cells. There is concern among many scientists that introducing a gene that codes for antibiotic resistance into the food supply could cause antibiotic resistance in the humans and animals who consume those foods, and in at least one case it has clearly been shown that a transgene from GE soya can survive passage through the small intestine and can transfer its DNA to the microflora of the small intestine[59]. In a report titled "The Health Effects of Genetically Engineered Crops On San Luis Obispo County"[60], the authors wrote that "Therefore there is horizontal gene transfer from plant material to gut bacteria and if for some reason there is a selective advantage for those bacteria expressing the gene (for example, during a course of antibiotics), they could become the dominant population within the gut. Since plant DNA also can be taken up by and integrated into the cells lining the intestines and other tissues (Einspanier et al., 2001; Schubbert et al., 1994; Schubbert et al., 1997; Schubbert et al., 1998), the possible health consequences of this transfer cannot be ignored."

Antibiotic resistance is already becoming a major problem worldwide[61], and while some of it can be attributed to overuse of antibiotics in the healthcare industry, a lot of it also has to do with the indiscriminate use of antibiotics in intensive animal farming[62], and genetically modified organisms may very well play a big roll in it as well.

Promoters reside at the start of a genetic sequence and are the gene's "on/off switches" which tell the transcribing enzymes when to produce certain proteins based on the organism's needs. Viral promoter on the other hand are "on-only" switches which continually churn the desired protein, irrespective of the organism's needs. The viral promoter is included in the gene cassette to ensure that the natural epigenetic mechanisms within the plant cell do not shut off the newly introduced gene, and that the new gene remain active.

The terminator sequence tells the transcribing enzymes where along the genetic code to stop the transcription. In the Book Altered Genes, Twisted Truth[63] the author explains the roles of promoters and terminator sequences in a very intuitive, easy to understand way. He states that "the terminator sequence acts like an instruction that tells a computer's printer to stop after the twelfth page of a very long document, while the viral promoter acts like an instruction to keep churning out copies of that twelve-page section." In other words, the gene sequence under the control of the promoter and terminator are stuck in an infinite loop of expression.

The modified cells are then cultured in order to propagate the newly engineered cell into a plant, but in order to do that, the genetic engineer has to introduce a growth medium into the culture, as well as induce a genomic shock in order to force the cell to accept and propagate the new gene.   All of those processes induce genetic mutations, causing genes to jump around from one position to another (a process called transposition), and causing the turning on and off of other genes.

It is important to note that even if one batch is tested for safety and is found to be safe, you could not extrapolate that data to all GMOs, even of the same crop, because based on where the inserted foreign genetic material is incorporated along the length of DNA, it will express different behaviors because of its interactions with its neighboring genes. In one location it may cause the production of a certain allergenic protein, and in another location it will not. An alteration to the genetic sequence could be enough to change the shape of a protein, which in turn could change a harmless protein to a toxin, such as with the case of the prion protein causing the "mad cow disease" (bovine spongiform encephalopathy)[64]. In addition, it has been shown that different environmental conditions and stresses will cause the genes to express at different levels[65,66] and even activate cryptic pathways[67], which could lead to the production of toxins that have not formerly been observed in the particular plant variety. In other words, in the lab or in a certain field, a gene may express a low level of toxicity of a certain chemical, but when exposed to high heat or another environmental condition in another field, the levels of that toxin which are expressed by the cells of the plant may be much higher, or may differ completely.

So now that you have a little background on what GMOs are and why they are used, let's look at what is already known, and some other concerns that need to be investigated further. Before we do that, first I would like to point out that many people in the media like to say over and over that we really don't know what the effects of GMOs are on people's health and we need to perform further studies – that is absolutely incorrect... There have been many scientific studies done by both the GMO companies themselves and by independent researchers that prove that GMOs are harmful and I will give you references to as many of those studies as I can so that you can be informed, or at least be aware when the deniers start spreading their misinformation. Also, some well-prepared deniers, mostly those who are paid by the GMO industry to act as independent GMO proponents, will make references to "thousands of studies that prove the safety of GMOs" – you will find out from reading this chapter that those studies that those deniers are referring to not only have nothing to do with food safety of GMOs for the most part, but some of the studies that they will be referring to actually show harm caused by GMOs and their associated herbicides and pesticides. They simply throw out a large number of studies to make their case look strong, and they rely on people not actually having the time to read the large volume of studies. If people did (and some have) they will realize that those deniers are full of it. They will also employ argumentum ad hominem in attempt to discredit good scientists and good science.

2.2   A BRIEF HISTORY OF GMOs

Genetically engineered seeds and crops were approved by the FDA for use in foods in world markets, and became commercially available in 1996, in spite of the warnings of the FDA's own scientists that genetic engineering is different from conventional breeding and poses special risks, including the production of new toxins or allergens that are difficult to detect.[68-73]   (Also see FDA memos starting on page 136). Although 1996 saw the first introduction of a genetically modified whole food product - Calgene's Flavr Savr tomato - it was not the beginning of the GMO venture, or the first introduction of a GMO food product. The genetic engineering venture started in the 1970's. In 1982 the FDA approved an insulin product produced with genetically engineered microbes. In 1984, Showa Denko K.K., a Japanese chemical manufacturer genetically altered a bacterium used in the production of l-tryptophan, and by 1989 they had made three additional genetic alterations to their bacteria. Those alterations lead to a metabolic issue with the bacteria, which caused it to produce a potent toxin, leading to the eosinophilia-myalgia syndrome (EMS) epidemic in the U.S. and abroad. This will be discussed in more detail on page 70. Then, in 1990, the FDA approved Pfizer's GMO-derived Chymosin for human consumption. Chymosin is used in cheese production, comprising 80% to 90% of all cheese produced in the U.S. and the U.K.

According to a 2014 USDA report titled "Genetically Engineered Crops in the United States", "More than 15 years later, adoption of these varieties by U.S. farmers is widespread and U.S. consumers eat many products derived from GE crops—including corn-meal, oils, and sugars—largely unaware that these products were derived from GE crops"[74].

Additionally, the report states that in 2013, 196 million acres (about half of the total land used to grow crops in the United States) was used for growing GE corn, cotton, and soybean. In 2013, 90% of corn, 90% of cotton and 93% of soybean planted in the U.S. was genetically engineered. Worldwide, in 2012 approximately 420 million acres of GE crops were planted in 28 countries.

Although GE seed companies have promised reduced reliance on herbicides and pesticides when their seeds are used, nature has been able to adapt and develop resistance to the pesticides within the plant, as well as to the various herbicides that are used in conjunction with herbicide tolerant (HT) crops. "The adoption of HT crops has enabled farmers to substitute Glyphosate for more toxic and persistent herbicides. However, an over reliance on Glyphosate and a reduction in the diversity of weed management practices adopted by crop producers have contributed to the evolution of Glyphosate resistance in 14 weed species and biotypes in the United States."[74] Between 1996 and 2011 GM herbicide-tolerant crops have led to a 527 million pound increase in herbicide use in the United States alone[75]. Roundup ready crops have led to massive increases of glyphosate use worldwide[75-80].

The lax, so-called "approval process" of GMOs, herbicides and pesticides sets a dangerous precedence. As demonstrated over and over by the authorities' raising of the "safe limits" of herbicides[81] in response to the need for increased herbicide use to combat herbicide resistance, it is only a matter of time before GMO companies produce increasingly toxic crops/chemical combinations in response to herbicide resistance, and resistance to the pesticides produced within the cells of the plant. The biotech industry has forced their fallacious "substantial equivalence" policy and the application of the "Generally Recognized as Safe" (GRAS) status to GMOs on U.S. and foreign governments the world over.

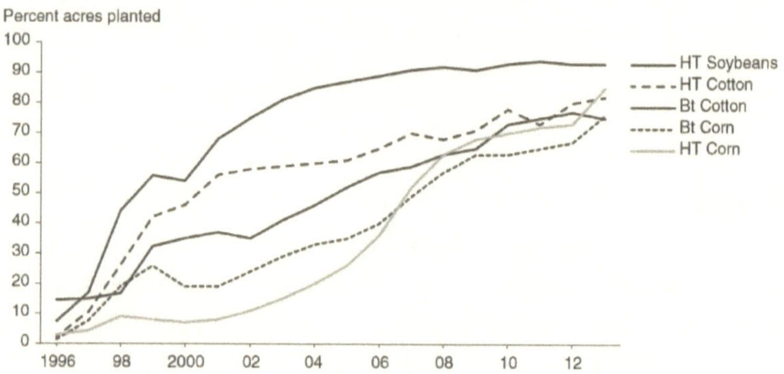

Bt crops have insect resistant traits; HT crops have herbicide tolerance traits.
Data for each crop category include varieties with both Bt and HT (stacked) traits.

Source: U.S. Department of Agriculture (USDA), Economic Research Service (ERS). 2013. *Adoption of Genetically Engineered Crops in the U.S.* data product.

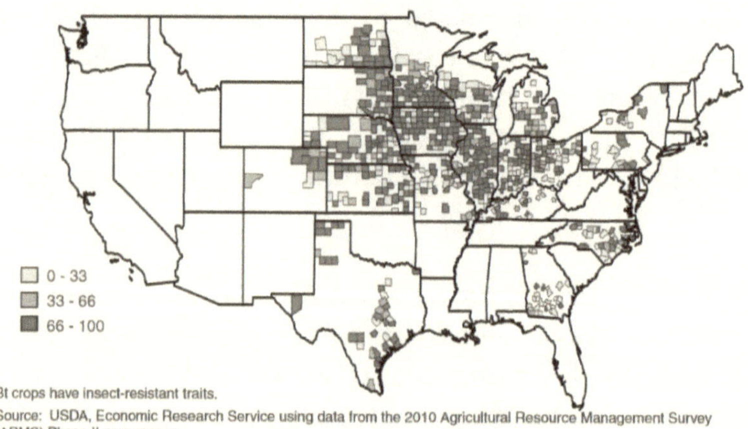

Bt crops have insect-resistant traits.

Source: USDA, Economic Research Service using data from the 2010 Agricultural Resource Management Survey (ARMS) Phase II corn survey.

The graph on the following page illustrates a very important point, which is that above all possible reasons, most farmers in the U.S. have adopted GMO crops due to greed. They were willing to overlook the mounting evidence that shows that GMOs are harmful to humans, animals and the environment for the promise of increased yields and more profits.

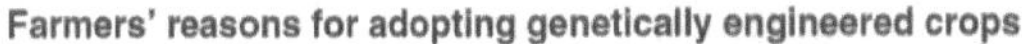

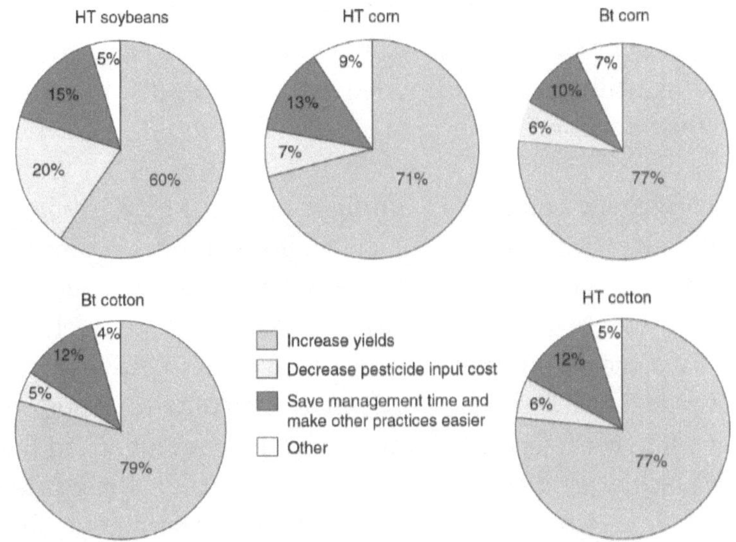

Bt crops have insect resistant traits; HT crops have herbicide tolerance traits.
Sources: USDA Economic Research Service using data from Agricultural Resource Management Survey (ARMS) Phase II surveys: 2010 for corn, 2007 for cotton, and 2006 for soybeans.

Ironically, studies have shown that GE seeds have not increased crop yields, and in some cases even caused a drop in yields. According to a report titled "Failure to Yield – Evaluating the Performance of Genetically Engineered Crops"[82], "commercial GE crops have made no inroads so far into raising the intrinsic or potential yield of any crop. By contrast, traditional breeding has been spectacularly successful in this regard; it can be solely credited with the intrinsic-yield increases in the United States and other parts of the world that characterized the agriculture of the twentieth century."

Additionally, the report states that "Several studies have actually found that background genetics is often more critical than the transgene for determining yield (Jost et al. 2008; Meredith 2006). But when high-yielding varieties also contain a transgene, higher yield may be inaccurately attributed to GE". Furthermore, "the record of GE has not kept pace with yield increases accomplished by other means, such as traditional breeding or newer methods that enhance selective breeding with molecular-marker technology such as marker-assisted selection."

In many poor counties in South America, Africa, India and elsewhere, GMO companies have bought up or otherwise forced seed suppliers to only offer GMO varieties.[83] Farmers wishing to grow certain crops, such as corn, soy, cotton or canola in those countries have no choice but to buy expensive GMO seeds and the herbicides associated with them, year after year. Most farmers in those countries cannot afford those GMO seeds and herbicides and end up incurring large amounts of debt as a result. Thousands of farmers in India have committed suicide as a result of GE crop failures and the increasing prices of seeds and herbicides[84,85].

In a 2003 study on consumer acceptance of GMOs, the authors concluded that "consumers' willingness to pay for a food product decreases when the food label indicates the food product is genetically modified. The evidence shows consumers were willing to pay a 14% premium for food items they perceived as not genetically modified."[86] In the U.S., misinformation campaigns and blocking of good science has led to most people not being aware of the dangers of GMOs.

Although the USDA report[74] was useful in shedding light on how widespread the use of GMOs are, especially in the United States, it is disturbingly apparent that not only is there no mention of the hundreds of studies that show sdverse health effects from GMOs and the herbicides used along with them to humans, animals and the environment, but also that tax funds were used to compile market research data that can only benefit the biotech industry and not the public. In this sense, the USDA has become a market research firm for the biotech industry, at no cost to them.

As you will ascertain from reading the rest of this chapter, Genetic engineers look at biological systems as "Newtonian machines" whereby they can change out the parts of the machine to change the function. However, even with machines, simply changing out one part for another part with differing function could lead to downstream, unintended implications. In biological systems however, the number of components and interactions between them are infinitely greater and more complex, and much, much less understood. Not only are genetic engineers not able to predictably insert foreign genes without causing unwanted downstream effects and side reactions, but they are not even able to insert more of the organism's native genes without the same undesired outcomes occurring. This is because:

1. The process of inserting the desired gene into the host organism is random, destructive, and causes unintended alterations to the host DNA. The complex interactions between genes are disturbed through reconfiguration or the reordering of genetic information, and/or deletion, transposition or turning on or off of the host genes. According to a published article by Jonathan R. Latham, at al., "Transgene insertion is infrequently, if ever, a precise event. Mutations found at transgene insertion sites include deletions and rearrangements of host chromosomal DNA and introduction of superfluous DNA... These genome-wide mutations can number from hundreds to many thousands per diploid genome."[87]

2. Genetic and epigenetic systems have defense mechanisms that disable foreign genes and prevents them from functioning in the organism, so genetic engineers need to disable these natural defenses in order to enable the inserted genes to function. Additionally, they need to insert a viral promoter to force the newly inserted gene to function continually, regardless of environmental/epigenetic inputs and the physiological needs of the organism, which taxes the energy systems of the cell and causes disturbances, alterations, dysfunction and disease. Imagine having an incessant hiccup that goes on and on, and never stops. This condition will in short order overtax your muscles and cause them to fatigue, which will cause them to overproduce lactic acid leading to intense pain. Eventually, in extreme cases, if nothing is done to stop it you will die from exhaustion or a heart attack.

3. The process of inducing a genomic shock to force the host organism to accept the foreign genetic material also causes mutations, transpositions and turning on and off of some of the host organism's native genes.

4. The process of separating the altered genes from unaltered genes causes mutations through the introduction of antibiotics or herbicides into the medium[88], and

5. The tissue culturing process to turn the altered cells into viable plants that could be transferred to soil likewise causes mutations[87] mediated by the growth medium that is introduced to the altered cells.

So, let's jump right into the heart of the matter and discuss the findings that have come from numerous scientific, toxicological studies on GMOs.

2.3   HUMAN AND ANIMAL HEALTH

"People were saying in the industry, in the regulatory agencies, that if the American people want progress they're going to have to be the guinea pigs."

Biologist Dr. Philip Regal Ph.D in videotaped testimony before a New Zealand commission[89]

"Someday we shall look back on this dark era of agriculture and shake our heads. How could we have ever believed that it was a good idea to grow our food with poisons?"

Jane Goodall, primatologist, ethologist, anthropologist, and UN Messenger of Peace[90]

There are a few reasons why animals are included in this section. Firstly, food additive and drug testing is performed on animals before it can be performed on humans, so for that reason we have the most pertinent data specifically for animals. Secondly, I have pets and I love them very much, and so do many other people around the world. We buy pet food for our pets, but we don't really know, just like with human food, where it came from and if it's natural and good for their health. And lastly, the majority of GMO crops are consumed by farm animals. Unlike human diets, farm animals consume a large amount of only a few crops, of which all may be from GMO sources. A small increase in the level of toxins in those crops, even if it is a toxin that is native to the plant, may be significant in a farm animal's diet. Additionally, many of those farm animals end up on the dinner plate and many others are used for their milk and other fluids which are used for human consumption and medical purposes. There is also the issue of animal suffering that is caused by diseases and disorders caused by GMOs and the herbicides and pesticides used along with them.

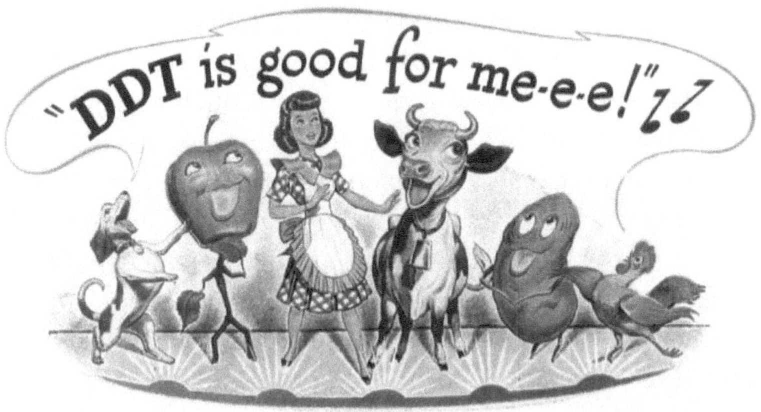

Part of a 1947 full page DDT add by Penn Salt Chemicals[91]

DDT, which is now banned in the U.S. [92] causes damage to the nervous, immune, endocrine, and neurological systems, as well as cancers and liver damage, reproductive harm and birth defects.[91,93] It is no surprise that the chemical companies whom manufactured DDT sued the federal government as a result of the ban[92], showing their complete disregard for human life and environmental health when profits are on the line.

In looking at the "guinea pigs" quote above, recalled by Philip Regal[89], the Nuremberg Code comes to mind, which states that "The voluntary consent of the human subject is absolutely essential."[94] In this regard, and in many other cases, such as the Tuskegee Syphilis experiment[37] and the St. Louis radiation experiment[38,39], the U.S. has repeatedly violated this code.

With this in mind, let's look at some studies that have shown negative health effects resulting from GMO consumption:

2.3.1   RNA and GE Plant Toxins in Human Tissues and Organs

In a study performed in Canada, where GMO use in food products is not as high as it is in the U.S. and where consumption of corn is not as high as some other parts of the world, it was found that "Cry1Ab [Bt] toxin was detected in 93% and 80% of maternal and fetal blood samples, respectively and in 69% of tested blood samples from non pregnant women."[95] Because those woman did not have a high intake of corn and soybeans in their diet, the researchers postulated that the Bt toxin must have come from the milk and meat of animals that did consume large amounts of GM corn and soybean on a daily basis, and the toxin survived the digestion process and ended up in the milk and meat, which was consumed by people. In other studies it was demonstrated that GM DNA from animal feed was found in meat and fish that are consumed by people[96-99]. Additionally, it has been shown that plant MicroRNA survives digestion in mammals and enters into the bloodstream, depositing itself in the liver, thereby altering liver function by binding to the LDL receptor adapter protein 1 (LDLRAP1) and preventing the removal of LDL cholesterol from the blood[100]. What this says is that contrary to what the GMO companies like to reiterate, DNA and RNA from GMOs do enter the bloodstream intact, and do alter organ function. The study[100] further states that "MiRNAs have been widely shown to modulate various critical biological processes, including differentiation, apoptosis, proliferation, the immune response, and the maintenance of cell and tissue identity". Additionally, "Dysregulation of MiRNAs has been linked to cancer and other diseases".

Jeffrey Smith of the Institute for Responsible Technology stated in an article on Dr. Mercola's website[101] that "The Bt-toxin produced in the GM plants is probably more dangerous than in its natural spray form. In the plants, the toxin is about 3,000-5,000 times more concentrated than the spray, it doesn't wash off the plants like the spray does, and it is designed to be more toxic than the natural version." Natural Bt toxin has been used safely for many years and is even allowed in organic agriculture. Bt toxin in its natural form is quite different than the Bt toxin that is produced in the GE Bt crop[67,102,103,104]. One of the biggest differences is that in nature, Bt toxin rapidly breaks down in contact with sunlight, and the only way to ingest this natural form of Bt toxin is by ingesting the soil that contains it, or an infected site on the plant's stalk, which is extremely unlikely. Bt toxin from GE Bt crops on the other hand is present in every cell of the plant in its pre-activated form, which makes it a certainty that it will be ingested by humans and animals who eat Bt crops. So comparing GE Bt toxin use to naturally occurring Bt toxins in the soil or the form which is used on non-GE crops is baseless.

2.3.2   <u>Tissue and Organ Damage in GMO Fed Pigs</u>

In another study[105], a team of Australian scientists and U.S. researchers conducted an experiment on 168 newly weaned pigs, both males and females, in a commercial U.S. piggery. They split the pigs into two groups of 84. They fed one group a diet of GE corn and soy and the other group an equivalent diet of non-GE feed. All of the pigs were reared and fed under the same conditions.

22.7 weeks later, the pigs were slaughtered and autopsied by veterinarians who were not told which pigs fed on which diet. The researchers found that 32% of the pigs that fed on a GE diet had a higher rate of severe stomach inflammation, compared with 12% of the pigs in the non-GE group, and of those, the severity of inflammation was 2 to 4 times worse in the GE fed group as compared with the non-GE fed group. The reason this is significant is because inflammation of the stomach can lead to malabsorption of nutrients, stomach bleeding, gastric cancer and many other problems, and because the immune system is in the gut, many other illnesses stem from inflammation of the digestive tract. In addition, the uteri of GMO fed females were 25% heavier than those in the non-GM group. "such a biologically significant difference in uterine weights may reflect endometrial hyperplasia or carcinoma, endometritis, endometriosis, adenomyosis, inflammation, a thickening of the myometrium, or the presence of polyps."

Furthermore, "the concentration of GGT, which is a measure of liver heath, was 16% lower in GM-fed pigs than non-GM-fed pigs"

The authors remarked that "Even though pigs are physiologically similar to humans, particularly for gastrointestinal observations, very few toxicology studies have been conducted on them for GM crops (Walsh et al., 2012a). In doing this study, we not only used animals that were physiologically similar to humans, but we also weighed and internally examined organs and took blood for biochemical analysis. We further used a large enough sample size (168 pigs, 84 per group) to be able to determine statistical significance for key toxicological outcomes. We also used GM crops that are planted in significant quantities in the USA (Ht soy, and Ht and Bt corn) and hence are commonly eaten by pigs and humans in the USA. We further fed these crops as a mixed diet. Mixed diets commonly occur for pigs and humans. This study therefore reflects the effects of eating GM crops in the 'real world'. To our knowledge, this is the first study of its kind conducted."

One important fact to keep in mind is that a pig's natural lifespan is 8 years. 22.7 weeks of a pig's life is equivalent to 4.3 years of a human's life. Imagine feeding your child GMO formula, GMO cereal, GMO corn – and by the time they reach the age of 4 they are already chronically ill. Pigs' and humans' digestive systems are very similar to one another as stated by the study's authors.

A report by Food Democracy Now! and The Detox Project exposed the very high concentrations of glyphosate and AMPA in America's most popular breakfast cereals and snacks. The results, obtained from testing conducted by a leading FDA-registered food safety testing laboratory showed levels of glyphosate to range from 8.02ppb to 1,125.3ppb, and levels of AMPA in two popular breakfast cereal to range from 14.5 to 26.4ppb[106]. The only safe limits set by European and U.S. governments are based on highly suspect industry studies, and based on what is known about the class of chemicals known as endocrine disruptors, which glyphosate and AMPA are, those limits; 0.3mg/kg-bw/day in the EU and 1.75mg/kg-bw/day in the U.S., are extremely high. Note that the U.S. "safe" level is nearly 6 times that of the EU.

2.3.3   Alteration of Gut Microbiome

Other studies have shown that GE foods modify the genetic makeup of bacteria in the stomach[59,107], and it has been suggested that this new acquired genetic material may cause gut bacteria to produce their own pesticide inside the body. GE foods have also been shown to cause alterations to the balance of and a reduction to the number of beneficial gut bacteria[108,109]. Again, gut bacteria are symbiotic organisms which are critical to our immune system[110], and many studies have even shown that gut bacteria control brain functions[111-117]. In addition, studies have shown that harmful, pathogenic gut bacteria are highly resistant to glyphosate, which is used on nearly all GMO crops, as well as many conventional, non-GMO crops, while beneficial gut bacteria are moderately to highly susceptible to glyphosate[118]. A disruption in the balance of gut bacteria (including a reduction of the beneficial bacteria in the intestinal tracts) leads to inflammation of the intestinal tract, permeability of the intestinal walls, autoimmune disease, liver toxicity, lymphatic disease and cancer. The increase in food allergies to hard to digest foods, like gluten-containing grains are actually caused by the destruction of the gut, which makes breaking down those foods impossible, leading to partially-digested and undigested proteins leaking into the lymphatic system, where they trigger an immune response.

2.3.4   The Pervasiveness of Toxicity

Now, let's go back to a statement that I made earlier and employ some logical thinking. I said that in GMO crops, every cell of the organism contains the modified genetic code and the expression of that code. Cells express a behavior based on their genetic code, or blueprint that they are reading, as well as in accordance with epigenetic mechanisms, so if a blueprint for pesticide production is selected within that cell, the cell will produce the pesticide, and so will every other cell in the plant. In nature, even though every cell has an identical and complete genetic code, the epigenetic mechanisms ensure that only codes which need to be expressed are expressed, based on the requirements of the cell and the organism at the particular point in time. The molecular and cell biologist Dr. Richard Strohman described the state of our knowledge into those mechanisms by stating that "The output from these [dynamic/epigenetic] networks change in response to signals from the body and from the environment. And some of these changes feed back to DNA to regulate gene expression. The key concept here is that dynamic/epigenetic networks have a life of their own - they have network rules - not specified by DNA: and we do not understand these rules."[119]

In GMOs, this natural epigenetic mechanism is overridden by the use of a viral promoter, which ensure that the code is expressed continually, regardless of the needs of the organism, and since this promoter is attached to the inserted foreign code, it is present in every cell, and every cell expresses that code. So what does this mean to you? Since the pesticide is inside the cell of the plant, you cannot wash it off[101], and since it is in every cell, it is present at much higher amounts than would be present in nature. You can wash your vegetables until you're blue in the face, but the pesticide is inside every cell and is not coming off. Additionally, since our state of knowledge surrounding epigenetic mechanisms is at best limited, suppressing or altering those mechanisms in products destined for supermarket shelves is irresponsible at the very least.

Dr. Richard Lacey M.D., Ph.D earned both a B.A. in biochemistry and an M.D. from the University of Cambridge and a Ph.D. in genetics from the University of Bristol. He is a member of the Royal College of Pathologists since 1971, and a Professor of Medical Microbiology at the University of Leeds since 1983. He has been on Emeritus status since 1995. In 1989-1990, he warned against the practice of feeding cattle rendered meat from sheep and other animals, predicting the mad cow epidemic before it occurred. He has also written several books on the topic of food safety and GMOs, as well as over 200 articles published in scientific journals.

In a 1999 Alliance for Bio-Integrity lawsuit against the FDA, Dr. Richard Lacey made the following statement:

"It is my considered judgment that employing the process of recombinant DNA technology (genetic engineering) in producing new plant varieties entails a set of risks to the health of the consumer that are not ordinarily presented by traditional breeding techniques. It is also my considered judgment that food products derived from such genetically engineered organisms are not generally recognized as safe on the basis of scientific procedures within the community of experts qualified to assess their safety." [120]

He further stated that "Recombinant DNA technology is an inherently risky method for producing new foods. Its risks are in large part due to the complexity and interdependency of the parts of a living system, including its DNA. Wedging foreign genetic material in an essentially random manner into an organism's genome necessarily causes some degree of disruption, and the disruption could be multi-faceted. Further, whether singular or multi-faceted, the disruptive influence could well result in the presence of unexpected toxins or allergens or in the degradation of nutritional value. Further, because of the complexity and interactivity of living systems—and because of the extent to which our understanding of them is still quite deficient—it is impossible to predict what specific problems could result in the case of any particular genetically engineered organism. Prediction is even more difficult because even when dealing with one variety of a food-producing organism and one particular set of foreign genetic material, each insertion event is unique and can yield deeply different results".

Recent developments have improved the accuracy of gene insertion using the CRISPR/Cas9 method. However, this process also uses a bacterium (Streptococcus pyogenes) to infect the host DNA, the inserted DNA is still disruptive in an environment it is not designed for, viral promoters and terminator sequences are still used, and the mutagenic and destructive genomic shock, antibiotic isolation, and tissue culturing processes are likewise implemented. All this, coupled with the fact that the state of our knowledge of genetic and epigenetic mechanisms is still in its infancy, genetic engineers would still not be able to predict or prevent adverse effects from occurring, or even be able to detect most of them when they do occur. For instance - the most researched genome in the history of DNA research is that of the Drosophila (fruit fly). Scientists were under the impression that they knew everything that there is to know about the fruit fly's genome, but in 2014 they received a rude awakening when it was discovered by a consortium that includes scientists from Indiana University that the genome of the fruit fly contained "1,468 new genes, of which 536 were found to reside in previously uncharacterized gene-free zones"[121]. "The paper shows that the Drosophila genome is far more complex than previously suspected and suggests that the same will be true of the genomes of other higher organisms. The paper also reports a number of novel, particular results: that a small set of genes used in the nervous system are responsible for a disproportionate level of complexity; that long regulatory and so-called 'antisense' RNAs are especially prominent during gonadal development; that 'splicing factors' (proteins that control the maturation of RNAs by splicing) are themselves spliced in complex ways; and that *the Drosophila transcriptome undergoes large and interesting changes in response to environmental stresses... Those environmental stresses resulted in small changes in expression level at thousands of genes; and in one treatment, four newly modeled genes were expressed altogether differently. In total, 5,249 transcript models for 811 genes were revealed only under perturbed conditions* [emphasis added]." This is critical as it relates to GMOs for the reason that combinations of environmental conditions which might stress the plant in ways which could result in unintended expressions of known toxin, or the expression of different toxins which are not native to the plant under normal conditions, or even toxins which are unknown to science, are incalculable and unfathomable. As much as I hate to quote Donald Rumsfeld, "there are known knowns; there are things we know we know. We also know there are known unknowns; that is to say we know there are some things we do not know. But there are also unknown unknowns – the ones we don't know we don't know."

Dr. Lacey further stated that "The mechanics and risks of recombinant DNA technology are substantially different from those of natural methods of breeding. The latter are typically based on sexual reproduction between organisms of the same or closely related species. Normally, entire sets of genes are paired in an orderly manner that maintains a fixed sequence of genetic information. Every gene remains under the control of the organism's intricately balanced regulatory system. The substances produced by the genes are those that have been within the species for a long stretch of biological time. (In cases where mating is between closely related species, there is generally close correspondence between the substances produced by each.) In contrast, biotechnicians take cells that are the result of normal reproduction and randomly splice a chunk of foreign genetic material into their genome. This always disturbs the function of the region of native DNA into which the material wedges. Further, the foreign genes will usually not express within their new environment without a big artificial boost, which is supplied by fusing them to promoters from viruses or pathogenic bacteria. As a result, these genes operate essentially as independent agents outside the host organism's regulatory system, which can lead to many deleterious imbalances. Moreover, this unregulated activity produces substances that have never been in the host species before and are usually very different from any that have—which could lead to problems even if production were at a low rather than a high level. There are several other major differences between genetic engineering and traditional breeding, all of which could, as can the above-mentioned ones, induce the presence of unpredicted toxins or allergens or the degradation of nutritional value... Consequently, whereas we can generally predict that food produced through conventional breeding will be safe, we cannot make a similar prediction in the case of any genetically engineered food."

He concludes that "Therefore, the only way even to begin to assure ourselves about the safety of a genetically engineered food-yielding organism is through carefully designed long-term feeding studies employing the whole food; and it would be necessary to test each distinct insertion of genetic material, regardless of whether the same set of genetic material in the same type of organism has previously been tested... Even if the most rigorous types of testing were performed on each genetically engineered food, it might not be possible to establish that any is safe to a reasonable degree of certainty, as is possible in the case of most ordinary chemical additives. However, we at least would be in a far better position than now to have greater confidence in these new foods."

He goes on to say that "I regularly attend professional conferences in my specialties and I keep abreast of the scientific literature. I also stay in communication with many life scientists and health professionals... To the best of my judgment, neither genetically engineered foods as a general class nor any genetically engineered food in particular is generally recognized as safe among those experts qualified by training and experience to evaluate their safety... I base this judgment on two factors. First, although many life scientists (including some molecular biologists) claim that genetically engineered foods pose no unreasonable risk, I know of many well-qualified life scientists who do not think that their safety has been established. For instance, a recent official statement of the British Medical Association seriously questions the assumption that genetically engineered foods are in general as safe as those produced by traditional methods. In my opinion, the number of scientists who are not convinced about the safety of genetically engineered foods is substantial enough to prevent the existence of a general recognition of safety. Second, there is insufficient evidence to support a belief that genetically engineered foods are safe. I am not aware of any study in the peer-reviewed scientific literature that establishes the safety of even one specific genetically engineered food let alone the safety of these foods as a general class. Few properly designed toxicological feeding studies have even been attempted, and I know of none that was satisfactorily completed. Those who claim that genetically engineered foods are as safe as naturally produced ones are clearly not basing their claims on scientific procedures that demonstrate safety to a reasonable degree of certainty. Rather, they are primarily basing their claims on a set of assumptions that, besides being empirically unsubstantiated, are in several respects at odds with the bulk of the evidence."

He remarked on the FDA's policy as it relates to genetically engineered foods that "although it claims to be 'science-based', this claim has no solid basis in fact. The only way to base the claims about the safety of genetically engineered food in science is to establish each one to be safe through standard scientific procedures, not through assumptions that reflect more wishful thinking than hard fact."

The official policy of Monsanto, the largest GMO seed company in the world, is that the crops produced from their seeds are safe for consumption and therefore there is no need for testing. This policy is posted on their website. They reached that conclusion after their own scientists concluded that GMOs are harmful; those scientists were threatened with lawsuits and were silenced.

In addition to the Bt toxin expressed within the cells of the plant, the crops are sprayed with enormous amounts of herbicides. The herbicides leach into the vegetables and stays there where it too cannot be washed away. Studies in Canada and Europe have shown that levels of Glyphosate, which is the active ingredient in Monsanto's highly popular herbicide Roundup have been detected in the blood and urine of humans at dangerously high levels[95,122]. Other studies in the U.S. have found dangerously high levels of Glyphosate in breast milk of humans and animals[123], as well as in urine[123,124,125]. Yet another study in Canada showed that 93% of pregnant women who were tested had the insecticide Bt toxin that is present in the GMO plant, in their blood[95]. Those herbicides and pesticides contain many toxic chemicals including carcinogens. IARC, the world's leading cancer research organization, and the cancer research arm of the World Health Organization (WHO) have recently classified Glyphosate as a possible human carcinogen[126]. It is no wonder that over 14 million people worldwide get cancer every year. Over a 50-year period that equals to over 700 million people. That is twice the population of the U.S. and about 10% of the world's population.

GMOs and herbicides have now been linked to increased rates of infertility[127], obesity[53], endocrine disruption / hormonal imbalances[53,128,129-134], digestive problems[105], liver damage[100,135], kidney damage[53,135], birth defects[53], autism[127], cancers[51,52,53], allergic reactions, and many other diseases and disorders. As a matter of fact, GMOs have been shown to cause allergic reactions to other, normally non-allergenic foods in a process called immunological cross-priming[127,136].

According to Jeffrey Smith of The Institute for Responsible Technology, when livestock are switched from GM to non-GM soy or corn, with no other changes made, within days the animals are using less medicine, their behavior is different, and their death rate is reduced. The same effects have been reported by people who switch to an all-organic diet.

It is very important to note that Glyphosate goes hand in hand with GMOs. As a matter of fact, as of 2012, over 80% of all GM crops were engineered to tolerate one or more herbicide[137,138].

The biotech industry claims that Glyphosate can only attack plants because plants have a metabolic pathway called the shikimate pathway, and humans do not possess this pathway, and therefore there is no risk for humans. In biochemistry, a metabolic pathway is a series of chemical reactions occurring within a cell, where one reaction leads to the production of another chemical, which leads to the production of another chemical and so on. So, the claim is that since humans do not have the shikimate pathway, the human body will not recognize Glyphosate and therefore will not metabolize it. However, our gut bacteria do have this shikimate pathway, which means that they will be affected by Glyphosate, which of course will affect the human through degradation of the digestive system, the immune system, the brain, and many other systems in our bodies that rely on the byproducts that are produced by our gut bacteria.

Furthermore, Dr. Stephanie Seneff, a Senior MIT Research Scientist had researched Glyphosate and its effects extensively and has written papers on its numerous ill effects on the human body.   In one paper with the mouthful title "Glyphosate's Suppression of Cytochrome P450 Enzymes and

Amino Acid Biosynthesis by the Gut Microbiome: Pathways to Modern Diseases"[127], Dr. Seneff went into those ill effects and the science behind the mechanisms by which those ill effects occur, in great detail. Some of the diseases and conditions which Dr. Seneff claims are caused by Glyphosate, with supporting evidence for her conclusions, are obesity[53], cardiovascular disease, cancer[126,139,140], colitis, Alzheimer's disease[53], Parkinson's disease[53], autism[111], depression[141] and many others. In addition, and this is something that research scientists should pay very close attention to, Dr. Seneff states that the Cytochrome P450 enzyme, or CYP enzyme in short, which is abundant in the liver is responsible for among other things, detoxification. Glyphosate disrupts this enzyme, and therefore it effectively renders all other toxins more potent. Keep in mind that there are toxins in everything you eat, natural or otherwise. However, enzymes in our body break down those toxins and eliminate them. A disruption of those detoxifying enzymes will therefore cause ordinary food to induce allergic or toxic effects.

So when toxicological studies with Roundup-Ready GMOs are performed, they should always be combined with Roundup. Detoxification enzyme activity and microbiome health should be evaluated to identify potential deleterious effects on the body's ability to effectively detoxify.

There is an excellent interview by Jeffrey Smith with Dr. Seneff where they go into many of those findings and many more, and I highly recommend watching it. It is certainly a lot easier to understand than reading a scholarly article. You can find the video by searching "The Health Dangers of Roundup (glyphosate) Herbicide. Jeffrey Smith & Stephanie Seneff" on YouTube.

2.3.5 Genetic Extortion

In an effort to reduce the risk of GMOs escaping into the environment and disturbing natural ecosystems, GMO researchers have now been successful at modifying the genetic code of a bacteria to create a "safety switch"[142]. This modified code makes it impossible for the organism to sustain life without being fed a synthetic amino acid produced by the scientists, and which does not occur in nature. Although this sounds like a good step forward in protecting the ecosystem from unwanted contamination by GMOs, this advancement has alarming implications. One of the big arguments of opponents of GMOs is a process called Horizontal Gene Transfer (HGT), also referred to as Lateral Gene Transfer (LGT). In this process, the genetic material of one species is introduced into another, completely unrelated species. Genetic engineering using A. Tumefaciens is an example of the implementation of this HGT process in a lab, and although this process does occur in nature, it is normally associated with bacterial and viral infections, and even then, when compared with genetically engineered organisms, bacterial and viral infections in nature do not affect all the cells of the organism (human, plant, etc.). Vertical Gene Transfer (VGT) on the other hand is the natural process by which genes are transferred from parent to offspring through sexual or asexual reproduction.

It has been shown that intact snippets of DNA from plants can survive the digestion process and enter into the bloodstream. DNA from plants would not interact with human DNA because it is not compatible with human DNA, however, as mentioned before, since GE genes that are inserted into the GMO crops often times come from viruses and bacteria, they will affect the bacteria in the human digestive system, which outnumber human cells 10 to 1, and 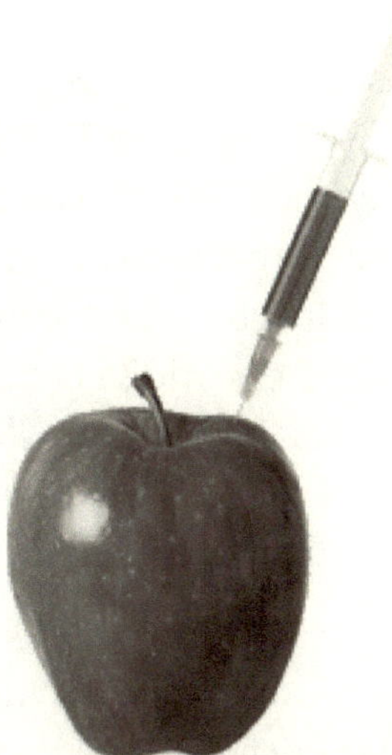 may affect human cells as well. It has been suggested in peer reviewed scientific studies that the Bt toxin producing gene inserted into Bt crops could potentially insert itself into the gut bacteria and cause the gut bacteria itself to produce the Bt toxin, effectively turning your stomach into a pesticide factory.

So, going back to the "safety switch"; if this genetic material inserts itself into the genetics of your gut bacteria, in the absence of the synthetic amino acid provided by the biotech company, which surely would be a trade secret, your gut bacteria could all die off, which would be the end of you. Not only is this an unintended risk, but in the hands of power-grabbing governments and corporations, it could be used as a weapon on people, entire nations, and the entire world to hold ultimate power over them.

2.3.6   Genetic Scrabble

One scenario that I have not heard anyone talking about, and which potentially throws a big monkey-wrench into the whole GMO debate is, assuming that the claims by GMO companies are correct that they rigorously test GMOs for safety, which as you just read is completely false, what would happen if a Monsanto plant cross-pollinates with a DuPont Pioneer plant, or a Syngenta plant? What would be the genetic outcome of the hybrid? What would be the nutritional or toxicological profile of this hybrid? Would you even know that you have a hybrid in your field before the crop is sold and transported around the world? I could not come up with a single reference which states that any GMO company tests every combination of every GMO crop cross-pollinating with one-another, and would that even be possible or financially feasible? I think not...

> *"One thing that surprised us is that US regulators rely almost exclusively on information provided by the biotech crop developer, and those data are not published in journals or subjected to peer review... The picture that emerges from our study of US regulation of GM foods is a rubber-stamp 'approval process' designed to increase public confidence in, but not ensure the safety of, genetically engineered foods."*
>
> David Schubert, professor and head, Cellular Neurobiology Laboratory, Salk Institute, commenting on the findings of a review of GMO regulation that he co-authored[67,143]

2.3.7   The EMS Epidemic

The following case predates the introduction of GE food crops, however it is a case of a genetically modified bacteria used in a supplement that has gone terribly wrong.

In mid to late 1998 an epidemic broke out across the United States and several other countries of a new disease that included such symptoms as swelling of the arms and legs, extremely severe joint and muscle pain (myalgia), extensive skin rashes, significant breathing problems, congestive heart failure and complete paralysis requiring a respirator to breath. In addition, it was discovered that the levels of white blood cells called eosinophils were highly elevated in individuals who exhibited those symptoms. Eosinophils typically fight infections and control mechanisms associated with allergies. Eosinophil levels in individuals exhibiting those symptoms went up from a normal level of 100 to 200 cells per microliter of blood to 4,000 and in some cases even much higher. During severe allergic reactions eosinophil levels could rise to 1,000 or more, but those individuals whom contracted this new disease had levels which were much higher. At those high levels eosinophils attack normal tissue which leads to severe damage and pain. Due to the high levels of eosinophils, accompanied by myalgia, the new disease was labeled Eosinophilia-Myalgia Syndrome (EMS).

At first, the source of the outbreak was unknown. It took several months to trace the new disease to a supplement called L-tryptophan – an amino acid critical to life and which also occurs naturally in various food sources. It took another several months to trace the source of this supplement to a single Japanese manufacturer named Showa Denko K.K. During the ensuing months, it was discovered that the source of the EMS outbreak was attributed to contaminants in the supplement caused by the manufacturing process. The purity standards set by the United States Pharmacopeia Convention put the maximum level of contaminants acceptable for supplements at 1.5%. Although there were 60 contaminants found in Showa Denko's L-tryptophan, which was very high, the total amount of contamination present was within the allowed limit. Therefore, whatever caused the outbreak had to be extremely toxic.

The manufacturing process by which L-tryptophan is obtained involved a fermentation process using bacteria. Upon further investigation, it was determined that Showa Denko has made a change to their manufacturing process by employing a new bacterial strain which was genetically engineered to produce higher amounts of L-tryptophan. Investigators discovered that this new genetically engineered bacterium produced an unforeseen novel toxin that circumvented all of the filtration steps in the manufacturing process and made its way into the final product, thereby shattering the biotechnology industry's assertions that the genetic modification process is inherently safe and cannot produce toxic effects.

Although the official number of EMS affected individuals was reported to be around 1,500 with 80 deaths, the CDC has stated that due to its lack of sensitivity in case definition, it has calculated that the actual number of affected individuals in the United States was somewhere between 5,000 and 10,000.

In order to protect the biotech industry, industry scientists, as well as the FDA and CDC attempted to prove that the EMS epidemic was caused by anything and everything other than the genetically modified organisms. They found that the Showa Denko L-tryptophan contained two substances; IMT and EBT, that were not found in other L-tryptophan supplements and were quick to blame the epidemic on those contaminants, even though they had no evidence to back up their claims. As a matter of fact, subsequent tests on EMS affected patients revealed that some of those patients did not even have those contaminants in their bodies. They then shifted their attention to the fact that Showa Denko had reduced the amount of charcoal in their purification process, which they claimed had let the toxin through into the final product. However, this also ignored the fact that after Showa Denko discovered that their product was causing people to get ill they reverted back to previous charcoal levels, which had reduced the EMS occurrences, but did not eliminate them. At the same time, out of all of the manufacturers of L-tryptophan, Showa Denko's product was the only one to have caused occurrences of EMS.

The biotech industry then had discovered that prior to the outbreak, and prior to Showa Denko's switch to the genetically engineered "Strain V", there had been 12 reported cases of EMS in the United States, and they were quick to point to that fact as proof that it could not have been the genetically engineered strain. Once again, they failed to mention that before "Strain V" there were "Strain I, II, III and IV". "Strain I" was the original, non-GE form of the bacteria. However, II, III and IV were earlier strains of genetically engineered bacteria which were engineered for successively higher outputs of L-tryptophan. When the 12 cases of EMS occurred, the affected individuals filed a lawsuit against Showa Denko and it was discovered that "Strain IV" had caused the illness. Showa Denko quickly reverted back to Strain III. At the same time, the attorneys for the patients notified the FDA, so the FDA knew well in advance of the outbreak, but chose to suppress that information in order to protect the biotech industry.

Showa Denko then further manipulated the genetics of the bacteria and came up with "Strain V", which was the cause of the epidemic. It is also worth noting again that no cases of EMS arose from the use of any other L-tryptophan supplement manufactured by any other source, and no new cases of EMS occurred after the use of the GE bacteria strains were halted. It is also noteworthy that no other L-tryptophan manufacturer used genetically engineered bacteria in their process. It was therefore clear that it was the genetic manipulation of the bacteria that had caused the toxin to form in the L-tryptophan, which caused the EMS outbreak. Even in the face of this evidence, to this day, the biotech industry, the CDC and the FDA continue to deny that the genetic manipulation had caused the toxic outbreak.

It is evident therefore that although GE strains II and III did not present an acute problem, or at least none was reported, and although long term chronic affects were not evaluated, strains IV and V did lead to the creation of novel toxins, which even though rigorous filtration processes were employed to eliminate contaminants, and even though the resulting contamination levels in the final product were extremely low, those novel toxins were so potent as to cause severe, irreversible damage to the human body, and in many cases, death. It is also entirely possible that strains II and III did produce a minute level of the toxin as well, but were sufficiently filtered out, or as stated before, did not cause acute reactions. It should therefore be immediately obvious to even the least educated person that if a product made with GE organisms, which undergoes rigorous filtration can nevertheless induce such toxic effects, that therefore plants that are genetically engineered, and which do not go through a filtration process before being sold to consumers could very well have highly harmful and even deadly toxins within them, and therefore rigorous toxicological and ecological testing by qualified third party laboratories must be conducted in advance of any release into the environment, and in advance of release to the market, as well as every time a genetic manipulation is generated, whether it is a reproduction of the same strain (since the gene insertion process is not controllable or repeatable) or a new strain. Just as FAA regulations require that all aviation products undergo qualification testing by third party laboratories in order to protect life and property, so should the FDA in regards to genetically modified organisms and food additive, which they currently do not.

Had the effects of "Strain IV" and "Strain V" taken a longer time to manifest or manifested as conditions or diseases which were more prevalent at the time, the contamination would have most likely gone undetected. It therefore leads one to wonder how many food additives and/or genetically modified organisms lead to illnesses which are considered common, genetically inherited, or to chronic conditions, such as multiple sclerosis, dementia, and cancer. Of course, one does not have to wonder, because there is a plethora of peer reviewed published studies on GMOs as well as many food additives that prove their toxicity, yet the FDA allows them to be used in and on our food supply, in vaccines and in medications, in a clear violation of the law, for the sake of continued profits. Or perhaps for more sinister reasons…

According to a report by the American College of Rheumatology[144], in regards to occurrences of EMS "no new cases have been published since the FDA ban [on l-tryptophan] was lifted in 2005."

The EMS incident is a clear example of what happens when an organism is forced to produce a substance in excess of what is normal. Even though the genetic alteration did not introduce any foreign genes, and instead inserted additional copies of the organism's native genes, the mere act of overproducing a substance was seen by the organism as a dysfunction, which lead to over-stressing of its system and the production of a novel toxin. Natural systems have an innate balance of energy distribution, and when this balance is disturbed, through overproduction, underproduction, introduction of a new gene or metabolic pathway, etc., unpredictable effects inevitably occur.

The American Academy of Environmental Medicine makes the following statement on their website[145]:

"With the precautionary principle in mind, because GM foods have not been properly tested for human consumption, and because there is ample evidence of probable harm, the AAEM asks:

- Physicians to educate their patients, the medical community, and the public to avoid GM foods when possible and provide educational materials concerning GM foods and health risks.

- Physicians to consider the possible role of GM foods in the disease processes of the patients they treat and to document any changes in patient health when changing from GM food to non-GM food.

- Our members, the medical community, and the independent scientific community to gather case studies potentially related to GM food consumption and health effects, begin epidemiological research to investigate the role of GM foods on human health, and conduct safe methods of determining the effect of GM foods on human health.

- For a moratorium on GM food, implementation of immediate long term independent safety testing, and labeling of GM foods, which is necessary for the health and safety of consumers."

2.4   **THE ENVIRONMENT**

> *"Monsanto is able to ignore the human and environmental damage caused by its products, and maintain its devastating activities through a strategy of systemic concealment: by lobbying regulatory agencies and governments, by resorting to lying and corruption, by financing fraudulent scientific studies, by pressuring independent scientists, and by manipulating the press and media. Monsanto's history reads like a text-book case of impunity, benefiting transnational corporations and their executives, whose activities contribute to climate and biosphere crises and threaten the safety of the planet."*
>
> Andre Leu, president of IFOAM and a member of the RI Steering Committee[146]

GMO crops also pose a risk to the environment on many fronts. Pollen from GMO crops is spread through pollinators and wind and fertilize other plants and trees. This pollen contains the modified genetic code, which then introduces this code to other plants. It is completely uncontrolled when grown in open air farms and once the environment has been contaminated, there is no way to recall the modified genes. As a matter of fact, the FDA, USDA, and EPA allow GMO developers to test their crops in open air farms without any data showing whether or not the variety under test is safe for the environment or human / animal consumption. In a testimony before Congress, Robert E. Brackett, Ph.D., Director of the Center for Food Safety and Applied Nutrition stated that the "FDA encourages developers to submit protein safety information *once field testing reaches a stage of development such that there could be concerns that new non-pesticidal proteins produced in the field-tested plants might be found in food or feed* [emphasis added]."[147] Would it not be prudent to gather this information before open air field trials begin? With cross-contamination of wild species, as well as traditionally grown crops in neighboring farms, which has occurred numerous times - if an outbreak of a gene coding for a potent toxin escapes the confines of the field trial, there will be no way to curtail it after the fact. Chemical and even radiological pollutants break down over time through physical and biological mechanisms, but GMOs are living organisms which reproduce and multiply. Once in the environment, they cannot be recalled.

In a recent study[148], published in December 2015, that aimed to "evaluate evidence that feral transgenic plants spread transgenes" and "determine environmental and agricultural production factors influencing the location of feral alfalfa, especially transgenic plants", the researchers found that 27% of feral (wild) Alfalfa in areas bordering GMO alfalfa fields contained the GE gene. "Our study confirms that genetically engineered alfalfa has dispersed into the environment". Alfalfa is a very important crop which is used extensively for animal feed. What this study reveals is that GMO alfalfa and conventional or organic alfalfa cannot co-exist, and that since alfalfa is an insect-pollinated crop, and many pollinators have far-ranging foraging grounds, the possibility of cross-contamination is great. Alfalfa is a very important crop for organic meat and milk production - it is the main food source for many organically raised cattle and contamination of this crucial crop would be devastating to organic farmers[149].

In Mexico, which has the largest biodiversity of corn in the world, GMO corn seeds have been banned due to the finding that natural crops are being contaminated by GMOs. Monsanto is now using NAFTA to get around Mexican law in an effort to contaminate all of Mexico's corn crops. Once those crops are contaminated, Monsanto legally owns them, which is a topic I'll discuss further under "Economic Impact". In Hungary, the government burned down all GMO fields and banned the future use of GMOs. More and more European countries, as well as other countries around the world are either severely limiting and labeling GMOs or outright banning their cultivation and use. Since the World Health Organization's report on Glyphosate was published, even more countries are banning Roundup, which by extension will limit the use of GMOs.

Additionally, Monsanto, and other companies are developing GMO trees in order to reduce the amount of lignin in the tree. Lignin is what gives trees their structural integrity, but in paper production, the lignin has to be removed from the wood before it can be used to make paper, and this removal process is expansive. If widespread cross-pollination occurs, a domino effect could ensue which could wipe out entire forests. The removal of lignin also causes trees to decompose quicker than normal, which disturbs the natural balance.

"In 2002 China's State Forestry Administration approved GM poplar trees for commercial use. Subsequently 1.4 million Bt (insecticide) producing GM poplars were planted in China. They were planted both for their wood and as part of China's 'Green Wall' project, which aims to impede desertification. Reports indicate that the GM poplars have spread beyond the area of original planting and that contamination of native poplars with the Bt gene is occurring. There is concern with these developments, particularly because the pesticide producing trait may impart a positive selective advantage on the poplar, allowing it a high level of invasiveness."[150]

In another instance, ArborGen, a tree seedling producer, altered the Loblolly pine variety by inserting genetic material from the American sweetgum tree, Monterey pine, Mouse ear cress and E. coli bacteria.[151]

The Center for Food Safety voiced its concern over potential environmental impacts, claiming that "changes in wood density could affect decomposition rates and forest species."[151]

ArborGen's Loblolly pine is not regulated by the USDA because the USDA claims that since it is not engineered with plant pathogens, it is not a regulated article and can be freely cultivated without undergoing environmental studies.

One of the most alarming effects of growing GMOs is the need for an increasing amount of herbicides[152,153], due to the development of herbicide resistance in the targeted weeds. As a result of increased herbicide and pesticide use, soil bacteria and other beneficial organisms are also dying off. Minerals in the soil and the crops are being depleted as well[154], and soil-borne diseases are promoted. As a result, the crops themselves have a depleted nutrient value[155], and long term, the soil will not be able to support any crop at all. On February 26, 1937, Franklin D. Roosevelt stated in a letter to all State Governors on a Uniform Soil Conservation Law that "The Nation that destroys its soil destroys itself". In a 2012 report, Bill Freese, science policy analyst at the Center for Food Safety stated: "Increasingly toxic herbicide cocktails will be used on multiple herbicide-resistant (HR) crops, spawning weeds with multiple resistances. The chemical arms race with weeds triggered by these HR crops entails an ever-escalating spiral of pesticide use and pollution, and attendant adverse impacts on public health and the environment."[156]

A 2006 Cornell University study states that by 2050, 30% of the land that is currently cultivated would be unfarmable.[157] Dr. Don Huber of Purdue University and other scientists have identified over 40 plant diseases that are on the rise in the U.S. due to overuse of Glyphosate.[154] Glyphosate has been used to such an extent that it is no longer effective against most weed varieties, so Monsanto and other companies are now combining Glyphosate with 2,4-D and Dicamba to combat herbicide resistance. If you recall, 2,4-D is the main ingredient in a chemical called Agent Orange, also developed by Monsanto and Dow Chemicals, and used during the Vietnam War to clear out enormous swaths of jungle vegetation and food crops. 2,4-D and its breakdown products are toxic, and due to the manufacturing process of 2,4-D, it is commonly contaminated with Dioxins. Dioxins are a class of chemicals, which include PCBs, which bioaccumulate and are extremely toxic. Dioxins are responsible for the alarming number of birth defects occurring in Vietnam to this very day, and among military personnel who were exposed to it during the war. Besides the obvious problem with using 2,4-D as a pesticide, which is already approved in the U.S. by the FDA, USDA, and EPA, weeds will inevitably form resistance to 2,4-D as well, which will mean that farmers will have to increase the dosage again and again. Eventually weeds will become completely resistant to 2,4-D, as is the case with every other pesticide used in the past, resulting in the use of increasingly toxic chemicals introduced into the food supply.

According to a study by the U.S. Geological Survey[158], "Seven compounds in 1995 and 5 in 2007 were detected in ≥50% of both air and rain samples. Atrazine, metolachlor, and propanil were detected in ≥50% of the air and rain samples in both years. Glyphosate and its degradation product, aminomethyl-phosphonic acid (AMPA), were detected in ≥75% of air and rain samples in 2007 but were not measured in 1995." Although most of those chemicals were detected both in 1995, prior to the introduction of GMOs, and in 2007, the concentrations in the rain and air samples were many times higher in 2007.

GMOs and herbicides, such as Glyphosate and neonicotinoids, produced by Monsanto, Syngenta, Bayer CropScience and Dow Agrosciences have also been linked to Colony Collapse Disorder and the deaths of millions upon millions of bees and monarch butterflies which are crucial to pollination and the survival of the food supply.

Albert Einstein was quoted as saying "If the bee disappeared off the surface of the globe, then man would have only four years of life left. No more bees, no more pollination, no more plants, no more animals, no more man."

2.5   ECONOMIC IMPACT

According to current patent law, companies like Monsanto, Dow, DuPont, Syngenta, Bayer and BASF and others can patent and own the rights to a modified gene. This has numerous implications. Let's explore one scenario: farmer "A" is a GMO farmer that purchases his seeds from Monsanto. Down the road, farmer "B" grows natural crops. During the growing season, pollen from the GMO crops of farmer "A" get blown in the wind and lands on the crops of farmer "B". Unbeknownst to farmer "B", his crops now contain the patented modified gene. Monsanto can now sue farmer "B" for using their patented gene without license and take over his farm. Sadly, Monsanto has done this hundreds of times. They have even hired investigators to illegally trespass on farmers' lands to test their crops, and the courts, which are in Monsanto's pocket, sided with them.

There is an excellent documentary which discusses exactly this topic, which is available on YouTube in its entirety, called "David versus Monsanto"[159]. It is very upsetting to watch, but I highly recommend watching it.

Let's look at another possible scenario. ArborGen creates a genetically modified tree. The pollen from this tree goes up in the air and lands in Yellowstone National Park and genetically alters the trees in the park. ArborGen can now go to the U.S. government and say, your trees contain our patented gene and under U.S. law we now own those trees. They can then go in and cut down all the trees and the government or anyone else is powerless to stop them.

In India, thousands of farmers committed suicide after having crop failure due to a defective Monsanto seed. In the U.S. and elsewhere farmers have been bankrupted after being sued by Monsanto.

In Africa, many promises for increased yield ended in disaster. After much media coverage about how Monsanto was going to save millions of people in Africa with their new virus-resisting sweet potato in Kenya, and with their virus-resistant cassava – a staple crop in Africa, which they promised would increase yields by as much as ten times[160], the GMO sweet potato and cassava performed poorly after succumbing to the virus they were designed to resist[161,162,163]. Meanwhile in Uganda, a conventional breeding program has produced a virus-resistant, high-yielding sweet potato which produced roughly 100% higher yields and at a fraction of the time and cost of Monsanto's GMO variety[164], and a new variety of cassava developed by the International Institute of Tropical Agriculture (IITA) has produced a virus and drought resistant variety that has 6 to 10 times higher yields[165] than other varieties grown in those regions. This high-yielding cassava has been successfully implemented across Africa.

In a statement signed by 24 delegates from 18 African countries to the UN Food and Agricultural Organization in 1998, the delegates stated – "We strongly object that the image of the poor and hungry from our countries is being used by giant multinational corporations to push a technology that is neither safe, environmentally friendly nor economically beneficial to us. We do not believe that such companies or gene technologies will help our farmers to produce the food that is needed in the 21st century. On the contrary, we think it will destroy the diversity, the local knowledge and the sustainable agricultural systems that our farmers have developed for millennia, and that it will thus undermine our capacity to feed ourselves."[166]

Monsanto are also developing seeds that produce sterile plants. This means that the plant will not produce seeds (or viable seeds) and the farmers will have no choice but to come back to them every growing season to buy new seeds. Coupled with their goal of contaminating and dominating the world food supply, in the future there will be no need for wars (not that I agree with wars). You would just stop the supply of seeds to the country of your choice and starve your enemy. Fortunately, GMOs are already banned in dozens of countries all over the world[167], and that number is growing. There are now more countries that have officially banned GMOs than countries that cultivate them[167].

Another fallacy perpetrated by the GMO industry is that without GMOs we couldn't possibly feed the growing world population. One of their promises, which has been scientifically disproved as shown in the examples above, is that GMOs produce higher yields than conventional crops. Not only is that not true, but it has been demonstrated that there are many organic and sustainable practices that produce up to 10 times the output of an average farm per acre of land. Additionally, the rate of current food production can feed 11 Billion people. This food shortage fallacy was perpetrated by the biotech industry to promote their supposedly "higher yielding" crops.

As a matter of fact, the following is a statement made by Steve Smith, head of GMO company Novartis Seeds UK (now Syngenta) at a public meeting on a proposed local GMO farm scale trial in Tittleshall, Norfolk, UK on March 29, 2000:

"If anyone tells you that GM is going to feed the world, tell them that it is not... To feed the world takes political and financial will."[168]

So if there is no food shortage, then why are so many going hungry? It turns out that the reason is access. In other words, certain areas of the world are being starved for political and financial reasons. Another problem is knowledge - knowing what to plant where, and when to plant it. Knowing how to tend to the soil, etc.

2.6   A GAME OF GMO PING PONG

According to Phil Angell, Monsanto's former director of corporate communications, "Monsanto should not have to vouchsafe the safety of biotech food. Our interest is in selling as much of it as possible. Assuring its safety is the FDA's job."[169]

This is a little bit of a problem when the people in the FDA who are in charge of evaluating biotech (GMO) products are former employees of Monsanto, and people with direct connection to the GMO industry control or have enormous influence over so many governmental agencies, in the U.S. and globally. As a result of this, the GMO industry and the governments they control and/or influence set up a system where they are both responsible and not responsible simultaneously, and nothing gets done on behalf of consumer safety.

Here are the statements made by the FDA (U.S. government's Food and Drug Administration, responsible for food safety) and EFSA (the European Food Safety Authority):

"Ultimately, it is the food producer who is responsible for assuring safety." – US Food and Drug Administration (FDA).[170]

"It is not foreseen that EFSA carry out such [safety] studies as the onus is on the [GM industry] applicant to demonstrate the safety of the GM product in question."– European Food Safety Authority (EFSA).[171]

According to a report by William Freese and David Schubert, "The FDA has left it up to the biotech industry to decide whether or not a transgenic protein is GRAS [Generally

Recognized as Safe], and so exempt from testing (FDA Policy, 1992). The FDA has yet to revoke an industry GRAS determination and require food additive testing of any transgenic crop"[67]. As a matter of fact, according to FDA regulations, the company developing the GE crop is not even required to notify the FDA of its intent to market the new crop. "Under voluntary consultation, the GE crop developer is encouraged, but not required, to consult with the FDA. The company submits data summaries of research it has conducted, but not the full studies. That is, the FDA never sees the methodological details, but rather only limited data and the conclusions the company has drawn from its own research. As one might expect with a voluntary process, the FDA does not require the submission of data. And in fact, companies have failed to comply with FDA requests for data beyond that which they submitted initially (Gurian-Sherman, 2003). Without test protocols or other important data, the FDA is unable to identify unintentional mistakes, errors in data interpretation or intentional deception, making it impossible to conduct a thorough and critical review."[67]

"contrary to popular belief, the FDA has not formally approved a single GE crop as safe for human consumption. Instead, at the end of the consultation, the FDA merely issues a short note summarizing the review process and a letter that conveys the crop developer's assurances that the GE crop is substantially equivalent to its conventional counterpart [the concept of Substantial Equivalence]. The FDA's letter to Monsanto regarding its MON810 Bt corn is typical:"[67]

"Based on the safety and nutritional assessment you have conducted, it is our understanding that Monsanto has concluded that corn products derived from this new variety are not materially different in composition, safety, and other relevant parameters from corn currently on the market, and that the genetically modified corn does not raise issues that would require premarket review or approval by FDA. ... as you are aware, it is Monsanto's responsibility to ensure that foods marketed by the firm are safe, wholesome and in compliance with all applicable legal and regulatory requirements"[67,172].

The Revolving Door Between the Biotech Industry and The U.S. Government:

Michael R. Taylor

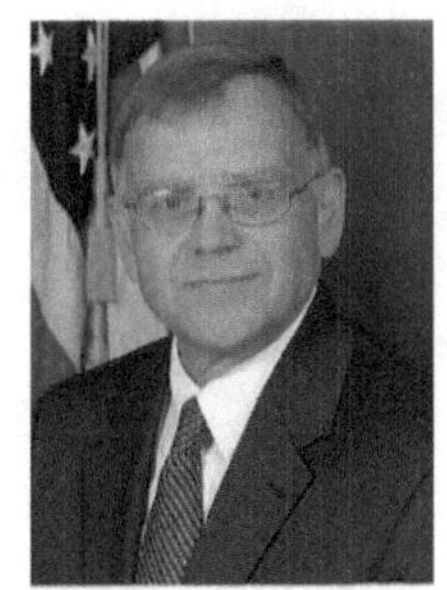

1976 – Attorney for FDA, executive assistant to the FDA Commissioner
1981 – Attorney at King & Spalding, representing Monsanto
1991 – Deputy Commissioner for Policy, FDA
1994 – Administrator of the Food Safety & Inspection Service, USDA
1998 – V.P. of Public Policy, Monsanto
2009 – Senior Advisor to FDA Commissioner
2010 – Deputy Commissioner for Foods, FDA

Michael Taylor was instrumental in various pro-GMO policies that kept the public blind, and kept biotech profits soaring.

2.7 RELIGIOUS BELIEFS

I personally believe in banning the open farming and inclusion of GMOs in the food supply for the time being until at least a large majority of the scientific community, and the public agree that GMOs are safe for humans, animals and the environment. I am not against GMOs, I'm against toxins. But let's explore another angle for a moment...

GMO proponents claim that people who object to GMOs based on religious beliefs are doing so based on ignorance of scientific facts. Ignoring for a moment the fact that there are many scientists who are also religious, or identify with a religion, this is completely irrelevant. Religions are not based on scientific principles, but on faith, and the Constitution guarantees freedom of religion without the precondition of scientific literacy. Although I do not believe that religion should inhibit scientific development, I do believe that people who hold religious beliefs should have the freedom to practice those beliefs and therefore information that may be pertinent to those beliefs should not be kept from them. Besides, those scientists who claim that GMOs are no different then crops generated through conventional means are not using science to back up their claims, but rather propaganda, misrepresentations of facts, and pure lies.

The Alliance for Bio-Integrity, in preparation for their lawsuit against the FDA, had assembled an impressive set of plaintiffs, which included nine well-credentialed life scientists as well as a coalition of religious representatives, which included "seven ordained priests and ministers from a broad range of Christian denominations (including Episcopalian, Lutheran, Baptist, and Roman Catholic); three rabbis (Orthodox, Conservative, and Reform); the chancellor of the Americas Dharma Realm Buddhist University; and a thousand-member Hindu organization from Chicago. These plaintiffs stated that in their view, the manner in which biotechnicians are reconfiguring the genomes of food-yielding organisms is a radical and irreverent disruption of the integrity of God's creation – and that they felt obliged to avoid consuming the products of such interventions as a matter of religious principle. They alleged that by failing to require proper labeling, the FDA was unavoidably exposing them to these foods and preventing them from the free exercise of their religious beliefs.[63]

At the conclusion of the suit, not only did judge Kollar-Kotelly ignore the evidence brought before her, and the law in the process, but she also violated the constitutionally guaranteed Freedom of Religion and the Religious Freedom Restoration Act (RFRA) by ignoring the arguments and pleas of all of the religious leaders who joined the suit.

Rabbi Harold White, Director of Jewish Chaplaincy and Lecturer in Theology at Georgetown University (and a plaintiff) stated that "Everyone who believes the biosphere developed through the purposeful plan of a benevolent God should reject gene-altered foods to preserve the dignity of that plan. Since the dawn of life on earth, Divine intelligence has systematically prevented genetic transfers between widely differing species. Limited human intelligence should not rush to make them commonplace."[173]

If you are Jewish, or Muslim for instance, there are certain foods that your religion forbids you from eating, such as pork, crustaceans / shellfish, etc. If you prescribe to Buddhism, Hinduism, or Jainism, and you are a devout vegan, you cannot eat any animal products. At the moment, the GMO industry claims that they do not use DNA from animals in food crop modifications, but those experiments have already occurred. If there is no labeling of foods containing genetically modified organisms, should in the future a GMO manufacturer decide to use genes from a pig, for instance, you will have no way of knowing whether or not you are fully observing your religious beliefs.

2.8   PRO-GMO BIAS

So now, let's consider some of the pro-GMO studies out there and ask a question. How is it possible that so many research scientists find negative health effects from GMOs, yet other scientists do not? Companies like Monsanto contractually forbid farmers from selling their seeds or crops for the purpose of health safety studies. They also typically control very closely who they themselves give product to for the purpose of health safety studies.

The question becomes, are the seeds or crops that the GMO companies provide specifically for testing different from those that are produced for or by farmers for general use? One possibility is that they are, in one key respect different, and that key difference is herbicides. The GMO companies know that herbicides, like Glyphosate, 2,4-D, and others are toxic[35], as confirmed by many scientists and multinational health safety organizations like The World Health Organization and the International Agency for Research on Cancer. For the sake of argument, it may very well be that the GMOs themselves, in part or entirely, are not particularly toxic, although as was previously demonstrated, the genetic engineering process itself leads to the production of toxins and allergens, both intentionally (as in the case of Bt toxins) and unintentionally. In knowing this about herbicides, it is entirely possible that the GMO companies grow seeds and crops destined for testing in specially designated, herbicide-free plots. It is therefore possible that the researchers that did not find health risks got those herbicide-free seeds and crops directly or indirectly from the biotech companies that developed them, while the researchers who found negative health effects got their GMOs from crops grown in the typical way, with herbicides. In that case, and if it is the herbicides that are the problem, and if as a result, herbicide use will be discontinued, then there will be no need for herbicide resistant GMO crops, which constitute over 80% of all GMOs in use today.

2.9   THE SCIENCE OF NONSENSE

> *"The greatest enemy of knowledge is not ignorance, it is the illusion of knowledge."*
>
> Stephen Hawking, theoretical physicist, cosmologist, author and Director of Research at the Centre for Theoretical Cosmology; the University of Cambridge

The GMO industry and its scientists, government agencies with a directive to promote biotech innovation and products, many scientific organizations of which some have vested interest in the biotech industry, and universities who are reliant on grant money and who see a lot of that money coming from the biotech industry have done their absolute best to muddy the GMO waters; some intentionally and some through ignorance of the facts or refusal to accept the facts for fear that their research would be hampered by regulations or halted due to public pressure.

It is understandable that scientists would react in a defensive manner when their work comes under attack, especially by lay people who do not understand the science. However, as you have read and will continue to read, much of the concerns and push-back has come from highly qualified scientists who are, in most cases, more knowledgeable about impacts of genetic engineering on human, animal, and environmental health than the genetic engineers themselves, and even from genetic engineers who allowed themselves to look at the broader picture, and review the objections of other scientists and come up with their own conclusions that extreme caution needs to be adhered to when dealing with modifications of natural systems.

So much propaganda, twisting of truths, and outright lies have been thrust upon regulators and the public for such a long time, to protect the image and profits of the biotech industry, as was done for decades with the tobacco industry, that many prominent scientists, inside and outside the industry, are so confused about the facts that they start believing the lies.

Paul Joseph Goebbels who was a German politician and Reich Minister of Propaganda in Nazi Germany stated that "If you tell a lie big enough and keep repeating it, people will eventually come to believe it. The lie can be maintained only for such time as the State can shield the people from the political, economic and/or military consequences of the lie. It thus becomes vitally important for the State to use all of its powers to repress dissent, for the truth is the mortal enemy of the lie, and thus by extension, the truth is the greatest enemy of the State."

In the book "Altered Genes, Twisted Truth: How the Venture to Genetically Engineer Our Food Has Subverted Science, Corrupted Government, and Systematically Deceived the Public"[63], the author goes into great detail in explaining how the deception started and the collusion that was necessary to propagate the deception and keep the public, regulators and even the scientific community at large ignorant of the facts.

Let's discuss some specific examples of statements made by scientists and scientific organizations that are misleading or flat-out wrong;

2.9.1   National Academy of Sciences (NAS) on GMOs

A 2004 report by the National Academy of Sciences (NAS)[174] attempted to draw the erroneous conclusion that GMOs are no more unsafe and are sometimes safer than crops generated through conventional breeding. While that was the overall theme of the report, the following statement was quite contradictory to that theme:

"While there are a variety of methods for identifying and measuring specific changes that result from genetic engineering, as well as from conventional breeding techniques, such changes are not always easily discernible – particularly when they are unexpected outcomes of the process or when they result from latent expression of the genetic change or accumulated changes in functional effects in the modified organism."

This and other statements clearly demonstrate the need for a heightened level of scrutiny when it comes to GMOs, and even when it comes to crops generated through other mutagenic processes, such as through chemicals and radiation.

At the same time, the NAS and the Royal Society repeatedly made claims that natural breeding techniques have led to the production of novel toxins, however, there is absolutely no evidence that any novel toxin has ever been generated through natural breeding, and they certainly do not provide any data to back up their claims. Although natural breeding could, and in some cases, does cause the levels of toxins naturally present in a plant to increase or decrease, those toxins are known and are screened for, and therefore are weeded out. However, it is a lot more difficult to screen out a novel toxin, especially when it is unexpected or unknown to science, such as with the toxin that caused the EMS epidemic, as discussed earlier in the chapter.

In an article published by eight experts in the journal Plant Physiology, the authors stated in reference to natural breeding that "Although breeders recombine tens of thousands of genes with virtually infinite potential interactions, to our knowledge, there has never been a report of a completely novel toxin or allergen appearing in a genus as a result of conventional breeding ... Hundreds of thousands of varieties have been bred without the emergence of any novel allergens or toxins, indicating that the likelihood of such events is virtually zero"[175].

The NAS report further states that "unintentionally introduced changes in the composition of foods may be more difficult to identify and assess. Whether genetic engineering per se affects the likelihood of unintentionally introducing undesired compositional changes in food is not fully understood." Yet the biotech industry and some scientific bodies (including the NAS, from the gist you get from reading the rest of the report) would like the public to believe that genetic engineering is a well-defined and understood science, practiced with precision, and is easily predictable, the fact is. The exact opposite is true.

They then go on to contradict themselves by making the following statement – "through the breeder's selection process, the genetic lines that express undesirable characteristics are eliminated from further consideration, and only the best lines – those that express desirable characteristics with no additional undesirable agronomic characteristics, such as increased disease susceptibility or poor grain quality – are maintained for possible commercial release." There are two main issues to be addressed in this statement:

"...only the best lines – those that express desirable characteristics with no additional undesirable agronomic characteristics, such as increased disease susceptibility or poor grain quality – are maintained for possible commercial release."

In the earlier statement mentioned above, the NAS report stated that "...unintentionally introduced changes in the composition of foods may be more difficult to identify and assess." yet they can confidently state that *ONLY* the best lines with *NO UNDESIREABLE CHARACTERISTICS* are maintained for possible commercial release. Likewise, their statement that "...such changes are not always easily discernible – particularly when they are unexpected outcomes of the process or when they result from latent expression of the genetic change or accumulated changes in functional effects in the modified organism" paints the same picture that certainty cannot be achieved as to the safety of GMOs, and it is reasonable and responsible to assume that unintended outcomes will most likely result from such alterations. In drilling down further into this sentence, the following words speak volumes:

"...no additional undesirable agronomic characteristics..."

Agronomic characteristics are those that will affect the biotech company's bottom line. While the biotech industry can't even prevent those types of unintended, undesirable characteristics from escaping detection and manifesting after commercialization as was demonstrated earlier in this chapter, this and potentially acute toxicity are the only things that the biotech companies seems to concern themselves with, since chronic toxicity – the kind that takes years to manifest cannot be traced back to the GMO crop, especially with the absence of GMO labeling, which makes epidemiological studies nearly impossible to conduct.

In a most mind-boggling statement the report claims that "Genetic engineering methods are considered by some to be more precise than conventional breeding methods because only known and precisely characterized genes are transferred. In contrast, conventional breeding involves transferring thousands of unknown genes with unknown function along with the desired genes."

This statement is so ignorant and arrogant that it's hard to believe that it came out of the mouth of a scientist, and was endorsed by the National Academy of Sciences. Not only is that statement ignorant, but it effectively contradicts itself once more, and in a single breath. On the one hand, when associated with genetic engineering "…only known and precisely characterized genes are transferred…", and on the other hand "…conventional breeding involves transferring thousands of unknown genes with unknown function…" To explain away this statement we either have to assume that the NAS scientists are going by the outdated (even for 2004), erroneous assumption that genes are isolated packets of information that do not interact with one another, and so inserting a "known and precisely characterized gene" into the DNA comprised of many "unknown genes" will not affect the plant beyond the expression of the inserted gene, and they are genuinely ignorant to the fact that genes work in complexes and form interactions to produce many products that cannot be produced from a single gene, or they are outright lying.

Besides, are we to believe that genes only become safe when they are known to our puny minds? In the short time that humans have been studying and tinkering with the generic code, apparently, we have learned more about it than nature has in the previous billions of years of evolution on earth.

Just to drive this point home, the 35S promoter, which has been in use since the introduction of GMOs into the market, was thought to not have any protein-coding sequences. 16 years into its use in GMOs, in 2012 it was discovered that the

35S promoter contained a viral gene called gene VI. This begs the question; what else do genetic engineers not know about their creations that could lead to deleterious effects, to humans, animals, and the environment?

In Altered Genes, Twisted Truth[63], when making a comparison between software engineers and genetic engineers Steven Druker compared genetic engineers to hackers, but I would take it a step further and say that hackers are very knowledgeable in programming and how to manipulate computer systems, whereas genetic engineers know very little about the genetic code and even less about the system in which it works. I think a better analogy would be to liken genetic engineers to early day archaeologists, or tomb raiders who were more interested in the treasure than preserving history and learning from it.

Australian software engineer and information security expert Stephen Wilson stated in an article titled "We're not ready for genetic engineering"[176] that "If genomes are like programs then let's remember they have been written achingly slowly over eons, to suit the circumstances of a species. Genomes are revised in a real-world laboratory over billions of iterations and test cases, to a level of confidence that software engineers can't even dream of". Additionally, he wrote that "In software engineering, it is received wisdom that most bugs result from imprudent changes made to existing programs. Furthermore, editing one part of a program can have unpredictable and unbounded impacts on any other part of the code. Above all else, all but the very simplest software in practice is untestable. So mission critical software (like the implantable defibrillator code I used to work on) is always verified by a combination of methods, including unit testing, system testing, design review and painstaking code inspection. Because most problems come from human error, software excellence demands formal design and development processes, and high level programming languages, to preclude subtle errors that no amount of testing could ever hope to find. How many of these software quality mechanisms are available to genetic engineers? Code inspection is moot when we don't even know how genes normally interact with one another; how can we possibly tell by inspection if an artificial gene will interfere with the 'legacy' code? ... Can today's genetic engineers demonstrate a rigorous verification regime, given the reality that complex software programs are inherently untestable?"

With all engineering disciplines and fields of science, even when a lot of information is known, there are still unintended effects and failures. In contrast, very little is currently known about genetics and epigenetic mechanisms and therefore alterations to such mechanisms are highly risky, unpredictable, unreliable, and unethical to be thrust upon the public, especially without their knowledge.

To demonstrate the lack of understanding on the part of bioengineers of basic genetic interactions, William Freese and David Schubert sum it up quite nicely in their report[67]:

"Biotechnology companies rarely test the transgenic protein actually produced in their engineered crops. Instead, for testing purposes they make use of a bacterially generated surrogate protein that may differ in important respects from the plant-produced one... This is, however, a serious mistake in testing paradigms, since plants and bacteria are very likely to produce different proteins even when transformed with the same gene (for discussion, see Schubert, 2002). Testing a bacterial surrogate should not substitute for testing the plant-expressed proteins for the following reasons: DNA transfected into both plants and animals is incorporated randomly into chromosomal DNA and in doing so may disrupt the function of the chromosomal gene into which it is incorporated, contributing to the unpredictable nature of GE organisms. In addition, only part of the transfected DNA sequence maybe incorporated and expressed, and additional problems arise if a fusion protein is made from both transfected and host DNA. For instance, Monsanto and Novartis developed a glyphosate-tolerant sugarbeet line in which only 69% of one of the transgenes was incorporated, resulting in fusion with sugar beet DNA and production of the corresponding novel fusion protein (FDA Note, 1998). Even if precisely the same foreign DNA is expressed in bacteria and plant, the two organisms – which are kingdoms apart in biological terms – process proteins differently. For instance, bacteria are not known to add sugar molecules to proteins, while plants do [a process called glycosylation]. Glycosylation patterns influence the immune response to proteins, and glycosylation is considered to be a characteristic of allergenic proteins (SAP MT, 2000, p. 23). Other secondary modifications will certainly occur when proteins are expressed in foreign organisms or different cell types (Schubert, 2002). As a result, animal feeding studies and allergenicity assessments that make use of bacterial surrogate proteins or their derivatives may not reflect the toxicity or allergenicity of the plant-produced transgenic protein to which people are actually exposed."

2.9.2 The New Zealand Royal Commission on the EMS epidemic

Another case of outright lying by a prominent scientific institution came in the form of a report by the New Zealand Royal Commission on Genetic Modification[177]. The commission, in response to the EMS epidemic and the allegations that Showa Denko's genetically modified bacteria was to blame, stated in their report that "The United States courts decided that the manufacturing process rather than genetic modification was at fault."

Steven Druker, Executive Director of the Alliance for Bio-Integrity who has thoroughly investigated the incident stated that "In my conversation with [Don Morgan, an attorney in the Washington, D.C. office of Cleary, Gottlieb, Steen and Hamilton, which serves as worldwide counsel for Showa Denko and represented it in all the U.S. lawsuits]... I learned that over 2,000 of the lawsuits were settled out of court and that only three went to trial. Mr. Morgan stated that due to the nature of product liability law, the basic issue in these cases was whether Showa Denko's product had caused harm. He said the issue about whether the genetic engineering process played a role in causing the harm was not relevant and was never raised – and that none of the jury verdicts in any way touched on it. He seemed surprised that the Royal Commission would assert that the U.S. courts had decided the issue."[178]

Druker further stated in his response to the Royal Commission report that "the report did make yet another false assertion in reporting that out of the six EMS-related toxins found in the GE-derived tryptophan, three were not accurately identified until 1999. In fact, two of these were identified in 1998, while one remained unidentified until 2000. This is further indication of how lax the commission's fact-finding process was – and how long it can take to identify novel toxic substances even after they have killed people (in this case, up to eleven years)."

"Further, the report implies that the only people who got EMS were taking "high doses." In fact, people taking relatively low doses, even as low as 100 mg, also contracted EMS."

The report then goes on to blame the toxic contamination on the fact that Show Denko had reduced the amount of charcoal in its filtration process. Druker made the analogy that "To attribute the problem solely to the filtering system is like saying that a soldier's death was caused by a defective helmet while saying nothing about the bullet that pierced his helmet and then shattered his skull. If the reduction of charcoal allowed toxins to contaminate the final product, it was only because toxins had been produced." The report also ignores the fact that cases of EMS arose from batches that were manufactured before the amount of charcoal was reduced, as well as after it was restored, albeit to a lesser degree.

Additionally, the filtration process that Showa Denko employed was not unique in the industry, yet no cases of EMS arose from the products of any of the other l-tryptophan manufacturers, none of which employed genetically altered bacteria.

Their statements are especially egregious because the commission was not ignorant to those facts. As a matter of fact, they were presented with reports, testimonies and other evidence;

"The RC was clearly informed of these facts by several witnesses in their written submissions as well as their oral testimony. Further, my submission provided an excerpt from a memo by the biotechnology coordinator of the U.S. Food and Drug Administration (FDA) stating that the genetic engineering of the bacteria could not be ruled out as the cause of the EMS. I additionally informed the commission that many experts regard the bioengineering as the most likely cause. Moreover, I directed them to a recent paper by researchers at the University of Hamburg stating that the use of genetic engineering in producing tryptophan generates problematic byproducts and '...restricts the possibilities of an effective clean-up procedure.' I also noted that the issue of causation has not been definitively resolved because several factors initially prevented independent experts from examining the bioengineered bacteria and Showa Denko eventually destroyed them."[178]

The report makes many more inexcusable and scientifically unsubstantiated claims that fly in the face of the evidence presented to them and common knowledge about basic biology. Their one-sided view of genetic engineering and their convenient exclusion of many studies by many respectable and highly qualified scientists who have demonstrated deleterious effects of GMOs and the genetic engineering process, as well as the attacks on others who have shown the same, further demonstrates the fact that their favorable view of genetic engineering stem not from science-based conclusions, but rather from political and financial motives.

2.9.3   The Royal Society on Genetic Engineering

"during a BBC interview in 2000, the Royal Society's President, Sir Robert May (who for five years had served as the government's chief scientist), declared that genetic engineering is 'vastly safer' and 'vast, vastly more controlled' than conventional breeding. But although those bold claims were imbued with an aura of scientific respectability, they were not backed by solid scientific evidence."[179]

As was demonstrated earlier in the chapter, GMOs are neither safer nor more controlled. Although the assembly process of the gene cassette is a controlled and scientifically rigorous process, the insertion process into the host genome is anything but. Additionally, although the processes required to force the plant cell to accept the newly inserted genes and control mechanisms are likewise scientific and rigorous, the outcomes of those processes are unpredictable from the standpoint of unintended side reactions, mutations and other undesired effects. And lastly – the selection process of the mature genetically modified plant is mostly focused on superficial phenotypical changes and agronomic traits, and seriously lack in the area of toxicity and allergenicity testing. As demonstrated with the case of Showa Denko's genetically engineered bacteria, unintended toxins are very difficult to detect, especially when those toxins are novel and present in minute amounts. In that case, as stated before, minute amounts nevertheless led to an epidemic which caused widespread and severe health effects, which in some cases were permanent, and some of which lead to death. Although the superficial nature of the selection process is not a feature of the genetic engineering process, but rather the unwillingness of the biotech industry to rigorously test their products, it is nevertheless part and parcel of the genetic engineering venture.

Dr. Louis J. Pribyl of the FDA commented in his "Comments on Biotechnology Draft Document" that "breeders have not had to face the issue of new, powerful regulatory elements being randomly inserted into the genome. So there is no certainty that they will be able to pick up effects that might not be obvious, such as cryptic pathway activation." This letter is shown on page 140.

Worse still is the fact that when the biotech companies do find deleterious effects resulting from their products, they suppress this information and go forward with commercialization. This suggests that deleterious effects are very common, and therefore halting commercialization of products of a technology which regularly result in such effects would not be financially wise. The biotech industry's continued manipulation of all branches of U.S. and foreign governments, including the justice system, the FDA, the USDA, the EPA and many other organizations, including writing laws to protect themselves from litigation, and their continued opposition to labeling of GMOs further illustrates that they have something to hide.

The Royal Society's statement also makes it sound like natural breeding is an unsafe and uncontrolled process. As a matter of fact, nothing could be farther from the truth. Although natural breeding does sometimes lead to increases in toxins and allergens already native to the plant, which are known and screened for, there is absolutely no evidence that a plant bred through conventional means has ever led to the production of a novel toxin. Natural breeding is also limited by natural barriers which prevent unrelated plant species from being crossed. In actuality, those same barriers exist in the genetic engineering process, which is why genetic engineer have to resort to unnatural methods to force the host cell to incorporate the offending genetic material, just as surgeons have to suppress a patient's immune system when implanting a donor organ, otherwise the immune system would set out to attack the foreign organ.

This absurd claim of the biotech industry and their proponents that natural breeding is more prone to unintended alterations than are GMOs is completely false, and moreover, it is completely ignorant, because genetic engineering also involves breeding and natural reproduction to propagate the altered plant. In that case, and assuming their ignorant assertions, GMOs are doubly dangerous, because they incur unintended alterations from both the genetic engineering process and subsequent natural breeding process. In reality, the last paragraph is actually accurate, because as they naturally breed the altered plant, it's genome attempt to adapt to its new, foreign gene insertions, and as a result, mutations, transpositions, and other potentially deleterious alterations occur. This is not the case under normal conditions in nature, because in nature mutations occur in response to environmental stressors, such as drought, unusually extreme temperatures, or exposure to toxins or pests, and typically not under normal conditions.

Druker further wrote in an open letter to the Royal Society – "while these claims may have reflected an opinion shared by many other scientists, they clearly did not represent a consensus within the scientific community. By then, numerous well-credentialed scientists had expressed opposite viewpoints, including the majority of the experts on the US Food and Drug Administration's Biotechnology Task Force. And early the following year, an expert panel of the Royal Society of Canada released an extensive report declaring that (a) it is 'scientifically unjustifiable' to presume that GM foods are safe and (b) the 'default presumption' for every GM food should be that the genetic alteration has induced unintended and potentially harmful side effects."

2.9.4   More of the Same from the FDA Disinformation Campaign

In a June 2005 hearing before the Senate Committee on Agriculture, Nutrition and Forestry, Robert E. Brackett, Ph.D – director of the Center for Food Safety and Applied Nutrition made the following statement in reference to genetically modified organisms:

"In a 1992 policy statement on bioengineered foods, FDA announced that the Agency was 'not aware of any information showing that foods derived by these new [genetic engineering] methods differ from other foods in any meaningful or material way, or that, as a class, foods developed by the new techniques present any different or greater safety concern than foods developed by traditional plant breeding.' This 1992 statement and its scientific underpinnings still reflect FDA's thinking about bioengineered foods."[147]

This statement is an outright lie. Not only did the FDA's own scientists issue strong warnings about GMOs in internal memos prior to the 1992 policy (see FDA memos below), but the FDA has also received comments from many other well-credentialed scientists warning of health and environmental dangers.

The director went on to say that "Many of the foods that are already common in our diet are obtained from plant varieties that were developed using conventional genetic techniques of breeding and selection." This statement is very misleading and only stands to blur the distinction between natural breeding and genetic engineering, which are very different from one another. The director purposely uses the words "conventional genetic techniques" to make it seem as if the genetic makeup of those plants were directly altered, and therefore draws a parallel between genetic engineering and conventional breeding – a parallel which in reality does not exist. As a matter of fact, the FDA scientists' own memos clearly declare that there are major differences between traditional breeding and genetic engineering and that the standards which are afforded to foods derived through traditional means cannot be afforded to foods derived through genetic engineering.

He then claimed that "The new gene splicing techniques are being used to achieve many of the same goals and improvements that plant breeders historically have sought through conventional methods. Today's techniques can be used with greater precision and allow for more complete characterization and, therefore, greater predictability, of the qualities of the new variety. They give scientists the ability to isolate genes and introduce new traits into foods without simultaneously introducing undesirable traits. This is an important improvement over traditional breeding. Any genetic modification technique, including both traditional methods and bioengineering, could change the composition of a food in a manner relevant to food safety. But because of the increased precision offered by the bioengineered methods, the risk of inadvertently introducing detrimental traits is actually likely to be lessened."

As it has been demonstrated repeatedly earlier in the chapter, the genetic engineering process is random and unpredictable in its effectiveness and outcomes, thereby shattering the FDA's and industry's incessant propaganda relating to "precision" and "predictability". Likewise, the idea that genetic engineering can preclude the introduction of undesirable traits is asinine and ignores everything we know about genetics, and even worse, everything that we still don't know about genetics. Therefore, his claim of "important improvement over traditional breeding" is nothing but propaganda.

Let's not forget - the FDA's own scientists confirmed the unpredictable nature of the genetic engineering process and called for thorough testing of each transformation event as if it is a unique genetic entity, and cautioned that genetic engineering could lead to alterations in the amounts of known toxins and allergens, as well as the introduction of unknown toxins and allergens.

Brackett then back paddles with the following statements – "If safety concerns should arise, however, they would most likely fall into one of three broad categories: allergens, toxins, or anti-nutrients. FDA has extensive experience in evaluating the safety of such substances in food" and "Our authority under section 409 permits us to require premarket approval of any food additive and, thus, to require premarket approval of any substance intentionally introduced via bioengineering that is not GRAS [Generally Recognized as Safe]."

This would be a fairly convincing and reassuring statement, except for the fact that the FDA does not evaluate anything other than the GMO developer's own safety statement, and in nearly all cases, the FDA does not receive the full data package or any other supporting evidence to substantiate the developer's conclusions. "Requiring premarket approval" is a term used to give the impression of regulation, but in reality, the FDA only requires a statement from the developer that declares they have done all required testing (of which none are defined by law or mandate) and that they have concluded that the additive is safe – without requiring proof. Furthermore, the FDA does not give approval for the additive, but rather submits a statement to the developer which reiterates that the developer states that they have done all relevant testing and that they have concluded that the additive is safe, and that it is up to the developer to ensure that their product is safe.

Probably the most telling statement in his address is the following statement which validates the fact that in actuality, the FDA does not regulate GMOs in the least bit:

"In general, substances intentionally added to or modified in food via biotechnology to date have been proteins and fats that are, with respect to safety, similar to other proteins and fats that are commonly and safely consumed in the diet and, thus, are **presumptively** GRAS [emphasis added]. Therefore, they have not needed to go through the food additive approval process." As a matter of law, the Federal Food, Drug, and Cosmetic Act (FD&C Act)[180] does not give room for "presumptions" and requires that GRAS status be based on technical evidence of safety, which needs to be presented in peer-reviewed published studies which are readily available to the scientific community and for which there is wide acceptance within the scientific community.

"GRAS determinations cannot be based on unpublished research and must instead be based on peer-reviewed, published science."[181]

2.9.5   The Nicolia Review

Promoters of genetic engineering often refer to the so-called Nicolia review[182], which provides a list of about 1,700 studies that supposedly demonstrates the safety of GMOs. However, most of those studies are not health safety studies. Of the few that are, most are tests conducted on fish, cows, and other animals whose digestive systems are completely different from humans, and therefore cannot be used to infer safety for humans. The very few studies which were performed on rats (which are a better human analogue), in actuality demonstrate harmful effects to organs and tissues, even though the industry claims that they show safety. This is because, when harmful effects are detected, the industry writes them off as "not biologically significant". However, in reality, those effects are extremely biologically significant, especially considering that most of those studies are short to medium term studies. Additionally, many of those studies are invalid from the standpoint that the controls used were not from the parental line (isogenic) variety, and in some cases, were not even of the same type of plant. The reasons that it is of critical importance that when a genetically altered plant is tested, it is compared with its isogenic counterpart, grown and harvested at the same time and location, and exposed to the same environment is because:

1. This is the only way to discern whether any changes in composition are due to the genetic alteration. Different strains of the same plant contain different levels of toxins and allergens, as well as different levels of proteins, vitamins, minerals, and other constituents. So, when evaluating a genetically altered plant, it is necessary to compare it to the strain that it was derived from (the isogenic strain) in order to preclude any differences that are not a result of the genetic alteration. Likewise, in mechanical or electrical engineering, if you are trying to resolve a failure of unknown origin, it is a sound scientific principle to make the fewest changes possible at one time in order to arrive at the true cause of the failure. Making multiple changes all at once might resolve the failure, but you will most likely not determine the true cause of the failure, and you might create additional problems in the process.

2. Living organisms produce more or less of certain constituents depending on the environmental conditions that they are exposed to, and since all plants contain toxins, it is important to know that the toxins in plants intended for human and animal consumption are within acceptable levels. If I compare a GE crop which was grown under ideal conditions (environment "A") with another non-GE crop which was grown under a condition that caused it to produce a particular toxin in excess (environment "B"), then I might say that the GE crop is "substantially equivalent" to the non-GE crop if it contains the same levels of proteins, toxins, allergens, vitamins, minerals, etc. as the natural variety. However, I would be wrong. This is because, if I then grow the GE crop in environment "B", the levels of toxins might rise to an unacceptable level.

Since in the real world, crops are grown in a range of different environments, it is important to know that the levels of toxins, allergens, and other constituents produced are not excessive under the same conditions, and that when grown under extreme conditions, that those constituents will always fall within acceptable levels. For this reason alone, GE crops can never be deemed safe, unless they are tested across all possible growing conditions that the plant would be expected to be exposed to in agricultural use. As Dr. Pusztai stated in his review in regards to isoflavone content in GE vs. non-GE soybeans in a study conducted by Lappe et al. (1999), "while the variability of the GM samples was indeed considerable, conventional soybeans showed less variation in isoflavone content. As the isoflavone content of soybeans might affect human health, there needs to be more awareness of potential health problems due to this variability"[183]

Many industry studies, and studies performed by scientists who are pro-industry have fatal flaws in this regard; they use non-isogenic comparators, they use crops grown under differing conditions and differing locations, as well as crops grown during different times / growing seasons. One Royal Society report even attempted to debunk Arpad Pusztai's GMO potato study by comparing it with the results of GE sweet peppers, tomatoes and soya feeding studies[184], while at the same time faulting him for decrying that all GMOs are unsafe (which he did not say) by stating that "The work concerned one particular species of animal, when fed with one particular product modified by the insertion of one particular gene by one particular method. However skillfully the experiments were done, it would be unjustifiable to draw from them general conclusions about whether genetically modified foods are harmful to human beings or not. Each GM food must be assessed individually."[185] Yet, when the Royal Society refer to industry studies supposedly demonstrating safety, they have no qualms about making broad statements about genetic engineering's safety and that additional studies are no longer necessary because they have been proven to be safe. Keep in mind that many of those statements were made by many industry scientists prior to the introduction of GMO foods into the market, and prior to any safety testing.

2.10   THE WAR ON SCIENCE

"Traditionally, scientists regarded intellectual honesty as part of collegiality, and there was accountability if one was caught telling lies. Accordingly, liars were blackballed. But since the rise of genetic engineering, the situation in molecular biology has to a significant degree become inverted, and, when it comes to that technology, one gets blackballed for telling the truth."

Philip J. Regal, Ph.D, quote taken from "Altered Genes, Twisted Truth"[63]

2.10.1   The Séralini Study

One of the longest and most thorough studies that has ever been conducted on GMOs is a study by Gilles-Eric Séralini and his team[128,186], in which they demonstrated clearly that the GMO under test (Monsanto's NK603 Roundup tolerant Maize/Corn), the herbicide Glyphosate that the GMO is designed to be grown with, and the combination of the two, caused highly significant damage to multiple organs, by themselves, and in combination. Immediately following the peer reviewed publication of Séralini's study in the Elsevier Journal Food and Chemical Toxicology (FCT), both Séralini and the publisher came under intense fire from Monsanto, the maker of the GMO crop and herbicide that was tested, and the European Food Safety Authority (EFSA), who approved the GMO for use in food and animal feed in Europe. More than a year after the study passed the peer review process and was published in the journal, and shortly following the appointment of a former Monsanto scientist, Richard E. Goodman, to the journal's editorial board[187], Dr. A. Wallace Hayes, the editor-in-chief of the journal gave into pressure, and without a valid reason and under secretive conditions, retracted the study[128,188].

In the retraction statement[188], the journal stated that "there is a legitimate cause for concern regarding both the [low] number of animals in each study group and the particular strain selected" and that "no definitive conclusions can be reached with this small sample size regarding the role of either NK603 or glyphosate in regards to overall mortality or tumor incidence." They also claimed that since the strain of rats used are known to exhibit a high rate of tumors, they cannot be relied upon, and claimed that the results were "inconclusive, and therefore do not reach the threshold of publication for Food and Chemical Toxicology".

According to the Committee on Publication Ethics (COPE) Retraction Guidelines[189], which FCT are members of[190], the following considerations should be made before a publication is retracted:

- they have clear evidence that the findings are unreliable, either as a result of misconduct (e.g. data fabrication) or honest error (e.g. miscalculation or experimental error)

- the findings have previously been published elsewhere without proper crossreferencing, permission or justification (i.e. cases of redundant publication)

- it constitutes plagiarism

- it reports unethical research

Although the editor attempted to make claims that those conditions have been met in his retraction statement, his statements were baseless and fallacious.

- _Low number of animals in each study group:_

This statement assumes that the object of the test was to detect cancer. However, that assumption is incorrect. As a matter of fact, the term "cancer" never appears in the paper[128]. The object of the study was long-term toxicity, and as such, the number of rats used in the test were in accordance with testing guidelines for toxicological tests. The confusion (if you could call it that) arose from the fact that the paper reported on incidences of tumors in the rats, and although it was not a cancer study, study guidelines require that any incidences of tumors be reported, which Séralini did. "Tumors are reported in line with the requirements of OECD chronic toxicity protocols 452 and 453, which require all 'lesions' (which by definition include tumors) to be reported."[186] Nevertheless, the reason for a higher number of rats in cancer studies is to make the test more sensitive to low or unusual incidences of tumors, which makes Séralini's finding even more alarming. According to Steven Druker, "the purpose of using more rats is to decrease the likelihood that an unusual rate of tumor incidence will go undetected, not to guard against the wrongful imputing of significance to differences in tumor rates between groups of rats that aren't actually meaningful. Therefore, as several experts have emphasized, because Séralini's study was less sensitive than the standard tumor-detecting trial but nonetheless detected numerous tumors, its results are even more portentous than if a higher number of rats had been used."[63]

- _Particular strain of animals used:_

Séralini's study employed the Sprague-Dawley strain of rat. Not only is this strain of rat the appropriate strain for Séralini's long-term toxicology study, but in fact, it is the standard strain used in toxicology studies, and cancer studies as well, and is also the strain used by Monsanto in their 90-day maize feeding and glyphosate studies, as well as many other studies conducted on GMOs. If the Journal's claim were to be valid, countless other studies would have to be retracted as well.

- *No definitive conclusion can be reached:*

In an article in The San Diego Union-Tribune, David Schubert, molecular biologist and Head of Cellular Neurobiology at the Salk Institute wrote "The editors claim the reason was that 'no definitive conclusions can be reached.' As a scientist, I can assure you that if this were a valid reason for retracting a publication, a large fraction of the scientific literature would not exist."[191] Most publications do not offer conclusive results, but rather findings and hypotheses which leads to further studies, either confirming and disproving, and thereby furthering the science.

Fortunately, on the 24th of June, 2014 the study was republished in the journal Environmental Sciences Europe[186], and in another turn of events, as a result of a defamation lawsuit brought by Séralini, "On 6 November 2015, after a criminal investigation lasting three years, the 17th Criminal Chamber of the High Court of Paris passed sentence. Marianne magazine and its journalist were fined for public defamation of a public official and public defamation of the researchers and of CRIIGEN, which is chaired by Dr Joel Spiroux de Vendômois. The trial demonstrated that the original author of the fraud accusation, prior to Marianne, was the American lobbyist Henry I. Miller in Forbes magazine. Miller had previously lobbied to discredit research linking tobacco to cancer and heart disease on behalf of the tobacco industry. Since then he has tried to do the same in support of GMOs and pesticides, through defamation."[1] If it's bad, Miller has defended it[2]. Clearly, a despicable human being...

In response to the retraction, many scientists and organizations sent the Journal letters voicing their concerns and disapproval. In return, Wallace Hayes wrote a response to those concerns[192] where he attempted to clarify his position and reasoning for the retraction. However, his reasoning, beside being disingenuous, and although he claimed to have performed a thorough investigation, were complete fabrications. Once again Hayes claimed that Séralini's reached a supposed conclusion that "there is a definite link between GMO and cancer". However, once again, the term "cancer" does no appear even once in the paper[128]. Then he suggested that Séralini violated the recommendations in OECD Nos. 451 and 453 (guidelines for Carcinogenicity Studies and Combined Chronic Toxicity/Carcinogenicity Studies, respectively) by choosing to use 10 rats/sex/group rather than 50, entirely ignoring the fact that Séralini's study was a long-term toxicology study, and not a carcinogenicity study, and 10 rates was proper according to OECD guidelines for such a study. So, are we to believe that Mr. Hayes cannot read, or is he simply being dishonest?

In bowing down to the biotech industry, Mr. Hayes has not only disgraced Dr. Séralini and his team, but also himself and his Journal.

2.10.2   Arpad Pusztai's GMO Potato Study

Another example of industry attacks on good scientists and good science is when Arpad Pusztai, PhD, a world-renowned food safety expert, was tasked by the Scottish Agriculture, Environment and Fisheries Department (SOAEFD) to establish a method for risk assessment of GMOs, had found that not only were GMOs harmful to the health of the test animals, but they were more harmful than conventional crops which have been sprayed with the pesticide that the GM crop was engineered to produce on its own.[193,194] Dr. Pusztai, as well as other researchers have found that it is not the pesticide in the crop that has caused the health problems, but the genetic engineering process itself.

The project was conducted at the Rowett Research Institute in Aberdeen, Scotland, where Pusztai had been employed for 32 years. The Rowett Institute is one of the world's most prestigious nutritional research centers. The Scottish Crop Research Institute and the University of Durham School of Biology also participated in the study.

The tests, which were conducted on rats, evaluated the effects of a potato which was engineered to produce a pesticidal protein called "lectin", which is native to the snowdrop plant. Lectin is toxic to a variety of insects, but is completely safe for mammals, even at extremely high doses, so Dr. Pusztai, who is a leading authority on lectins had no reason to suspect that there would be any deleterious effects to the rats. Pusztai selected the lectin-producing gene from the snowdrop specifically for that reason, so that if any ill-effects were discovered, it would not be as a result of the toxin, but rather, the genetic engineering process itself.

Pusztai selected potatoes for his experiment specifically for the reason that potatoes can propagate asexually and do not require callus-inducing tissue culture, which on its own is known to cause genetic mutations, thereby further reducing the potential for adverse effects.

Pusztai and the Rowett Institute planned to commercialize the engineered potato, so they had every reason to ensure that the results of the tests would yield a safe product, but they didn't.

They had discovered that the GM potatoes caused a slower growth rate in the rats, problems with organ development, and also knocked out the immune system. Within 10 days, the rats that ate the GM potatoes also had precancerous cell growth in their digestive tract, smaller brains, livers and testicles, partial atrophy of the liver and damaged immune system. Those conditions did not manifest in either the parental potato, or the parental potato laced with lectin from the Snowdrop plant. Additionally, it was found that the two strains of potatoes that were engineered with the lectin-producing gene were different from each other in many key respects, yet both lines produced deleterious effects in the rats. The differences between the two lines of engineered potatoes were due to, as discussed earlier, the fact that each transformational even is unique, and even though the same genes were used, the place in which they were inserted along the potato's DNA could not be controlled, and therefore was different in the two lines.

At the time of Pusztai's findings, GM foods had already been on the market and there were plans to introduce a GM potato in the U.S. in the near future, so Dr. Pusztai thought that the public should be informed immediately. However, standard procedure dictated that research findings should not be communicated to the public until a study has been published in a scientific article or has been presented at a conference, which could take years. He couldn't let convention stand in the way of informing the public of a serious health risk which was happening present-time. Nevertheless, he felt that this was not his decision alone, so he sought the approval of the Rowett Institute's director, Professor Phillip James, which was happily granted.

In an interview on the British TV show "World in Action" which aired on August 10, 1998, Dr. Pusztai informed the public of the findings of his study and had urged for better testing standards. He warned of the health risks of GMOs and the fact that their safety had not been demonstrated.

As a result of the airing of the interview, Dr. Pusztai and the Rowett Institute found themselves in the spotlight. Professor James, who was delighted with all this attention, praised Dr. Pusztai and his research and how well he handled the interview.

"On the evening the programme went out, the Rowett Institute's director Professor Philip James congratulated Dr Pusztai on his appearance, commenting how well he had handled the questions. The following morning a press release from the Institute gave him further support, stressing that a 'range of carefully controlled studies underlie the basis of Dr Pusztai's concerns'. Yet within 48 hours, everything had changed. Dr Pusztai had been suspended by the Institute and ordered to hand over all his data. His research team was dispersed and he was threatened with legal action if he spoke to anyone. His phone calls and e-mails were diverted; his personal assistant was banned from speaking to him. He read in a press release issued by the Institute that his contract would not be renewed."[3]

What could have possible triggered such a sharp turn of events? In less than 24 hours, Pusztai went from hero to zero.

According to two employees and a senior manager, professor Robert Orskov OBE, who worked at the Rowett Institute for 33 years and is one of Britain's leading nutrition experts, "phone calls went from Monsanto ... to Clinton and then to Blair. 'Clinton rang Blair and Blair rang James,' says Professor Orskov."[3]

Dr. Pusztai's admonition had hit a nerve with the Biotech industry, and they could not let it stand. In return, they had destroyed his research, his career, and his life.

In 1999, Pusztai's house and old office at the Rowett Institute were both broken into and all his research papers were stolen[3].

In an interview with GM-Free Magazine, Dr, Puztai stated - "Other scientists often ask me why I went against the code of practice and spoke out before publication in a peer reviewed journal. I made my 150-second testimony on TV's World in Action because I had facts that indicated to me there were serious problems with transgenic food. It can take two to three years to get science papers published and these foods were already on the shelves without rigorous biological testing".[195] Besides, the industry doesn't seem to mind when their own scientists or the FDA publicizes research results ahead of publication, or even outright lies, when they are favorable to the Biotech industry.

Since then, Pusztai and his research has continued to be unjustly maligned, by supposedly prestigious scientists and scientific organizations, such as the Royal Society, by making statements that are both unsupported by scientific facts, and have no basis in logic. Not only did the Royal Society pass judgment on Pusztai's work based on an incomplete summary, which was prepared for use by scientists on the research team who were familiar with the details of the research, but the review panel at the Royal Society was not even qualified to review the study. One reviewer commented that too few rats were used in the study, being unaware that the number employed by Pusztai and his team was proper for the tests performed, and that this number has been employed in dozens of other studies by Pusztai, which have been peer reviewed and published in prestigious journals.

In response to the Royal Society's unjust attacks on Pusztai, the editor of one of the world's most prestigious journals; the Lancet, commented by calling the Society's report "a gesture of breathtaking impertinence to the Rowett Institute scientists who should be judged only on the full and final publication of their work."[196]

Likewise, Steven Druker wrote an open letter to the Royal Society[179] criticizing their "misleading statements in regard to GM foods that have created significant confusion and illegitimately downplayed their risks", and their "deplorable actions" against Dr. Pusztai, and called on them to issue a formal statement acknowledging the facts about GMOs and denouncing all of their lies. He concluded by stating that *"Unless you promptly take these steps, it will demonstrate that your commitment to promoting GM foods is stronger than your commitment to honoring the truth and upholding the integrity of science.* [emphasis in original]"

Three months after Druker had published his open letter to the Royal Society, they had responded in the same manner in which they had attacked Dr. Pusztai; making false assertions for which they themselves are guilty of. Their response stated that "The Royal Society bases its views on evidence, evidence that has been closely scrutinized by people with expert knowledge and that has stood up to that scrutiny. Personal opinions and unsubstantiated anecdotes are unhelpful to having a rational public debate on science and the use of new technologies."[73]

Never mind that in Steven Druker's open letter and in his 528-page book, as well as his many articles on the subject, he has presented many scientific facts, references to peer reviewed, published scientific studies, and accounts of dozens of well-respected scientists to back up his assertions, yet, the Royal Society saw it fit to insult him by claiming that his assertions were "Personal opinions and unsubstantiated anecdotes". This response illustrates the Royal Society's lack of desire for truly open and substantive scientific discussion. Their attitude is more indicative of an inquisition court than a scientific organization.

Shortly after the response to the Royal Society by the Lancet editor, the Lancet planned to publish a paper co-authored by Dr. Pusztai and a pathologist at the University of Aberdeen; Dr. Stanley Ewen, discussing one of the studies that detected abnormal cell growth in the rats' intestines. Being mindful of the controversy surrounding Dr. Pusztai's study, the journal's editor, Dr. Richard Horton had selected a team of six reviewers to review the paper - twice the usual number. Out of the six reviewers, only one individual who worked at a government-funded institute sided against publication.

At a later interview with the Guardian, "Dr Horton said he never expected what would follow from his decision to promote scientific debate by publishing both papers. He said there was intense pressure on the Lancet from all quarters, including the Royal Society, to suppress publication."[70]

Dr. Horton stated to the Guardian that he received a phone call from a senior member of the Royal Society which began in a "very aggressive manner". "he was threatened by a senior member of the Royal Society, the voice of the British science establishment, that his job would be at risk if he published controversial research questioning the safety of genetically modified foods. Richard Horton declined to name the man who telephoned him. But the Guardian has identified him as

Peter Lachmann, the former vice-president and biological secretary of the Royal Society and president of the Academy of Medical Sciences." [70]

Despite the pressure and threats, Dr. Horton maintained his integrity and published the paper as planned on October 16, 1999.[193]

2.10.3 Vicious Attacks on Dr. Oz

In an April 7, 2015 episode of The Dr. Oz Show[197], Dr. Oz discussed a report by the International Agency for Research on Cancer (IARC) that has concluded that glyphosate, the active ingredient in the world's most popular herbicide - Roundup is a probable carcinogen. As he usually does, Dr. Oz offered the promoters of glyphosate a chance to appear on the show to voice their position, as he did in his March 10, 2015 episode on GMO Arctic® apples[198]. He reached out to Monsanto (the maker of Roundup) as well as to the Grocery Manufacturers of America and CropLife America who support the use of glyphosate on food crops, to appear on the show and present their side, but they all refused. Instead Monsanto and CropLife America had submitted one-paragraph written statements that deny the findings of IARC, who are the world's eminent experts on carcinogenicity. In spite of their absence, Dr. Oz fairly presented the arguments from both sides.

As a result of this episode, the biotech industry had initiated a personal attack campaign against Dr. Oz, attempting to silence him and destroy his credibility. A letter signed by ten doctors and sent to Columbia University Medical School demanded that Dr. Oz be removed from his position at the University's Department of Surgery. Among other things, the letter stated that "Dr. Oz has repeatedly shown disdain for science and for evidence-based medicine, **as well as baseless and relentless opposition to the genetic engineering of food crops.** [emphasis added]"[72] Dr. Oz launched an investigation[71] into the identity and affiliation of the ten doctors, and what he found was very illuminating. All ten had big industry ties. One of the big names on the letter was Henry Miller. If that name sounds familiar it's because I've mentioned his misdeeds in the section discussing the attacks on Séralini. Miller fought smoking restrictions for the tobacco industry, has spoken in support of pesticides and GMOs for the agrochemical/biotech industries, has fought to defend PCBs in the face of horrific evidence of harm, and has defended other nasty, cancer causing, life destroying chemicals in support of various industries and their executives, who should have been jailed for crimes against humanity.

A second name on the letter is Dr. Gilbert Ross, who is also connected to Henry Miller, and also happens to be a convicted felon who spent four years in federal prison.

Regardless of your personal opinion of Dr. Oz, in this instance, the information he presented was not merely his opinion or point of view, but the scientific conclusion of the world's top carcinogenicity experts, which was based on years of scientific evidence written, compiled, and reviewed by hundreds of scientists around the world. Whatever gripe the industry or their shills have should be directed not at the messenger, but at the source of the information. Of course, in this instance, whatever they have to say on the subject is obviously not based on facts, as evidenced by the Biotech industry's very long history of subterfuge, fraud, death and destruction.

2.10.4 <u>U.S. Retaliates Against Other Nations</u>
<u>for Refusing GMOs</u>

In recent years there have been many leaked documents revealing the inner workings of world governments. In one such instance it was revealed by WikiLeaks that in late 2007, the United States ambassador to France and business partner to George W. Bush, Craig Stapleton sent a diplomatic cable requesting that "retaliation" be initiated against France and other EU nations who oppose GMOs, in favor of the biotech industry:

"Mission Paris recommends that that [sic] the USG reinforce our negotiating position with the EU on agricultural biotechnology by publishing a retaliation list when the extend 'Reasonable Time Period' expires. In our view, Europe is moving backwards not forwards on this issue with France playing a leading role, along with Austria, Italy and even the Commission. In France, the 'Grenelle' environment process is being implemented to circumvent science-based decisions in favor of an assessment of the 'common interest.' Combined with the precautionary principle, this is a precedent with implications far beyond MON-810 BT corn cultivation. Moving to retaliation will make clear that the current path has real costs to EU interests and could help strengthen European pro-biotech voices. In fact, the pro-biotech side in France -- including within the farm union -- have told us retaliation is the only way to begin to begin [sic] to turn this issue in France."[199]

Those are but a few examples of the many vicious attacks on scientists, foreign governments, and the media by the biotech industry and their shills, which include high-level government officials in all levels and branches of government.

In the book Altered Genes, Twisted Truth[63], Steven Druker made the following statement in regards to the dissemination of false and misleading information on the subject of GMOs:

"Our legal system recognizes that fraud can exist without overt falsehood and that its defining feature is deception. As one court stated: 'Acts constituting fraud are as broad and as varied as the human mind can invent. Deception and deceit in any form universally connote fraud.' Because the essence of deception is to cause a false impression in the minds of others, one can be guilty of it not only by employing misleading words, but also by withholding words. Therefore, according to the law, failing to reveal pertinent facts is a form of fraud, as is the attempt to hinder others from gaining or understanding them. So from the perspective of the legal system, a large number of scientists have clearly engaged in fraudulent behavior in order to promote genetically engineered foods. Whether or not they have intentionally lied, they have generated widespread confusion, and often delusion, about the facts; and they are therefore guilty of fraud. The misrepresentations that have surrounded GE foods are varied, ranging from blatant lies issued by FDA officials to nuanced distortions dispensed by university professors. But while the forms vary, they are all in some significant way deceptive – and have all been effective. And the individuals who have dispensed them should be held accountable."

2.11   THE APPEARANCE OF REGULATION

> *"This technology is being promoted, in the face of concerns by respectable scientists and in the face of data to the contrary, by the very agencies which are supposed to be protecting human health and the environment. The bottom line in my view is that we are confronted with the most powerful technology the world has ever known, and it is being rapidly deployed with almost no thought whatsoever to its consequences."*[200]
>
> Dr. Suzanne Wuerthele, U.S. Environmental Protection Agency (EPA) toxicologist

As you will see in the next section, FDA scientists had major concerns about GMOs prior to their release into the market - concerns that were ignored and swept under the rug by political appointees at the FDA who were more concerned with promoting an industry than with the health of the nation and the world. But let's take a few steps back...

In 1986, four executives at the Monsanto Company decided to pay a visit to Vice President George H. W. Bush at the White House. Although the Reagan administration was already promoting deregulation, Monsanto executives feared that deregulating GMOs right out of the gate will result in a public backlash, and might doom the industry, which had already cost investors billions of dollars. Monsanto wanted to give the public the appearance of regulation, but on their terms. "In the weeks and months that followed, the White House complied, working behind the scenes to help Monsanto ... It was an outcome that would be repeated, again and again, through three administrations. What Monsanto wished for from Washington, Monsanto — and, by extension, the biotechnology industry — got. If the company's strategy demanded regulations, rules favored by the industry were adopted. And when the company abruptly decided that it needed to throw off the regulations and speed its foods to market, the White House quickly ushered through an unusually generous policy of self-policing."[201]

According to industry shill Henry Miller, "In this area, the U.S. government agencies have done exactly what big agribusiness has asked them to do and told them to do"[201].

This "self-policing" policy reared its ugly head in the fall of 2000 when it was discovered that "certain taco shells manufactured by Kraft contained Starlink, a modified corn classified as unfit for human consumption, prompted a sweeping recall and did grave harm to the idea that self-regulation was sufficient"[201,202].

On page 3 of his "Comments on Biotechnology Draft Document", shown on page 142 of this book, Dr. Louis J. Pribyl, a toxicologist and microbiologist at the FDA, commented about unexpected effects by stating that "This is industry's pet idea, namely that there are no unintended effects that will raise the FDA's level of concern. But time and time again, there is no data to back up their contention". Many other scientists at the FDA reached the same conclusions and asked for rigorous testing of every insertional event, however, Monsanto had other ideas. Rigorous testing would mean high costs and delays in introducing their products to market. What's more, they had already known that what the FDA scientists were worries about was true, but they could not let their investments go down the drain. After all, the kinds of health effects that would result from GMOs are likely to be long-term health effects that would be nearly impossible to trace back to GMOs, like cancer or gastrointestinal disorders, so why bother shine the light on those pesky problems?

So on May 26, 1992, Dan Quayle, George Bush's Vice President, announced the Bush administration's new policy on bioengineered foods. "The reforms we announce today will speed up and simplify the process of bringing better agricultural products, developed through biotech, to consumers, food processors and farmers"[203] he proclaimed. "We will ensure that biotech products will receive the same oversight as other products, instead of being hampered by unnecessary regulation." [203] By "other products" of course, he meant natural crops that do not go through the regulatory process.

However, the FDA could not be completely eliminated from the equation, otherwise it would be obvious to the public that no regulation at all is being implemented, so the FDA has enacted a "voluntary consultation process", by which biotech companies developing genetically engineered products would consult the FDA. However, this consultation process is a ruse - a misdirection. The FDA claims that although it is a voluntary process, all genetically engineered products so far have gone through this consultation process. However, a closer inspection reveals why. In reality, the developer of the genetically engineered product has no obligation to provide any data to the FDA, and on all occasions, except for the Flavr Savr tomato, when the DFA had requested test data, the developer has either refused, or ignored the request. All the developer has to do is provide a statement which notifies the FDA that they had done all appropriate testing, and that they (the developer) had concluded that their product is safe for its intended use. In return, the FDA sends the developer a cookie-cutter "Agency Response Letter"[204-212] stating that it is the FDA's understanding that the developer has concluded that food and feed derived from their products are not materially different in composition, safety, and other relevant parameters from comparable food and feed currently on the market, and that the genetically engineered products do not raise issues that would require premarket review or approval by FDA. Essentially, the developer says "it's good" and the FDA says "if you say so...". In a few instances[206,207] the engineered products had significant compositional differences, but rather than require that the products be labeled as Genetically Engineered, Monsanto has agreed to give the oil derived from the product a slightly different scientific name - a distinction that would go unnoticed by even those consumers that do read labels.

2.12   THE FDA MEMOS

> *"in holding scientific research and discovery in respect, as we should, we must also be alert to the equal and opposite danger that public policy could itself become the captive of a scientific-technological elite."*
>
> Excerpt from Eisenhower's Farewell Address to the Nation; January 17, 1961[213]

The following pages contain the memos obtained through the lawsuits brought against the FDA by the Alliance for Bio-Integrity. It shows the objections of several of the FDA's scientists and their comments about the potential risks of genetic engineering. FDA executives had decided to break the law and ignore their own scientists' warning in their subsequent 1992 policy. The judge in the lawsuit against the FDA further broke the law by dismissing all of the evidence, including the FDA memos, ignoring all of the arguments made by the plaintiffs, and twisting the meaning of words and the law to fit her narrative.

Comments from Dr. Linda Kahl, FDA compliance officer, to Dr. James Maryanski, FDA Biotechnology Coordinator, about the Federal Register document "Statement of Policy: Foods from Genetically Modified Plants." Dated January8, 1992. (3 pages). Source: *www.biointegrity.org*

```
Jim -

     Here are my comments on the Federal Register document
"Statement of Policy: Foods from Genetically Modified Plants".

1.   What is the objective of this policy statement?  I see the
     following possibilities, based on what is in the document:

     a.   To respond to numerous requests to the agency to
          clarify our position with respect to the use of the new
          techniques of biotechnology, and specifically genetic
          engineering, to produce new cultivars of food crops.
     b.   To prepare a comprehensive agency policy with respect
          to new cultivars of food crops - regardless of whether
          those food crops are prepared by new or traditional
          methods.

     The current document (particularly the section on scientific
     issues and the appendix) is very schizophrenic in regard to
     the objective.  Some of this has been provoked by
     conflicting comments from multiple sources on previous
     drafts.  Some advice has been "the recommended actions
     should be the same for cultivars developed by new and
     traditional methods, because it is the product and not the
     process that is regulated".  Other advice has been "Do you
     realize that you are proposing regulations for an entire
     industry that has previously been virtually unregulated and
     has a history of safety" (i.e., traditional plant breeding).

     Therefore, perhaps the relevant question is not only what
     the objective of the document as a whole is, but what the
     objective of the Appendix is.  Should this in fact be
     "Points to Consider" for new methods of biotechnology, since
     guidance has been requested, and guidance on traditional
     breeding has already been given (GRAS symposium, CFR)?  Can
     the objective of the Appendix be "A" even if the objective
     of the policy statement is "B"?

     The June 1986 Coordinated Framework does not seem to be so
     concerned with traditional methods and makes no apologies
     for discussing only biotechnology.  It is very concerned
     with making it clear that no new legislation is needed.  It
     notes that the framework seeks to distinguish those
     organisms that need review and those that do not.  So why
     can't the current appendix deal only with new biotechnology?
     Why try to make it appear that we are discussing all
     modified crops?

2.   I believe that there are at least two situations relative to
     this document in which it is trying to fit a square peg into
     a round hole.  The first square peg in a round hole is that
     the document is trying to force an ultimate conclusion that
```


-((18952

there is no difference between foods modified by genetic engineering and foods modified by traditional breeding practices. This is because of the mandate to regulate the product, not the process.

a.   The processes of genetic engineering and traditional breeding are different, and according to the technical experts in the agency, they lead to different risks. There is no data that addresses the relative magnitude of the risks - for all we know, the risks may be lower for genetically engineered foods than for foods produced by traditional breeding. But the acknowledgement that the risks are different is lost in the attempt to hold to the doctrine that the product and not the process is regulated.

b.   I don't see how the acknowledgement of the fact that the risks are different compromises the position that it is the product that is regulated. The "Points to Consider" for products of genetic engineering must be different than the "Points to Consider" for products of traditional breeding - how can you expect a traditional breeder to have the most basic molecular data (e.g. DNA sequence of the inserted material) when he has no idea of the molecular identity of the genetic material being introduced? Are we to insinuate that practitioners of genetic engineering do not need to adhere to the most basic level of good laboratory techniques simply because the traditional breeding community cannot also provide that data?

3.   The second square peg in a round hole is that the approach of at least part of the document is to use a scientific analysis of the issues involved to develop the policy statement.

a.   In the first place, are we asking the scientific experts to generate the basis for this policy statement in the absence of any data? It's no wonder that there are so many different opinions - it is an exercise in hypotheses forced on individuals whose jobs and training ordinarily deal with facts.

b.   In the second place, I don't think that the scientific analysis as presented is complete. The scientific issues section of the document talks of the "possibility of unintended, accidental changes in genetically engineered plants" but I believe that in most cases the word "risk" is avoided. This is probably at least partly due to the fact that there is no data that could quantify risk. But if the scientific issues section of the document deals totally in hypotheses about "possibilities", why does it not address the fact that multiple events would have to

18953

occur in order for the "possibility of unintended, accidental changes in genetically engineered plants" to result in a danger to the public health. Surely the following series of events must all occur in order to present a danger to the public health: (1) The accidental change must activate a pathway for production of a toxin that was unanticipated, or for which there is no suitable analytical method. (2) This unanticipated toxin must be expressed at a high enough level to exert an effect. (3) This toxin must have serious adverse consequences to humans and/or animals that consume it. (4) The presence of this dangerous unanticipated toxin in amounts sufficient to cause a public health problem must not manifest itself in any other way, so that the first and only clue will be the "body count", so to speak.

c. I wonder if part of the problems associated with this approach - using scientific issues to set the stage for the policy statement - are due to the fact that the scope of technical experts assigned to the project did not include any whose usual job is risk analysis. This does not eliminate the problem with a lack of data, but if the molecular biology, chemistry, and toxicology experts are being forced to deal with hypotheses rather than data, why not the risk analysis experts?

4. Are there any alternatives to toxicology testing that could tip the scales to a level where the modified food can meet a safety standard of reasonable of no harm? My impression is that the limitation of the number of insertion sites to one is not sufficient - what does that actually tell you about safety? Could a recommendation that any new cultivars that are produced by genetic engineering only be used (at least for the present) after they have been crossed by traditional breeding into an established cultivar take us over the edge to where no tox testing is necessary? Is that what we expect the plant breeding community to be doing anyway? If so, then such a suggestion is not a burden.

5. If we don't get specific and substantial input from CVM on animal feed, should the objective be reduced to human food?

6. This is a minor comment in relation to the overall problems in the document, but there needs to be a decision as to whether we use one phrase exclusively to refer to certain issues/topics/procedures (i.e. to promote clarity), or if we use multiple terms to liven the document up. E.g. the document tends to use the phrase "new methods of biotechnology" in its entirety when applicable; but the document uses "traditional breeding practices", "conventional plant breeding", classical plant breeding",

Comments from Dr. Louis J. Pribyl re: the "Biotechnology Draft Document, 2/27/92." Dated March 6, 1992. (5 pages). Source: *www.biointegrity.org*

DRAFT

```
LOUIS J. PRIBYL                           3/6/92
          Comments on Biotechnology Draft Document, 2/27/92
```

-What has happened to the scientific elements of this document? Without a sound scientific base to rest on, this becomes a broad, general, "What do I have to do to avoid trouble"-type document. The examples do not supply the scientific rational that is needed. A scientific document is needed, because there is very little (even when things are called scientific) scientific information supplied. If the FDA wants to have a document based upon scientific principles these principles must be included, otherwise it will look like and probably be just a political document.
-This document reads like a biotech REDBOOK!! The initial intent of the document was to present scientific considerations and to avoid telling industry what tests to run and how to go about doing it, but the flow charts do just what (initially) was to be avoided.
-It reads very pro-industry, especially in the area of unintended effects, but contains very little input from consumers and only a few answers for their concerns, many of which would be answered by supplying the scientific grounding principles.
-The document is inconsistent, in that it says (implies) that there are no differences between traditional breeding and recombinant, yet consultations, and premarket approvals are being bantered around, when they have not been used for foods before. In fact the FDA is making a distinction, so why pretend otherwise.
-The unintended effects cannot be written off so easily by just implying that they too occur in traditional breeding. There is a profound difference between the types of unexpected effects from traditional breeding and genetic engineering which is just glanced over in this document. This is not to say that they are more dangerous, just quite different, and this difference should be and is not addressed.
-A lot of time is spent on selectable markers, which in reality will not be of much concern with the advent of several ways to disarm the marker gene. If the length of the section is any indication of the level of concern, then this is way out of proportion.
-The flow charts are just a version of the Redbook, hoops through which industry must jump, and not scientific considerations. Industry will do what it HAS to do to satisfy the FDA "requirements" and not do the tests that they would normally do because they are not on the FDA's list.
-Why should companies conduct tests as described in the flow charts if there are no differences between traditional foods and those produced by modern technology? And what are the regulatory grounds for all the "shoulds" that are spread throughout this document? If industry does not follow these "should" items is the FDA going to perform these tests and penalize the companies or does the Agency wait for something to go wrong and then act?

(19179

<u>Specific Comments</u>
-pg.3, line 24 (and elsewhere)- How many "first" examples will

2

have to be examined? First examples of what- new genes; new types
of modifications; genes from organisms from other kingdoms; first
submissions? Also in order not to be sued by the "first" group of
submitting biotech companies who will be required to submit data
when others later on will not, what will they receive for being the
guinea pigs? (After all even those who do not submit will also
have the implicit seal of approval from the FDA if the "follow" the
code of practice.)
-pg.6- (In order to bolster the idea of a scientific basis for this
document) please add something like this to line 4: "...these and
other documents, including scientific research in developing this
notice."
-pg.7, line 12- "...notice also discusses in detail current..."
Where is the detailed scientific discussions? This sentence has to
be revised considering that there are few really scientific details
presented.
-pg.7, line 14-17- The scientific considerations are NOT the Codes
of Practice. The scientific considerations are ideas which can be
discussed (proved or disproved).   The Codes of Practice are
guidelines (hoops) for industry to follow. They will not want to
discuss them scientifically since they will be viewed as the FDA
Guidelines for Plant Biotechnology. (Page 36, lines 10-12, "The
Codes of Practice identify specific situations where developers
should consult with FDA.")   These sound like practical
(regulatory), not scientific concerns.
-pg.7, line 18- "First" examples again, who decides when enough is
enough? Industry? FDA? Congress? Safety? The President? The
Council for Competitiveness?
-pg.7, line 24-...will not be challenged on legal grounds... If
there is no difference between traditional foods and genetically
engineered foods, then why would the FDA even bother to challenge
them; unless it is really saying that they are in fact different.
-pg.8, lines 9-10- Has any other whole food ever needed pre-market
approval? If not, then this is saying that the two ways of
producing foods are in fact different.
-pg.11, line 16- "Wide" crosses are defined as NOT between closely
related species or genera.
-pg.12, lines 20-23- Is it really feasible to think that breeders
would freely (without some sort of urging) backcross to get only
one chromosomal location, unless there was interference with the
desired outcome. And besides multiple copies inserted at one site
could become potential sites for rearrangements, especially if used
in future gene transfer experiments, and as such may be more
hazardous.
-pg.13, lines 10-12- If the idea of this sentence is to reassure
people that this process will require many crosses as a kind of
fail-safe system, it will fail.   There are already techniques
available that will transform formally hard to transform "elite"
lines. When those are used, there will be less backcrossing, and
therefore not as much concern about safety.
-pg.13, lines 13-16- One viewpoint is that once the technology
really catches on, that there will be less site-years put into

3

products, rather than more. This will mean less concern about safety, because of a false sense of "knowing what one is doing" and "its been done hundreds of times before without a problem, why check it now".
-pg.15-16, Unexpected Effects- This is industry's pet idea, namely that there are no unintended effects that will raise the FDA's level of concern. But time and time again, there is no data to backup their contention, while the scientific literature does contain many examples of naturally occurring pleiotropic effects. When the introduction of genes into plant's genome randomly occurs, as is the case with the current technology (but not traditional breeding), it seems apparent that many pleiotropic effects will occur. Many of these effects might not be seen by the breeder because of the more or less similar growing conditions in the limited trials that are performed. Until more of these experimental plants have a wider environmental distribution, it would be premature for the FDA to summarily dismiss pleiotropy as is done here.
-pg.38, line 8- "FDA has also been asked whether foods developed by with... (delete the word with).
-pg.42, lines 1-4- The potential for activating cryptic pathways has **NOT** "been effectively managed in the past by sound agricultural practices", because the breeders have not had to face the issue of new, powerful regulatory elements being randomly inserted into the genome. So there is no certainty that they will be able to pick up effects that might not be obvious, such as cryptic pathway activation. This situation IS different than that experienced by traditional breeding techniques.
-pg.45, Chart II, box that reads- "Is the host plant or related species a source of toxicants?" All plants produce toxicants, so the answer to this question is always YES. Many of these toxicants are directed against insects or other herbivores, and so there is little knowledge as to their effect on humans. At their native dose ranges, they might be benign, but if they are increased by unintended effects, their effect(s) are unknown. So to just say "No problem" would be premature and potentially unsafe.
-pg.46, Chart III, box that reads- "Is there clear evidence that allergens have not been transferred to host?" Since there are very few allergens that have been identified at the protein or gene level, this question can only be answered "No" when the gene comes from a plant which produces allergies. So the companies are going to have to consult FDA on tomatoes, peanuts, wheat, and every other plant which produces allergic reactions. Also the only definitive test for allergies is human consumption by affected peoples, which can have ethical considerations.
-pg.46, Chart III, box that reads- Donor a source of toxic substances? SEE ANSWER TO pg.45, Chart II.
-pg.46, Chart III, box that reads- "Evidence that the **donor** toxic..." **Donor** should read DONOR'S.
-pg.47, Chart IV, box that reads- "Newly introduced protein present in food from the plant?" This does not take into account, nor does the document as a whole, those introduced proteins

4

(enzymes) that while acting on one specific, intended substrate to produce a desired effect, will also affect other cellular molecules, either as substrates, or by swamping the plant's regulatory/metabolic system and depriving the plant of resources needed for other things. It is not prudent to rely on plant breeders always finding these types of changes (especially when they are under pressure to get a product out). No where is such an issue discussed or examined in this document.

-pg.47, Chart IV, box that reads- "Will the donor...processing in donor?" Since there are several possible answers for this one question coming from several sources, it should be split up into two separate questions. The first question should end with "...to levels in donor or other food?" and the second question (separate box) Should begin "Will the processing in new...?".

-pg.47, Chart IV, box that reads- "Will the introduced protein be a macroconstituent, or have a cumulative exposure due to use in many foods?" Should this read, "...or have <u>an increased</u> cumulative exposure..."?

-pg.48, Chart V, box that reads- "Has there been an intentional alteration...", what about <u>UNINTENTIONAL</u> alteration? These can and do occur, and could affect the food in subtle ways, that might not be picked up by traditional plant breeders, unless of course they are using biochemical carbohydrate testing procedures.

-pg.48, Chart V, box that reads- "Have any structure...that do not normally occur in carbohydrates?" The strict answer to this question all the time is "NO" because unless some brand new carbo combination is invented by the plant, any combination can be found in some organism somewhere on earth. Maybe it should read, "...that do not normally occur in <u>food</u> carbohydrates?"

-pg.48, Chart V, boxes that reads- "Consult the FDA", these two boxes should be made into one, because it would be more beneficial to the companies to consult after they have completely analyzed the product than after piecemeal analysis. It would be less work for the agency as well.

-pg.49, Chart VI, box that reads- "Is there a significantly altered ratio of omega-6 to omega-3 fatty acids?" Is this the only fatty acid ratio that the FDA will be concerned about, and what happens if this ratio is shown to be non-significant? "Ratios of critical fatty acids, ought to be examined.", might be a way around this problem.

-pg.56-57, lines beginning at 15 and ending on 5- This is a repeat of the material under the section called "a. Whole plants" on page 55, and it does not belong. There is much more appropriate material that should go here.

-pg.66, lines 12-16- If individual proteins are produced in significant quantities, so what. The document just stated in the line above (5-7) that "...the amount and quality of total protein in the diet, rather than of any particular protein, is of greatest significance." The logical reason for the statement beginning on line 12 is not obvious.

-pg.74, line 10 onward- The Toxicology section is going to be a problem. Industry will say it is too much and the

5

environmental/consumer groups will say it is not enough. A more complete presentation of the scientific concerns than is given in this document, as well as a more forceful show of reliance on the usefulness of molecular biology would have reduced this problem by spelling out the need for toxicity tests in limited circumstances. Better yet, a separate (Federal Register) presentation of the scientific concerns with an analysis of comments before ever producing flow charts of guidelines (as currently presented) would produce better understood guidelines.
-pg.78- This environmental section is quite important, but it should be separate or at least given a different label that indicates that it is separate. It could be shortened by being less wordy, without diminishing it's importance.
-pg.78, lines 20-25- "It may be reasonable...plant species into the ecosystem." A recent report in the Feb. 8, 1992 issue of New Scientist (pg.40-44), by C. Heron, implies that plants can form hybrid chains that include plants that are not often considered capable of making such hybrids. There are many things about hybridization that are not known that could cause the transfer of introduced genes into unintended species. This possibility should not be written off so easily.

Louis J. Pribyl, Ph.D.

19183

Memorandum from Dr. Mitchell Smith, Head of Biological and Organic Chemistry Section, to Dr. James Maryanski, Biotechnology Coordinator. Subject: "Comments on Draft Federal Register Notice on Food Biotechnology, Dec. 12, 1991 draft." Dated January 8, 1992. (2 pages)

Source: *www.biointegrity.org*

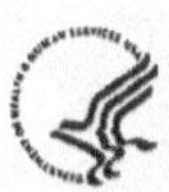

DEPARTMENT OF HEALTH & HUMAN SERVICES   Public Health Service

---

Memorandum

Date: 8 January 1992

From: Mitchell J. Smith, Ph.D.

Subject: Comments on Draft Federal Register Notice on Food Biotechnology *(Dec 12, 1991 draft)*

To: Jim Maryanski

Dear Jim,

My specific comments are delineated below, as requested. My general conclusion is that this issue turns the conventional connotation of *food additive* on its head. It also conveys the impression that the public need not know when it is being exposed to "*new food additives*," for lack of a better descriptor.

P28, L 10: Add "the extent of expression of the introduced DNA."

P31, L 3-7: Overly optimistic since one could argue just the opposite and be equally valid.

P33: Version # 1 is better.

P46, L 24: To call a "trait" a new substance misconstrues the scientific connotations of both, particularly the latter, which is usually interpreted to mean a physical component or chemical. In any event, just because the agency failed to evaluate 'new substances' introduced by conventional breeding gives it no reason to continue to do so now with new biotechnology. Moreover, on page 51 you go on to state that "Foods derived from genetically modified plants developed by classical plant breeding methods have been regulated by FDA primarily under the adulteration provisions of section 402 (a) (1) of the Act.

P53: The statement "(3) organisms modified by modern molecular and cellular methods are governed by the same physical and biological laws as are organisms produced by classical methods" is somewhat erroneous because in the former, natural biological barriers to breeding have been breached.

P55, L 6-7: The statement "to the extent that it is known" begs the question as to what degree of identification and toxicological evaluation is sought or prudent. In this instance ignorance is not bliss.

P60, L 9: You now use the normal connotation of *substance*, in contradistinction to a trait being a substance (P46, L 24).

P60, L 9: "Heavy metals" may require qualification since some, *e.g.*, iron, are both essential and toxic.

P63, L 23: Your distinction between "added" and "inherent" is fanciful. The two two are not dichotomous; thus the ambiguity is in your choice of language, not reality.

18960

P67, L 5-8: This contradicts P61, L 8-11!

P68, L 20: This should read that the *intended* changes . . .

P68, L 24: This should read that the substances *intended, per se,* . . .

P73, L 3 & P74, L 1: It is immaterial that the FDA doesn't believe methods of genetic modifications are material information important to consumers if regulations do indeed indicate that the former will be a material fact when consumers view such information as important.

P83, L 4: This is a very contestable issue for a variety of reasons, amongst which are that many plants will be engineered to be sterile . . .

P83, L 28-31: What degree of "monitoring," is actually being suggested?

P86: Version #1 is better, although both fail to address the interdependency between chemical analyses and toxicological testing.

P87, L 20-30 & P88, L 1-9: This section seems very arbitrary.

P90: Version #1 is better.

P92: Version #1 is better.

Sincerely,

Mitchell J. Smith, Ph.D.
Head, Biological and Organic Chemistry Section
NPIB, CDC, CFSAN

Comments from Dr. Carl B. Johnson on the "draft statement of policy 12/12/91." Dated January 8, 1992. (2 pages)
Source: *www.biointegrity.org*

```
1/8/92  Comments on draft statement of policy 12/12/91

p. 1
line 11-12 last part of sentence is redundant.  Any food subject to FFDCA is
already introduced into interstate commerce.  Antecedent is ambiguous; could be
either foods or new scientific methods.

line 16 "scientific information" is too vague.  "information on the chemical
composition" might be better.

p. 10  Clearly state that FDA is developing an inventory of future commercial
foods derived from plants developed by new biotechnology (see lines 14-15 "FDA
is using this inventory . . .") in order to identify the types of new plants
under development.

p. 27  B. Unintended events
p. 28   The nature of the unintended effects on gene expression may vary,
depending on:
 1. the site of integration in the genome of the host plant
 2. the number of integration sites
 3. the number of copies of the introduced DNA at each integration site
 4. the source and nucleotide sequence of all introduced DNA

p. 34
lines 9-17 appear to provide a justification for the use of tox studies in safety
assessment, citing as an example the inability of analytical or molecular methods
to detect the presence of a unknown toxin produced by activation of a previously
cryptic gene. However, lines 8-end of paragraph say that tox studies will not be
needed if DNA insertion is limited to only a single site of known genomic loca-
tion.  This discussion implies that pleiotropy (i.e., production of a unknown
toxin due to activation of a previously cryptic gene) will disappear or be
negligible if gene insertions are limited to a single copy at a known genomic
location.  Evidence should be provided to support this position.

p. 37
lines 10-15  Are we asking the crop developer to prove that food from his crop
is non-allergenic? This seems like an impossible task.  Perhaps we could ask for
evidence that the new variety is no more allergenic than conventional varieties.

p. 38
lines 2-4  As sequence data on known allergens increases, it may become
increasingly useful to utilize sequence data to screen for the presence of
potential allergens in food.

p. 87 Paraphrase of Version #2
If insertion of genetic material is restricted to a single known site in the
plant genome, then traditional toxicology studies will not be necessary to
provide adeqate assurance of safety with respect to the issue of unknown
toxicants.

                                   6
```

Comment: What if the inserted DNA is from a non-food source and encodes a protein product that is toxic to certain organisms (e.g., Bt toxin)? Wouldn't knowledge of the toxicity of this protein product be necessary to ensure safety? It is my understanding that pleiotropic effects are unpredictable, and may be triggered by gene insertion at a single site, as well as at multiple sites, in the plant genome. Restriction of foreign DNA insertion to a single site in the plant genome would reduce, but not eliminate the chance that the insertion event might trigger pleiotropic effects. This position is supported by the discussion on p. 28. The document does not present evidence that pleiotropic effects (e.g., alterations in biosynthesis of unknown toxicants) can be controlled by restriction of foreign DNA insertion to a single site in the plant genome. If such evidence exists, it should be summarized in the document.

Carl B. Johnson

7

Memorandum from Dr. Gerald B. Guest, Director of the Center for Veterinary Medicine, to Dr. James Maryanski, Biotechnology Coordinator. Subject: "Regulation of Transgenic Plants–FDA Draft Federal Register Notice on Food Biotechnology." Dated February 5, 1992. (4 pages) Source: *www.biointegrity.org*

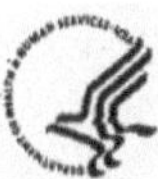

DEPARTMENT OF HEALTH & HUMAN SERVICES   Public Health Service

Memorandum

Date   February 5, 1992

From   Director, Center for Veterinary Medicine, HFV-1
            Through: Director, Center for Food Safety and Applied Nutrition, HFF-1

Subject   Regulation of Transgenic Plants - FDA Draft Federal Register Notice on
            Food Biotechnology

To   Biotechnology Coordinator, HFF-300

Thank you for sending us the draft Federal Register Notice on Food
Biotechnology (hereafter referred to as Notice), dated December 12, 1991. It
is obvious that you have had a major task in synthesizing the scientific and
regulatory issues.

In response to your question on how the agency should regulate genetically
modified food plants, I and other scientists at CVM have concluded that
there is ample scientific justification to support a pre-market review of
these products. As you state in the Notice, the new methods of genetic
modification permit the introduction of genes from a wider range of sources
than possible by traditional breeding. The FDA will be confronted with new
plant constituents that could be of a toxicological or environmental concern.
The Notice further describes unintended or pleiotropic effects that pose
unknown safety concerns. It has always been our position that the sponsor
needs to generate the appropriate scientific information to demonstrate
product safety to humans, animals and the environment.

A marked-up copy of the Notice with our comments will be provided to you
directly by the Center's scientists. Generally, I would urge you to eliminate
statements that suggest that the lack of information can be used as evidence
for no regulatory concern. Examples of statements to this effect occur on p.
30 and p. 64 of the Notice. Furthermore, we believe that much of the
detailed discussion on current scientific methods is not required in the
Notice and, in fact, may be misleading. Sponsors may assume that if their
transgenic product or methodology is not included in the Notice, that it is
exempt from regulation. FDA regulatory policy must encompass both
current and future techniques.

In addition to the human food safety and environmental concerns outlined
in the appendices to the Notice, CVM believes that animal feeds derived
from genetically modified plants present unique animal and food safety
concerns. We list some of these concerns below:

1)   Unlike the human diet, a single plant product may constitute a
significant portion of the animal diet. For instance, 50 - 75 percent of the
diet of most domestic animals consists of field corn. Therefore, a change in

18990

nutrient or toxicant composition that is considered insignificant for human consumption may be a very significant change in the animal diet.

2)	Animals consume plants, plant parts and plant byproducts that are not consumed by humans. For example, animals consume whole cottonseed and cottonseed meal, whereas humans consume only small amounts of cottonseed oil. Gossypol, a natural toxicant, is concentrated in the cotton seed meal during the production of cottonseed oil. Since plant byproducts represent an important feed source for animals, it is important to determine if significant concentrations of harmful plant constituents or toxicants are present in the transgenic plant byproducts.

3)	The use of antibiotic-resistance genes as selectable markers in transgenic plants must be reviewed to determine the effect on animal therapeutics. For example, the enzyme product of the *kan*^{r} gene, aminoglycoside 3' phosphotransferase-II, inactivates the antibiotic, neomycin, which is used in feed and drinking water of animals..

4)	Nutrient composition and availability of nutrients in feed are extremely important to the animal industry and animal health. Feed costs often represent 50 percent or more of the cost of producing animals. If a genetic modification made a higher percentage of a nutrient unavailable to the animal, it could have a major effect on animal health. For example, if an unintended effect of modification of soybeans was increased content of phytin, the amount of phosphorus available to the animal could be greatly reduced. Animal health problems could result unless the diet were supplemented with phosphorus.

5)	Residues of plant constituents or toxicants in meat and milk products may pose human food safety problems. For example, increased levels of glucosinolates or erusic acid in rapeseed may produce a residue problem in edible products.

Because of the target animal, human food and environmental safety concerns delineated above and in the Notice, CVM proposes the acceptance of a modification of the primary regulatory scheme outlined in the Notice. The CVM proposed regulatory approach is as follows:

1) Firms expecting to market transgenic plants, for use in animal feed should contact Director, Division of Animal Feeds (DAF), HFV-220, Office of Surveillance and Compliance, Center for Veterinary Medicine, 7500 Standish Place, Rockville MD. 20855.

2) Firms requesting a decision on the status of their genetically modified plant should submit a data package under 21 CFR 570.30. DAF can make three determinations on a submission: a) the modified plant is not substantially different from traditional varieties , b) a Food Additive Petition (FAP) for the modified plant should be submitted under 21 CFR 571.1, or a GRAS Affirmation petition should be submitted under 21 CFR 570.35 or, c)

not enough information was submitted for a conclusion to be reached. For consultation and protocol reviews, firms should establish Investigational Applications under 21 CFR 570.17. DAF will apply the same review time frames as for an FAP.

3) For modified plants that CVM decides are not substantially different from traditional varieties, CVM will publish a notice of such finding in the Federal Register.

4) For transgenic plants that serve as food for both animals and humans, a decision must be made as to whether CFSAN or CVM will administer the document. The decision should be based on the primary use for the product. The administrator at the primary Center will have the responsibility of forwarding the submission to the secondary Center for a consulting review. Investigational animals to be used for human consumption would be authorized either under 21 CFR 170.17 or 21 CFR 570.17 by the respective Center.

If you have any questions, please contact Dr. Bill Price at (301) 295-8724.

Gerald B. Guest, DVM

ATTACHMENT: REVISED FDA DRAFT FEDERAL REGISTER NOTICE ON FOOD BIOTECHNOLOGY

P. 74

G. TOXICOLOGY

4. Target animal safety feeding study.

Sponsors with products to be incorporated into animal feeds should conduct well controlled feeding studies in the target animal comparing the new plant variety to the conventional plant. The study should be of sufficient size and duration to provide adequate statistical power to detect adverse effects should they occur. Only the highest normal feeding level of the feed product from the new plant variety would have to be tested. Common animal study parameters should be measured, including feed and water intake, weight gains, and blood clinical chemistry profiles. Gross pathology should be performed on preselected animals consuming the new plant variety and the conventional plant diets. Animals that die during the study should be necropsied to determine the cause of death. Additional testing may be necessary if it appears that residues from constituents of the new plant variety pose a risk to humans consuming animal products. Further guidance can be obtained from the Center for Veterinary medicine upon request.

Additional FDA documents objecting to the use of antibiotic-resistant marker genes and safety questions raised by tests on the Flavr Savr Tomato™ – the first bioengineered plant that came to market, as well as additional evidence of improprieties in the formation of FDA policy on bioengineered foods can be found on the Alliance for Bio-Integrity website at www.biointegrity.org/.

2.13   ALTERNATIVE & SUSTAINABLE SOLUTIONS

First, let's bring light to the fact that GMOs and conventional, monoculture farming practices are unsustainable and damaging to the entire ecosystem. The approach that the biotech and chemical industries have taken to farming is the same approach that they have applied to medicine for years, and it is no surprise that the biotech industry, the chemical industry, and the pharmaceutical industry are really the same industry, and the same companies. Bayer, Dupont, Monsanto, and many others all produce medicines, industrial and agricultural chemicals, and GMOs. The philosophy that humans, and nature as a whole are machines, and that we can swap out or throw out the parts of that machine and alter or delete sections of its code, and expect the machine to work better is an arrogant and fallacious point of view, and the results of such points of view are painfully apparent in the amount of sickness in the world, and especially in developed countries, and the amount of destruction wroth on the environment - the animals, soil, air, water - the entire ecosystem.

It is time that scientists admit what they have known since the beginning of science, and beforehand, but refuse to confront for their own selfish reasons of fame, domination, and monetary gain. The fact that you cannot work with nature by working against nature. You cannot get rid of pests by growing thousands of acres of a single crop, year after year. You cannot cure disease by killing off the body's disease-fighting mechanisms. You cannot expect balance by creating an imbalance.

William Belknap, a pioneer in the field of bioengineered food stated that "It's not nice to fool nature. Sometimes you get slapped. And some people get slapped around a lot." [214]

Let's look at a few alternatives to the destructive and unsustainable current mainstream agricultural systems:

2.13.1 <u>Small farms are the answer to monoculture and mega-farms</u>

According to a report by the United Nations Environment Programme (UNEP) and the International Fund for Agricultural Development (IFAD) on smallholdings (small farms and gardens), "multiple studies have found that smallholdings are relatively more productive per hectare than large-scale plantations ... and are also more resource-efficient"[215]. "The variety and variability of animals, plants and microorganisms – at genetic, species and ecosystem levels – are necessary to sustain key functions of the ecosystem. Biodiversity needs to be carefully managed in smallholder cultivation practices. In general, the more diversified the agricultural land use, the more resilient the land is to climate change and other disturbances, and the more it can produce relative to energy, water and other costs. Diversity on the farm also helps maintain the genetic pools of plants and animals (UNEP 2012). Smallholders and indigenous peoples play a critical role in in situ conservation of crop genetic diversity, since local varieties are often more resilient than modern varieties. For example, during the spring drought in south-west China in 2010, most of the modern varieties were lost, while most of the landraces survived"[215].

The report additionally states that "Organic agriculture for smallholders leads to increased food production and increased benefits for the ecosystem services that support agricultural production: improved organic matter, reduced soil erosion and increased biodiversity. Producing organically also enables farmers to earn premium prices and tap into niche export markets. [215]" Even the Royal Society, whom have been on the side of GMOs for decades recognize that the current models of commercial agriculture are destructive and unsustainable, and they recognize the need for an intensification of sustainable models[216].

2.13.2 Conservation Agriculture

Conservation agriculture (CA) is a method of farming whereby the soil is not tilled, and cover crops or mulch are used to physically protect the soil from sun, rain and wind and to feed soil biota, reduce soil erosion, maintain soil fertility, improve soil moisture retention, and reduce pollution due to reduced pesticide use.

"The soil microorganisms and soil fauna take over the tillage function and soil nutrient balancing. Mechanical tillage disturbs this process. Therefore, zero or minimum tillage and direct seeding are important elements of CA"[215].

This agricultural method also increases yields, and diversifies the use of the land, allowing farmers to profit in off-seasons by renting the land for animal grazing.

2.13.3 Agroforestry systems

Agroforestry incorporates agricultural crops and/or livestock farming with fast growing trees and shrubs. besides maximizing the use of the land and increasing profits through fodder and non-timber forest products, benefits of agroforestry include suppression of weeds, which reduces or eliminates the need for herbicides, improved soil fertility and water retention through the increase of soil organic matter, nitrogen fixing and improvement of nutrient balances, and carbon sequestration, which mitigates climate change. The method also reduces soil erosion and improves water quality.

Additionally, "Farmers have frequently reported significant crop yield increases for maize, sorghum, millet, cotton and groundnut when grown in proximity to Faidherbia [a tree commonly found in agroforestry systems in sub-Saharan Africa]. [215]"

The return on investment in agroforestry systems has been shown to be very high[217,218,219].

2.13.4 Push-Pull Cropping Systems

"The push–pull technology is a strategy for controlling agricultural pests by using repellent 'push' plants and trap 'pull' plants. For example, cereal crops like maize or sorghum are often infested by stem borers. Grasses planted around the perimeter of the crop attract and trap the pests, whereas other plants, like Desmodium, planted between the rows of maize repel the pests and control the parasitic plant Striga."[220]

In additional to repelling unwanted pests, push-pull systems also attract beneficial organisms. "Companion plants attracting parasitoids that control the African witchweed, or Striga, have led to an increase in cereal yields (maize, sorghum, millet) from about 1 ton/ha to 3.5 tons/ha in places where the system is used. These plants can provide multiple additional benefits such as nitrogen fixation (in the case of legumes such as beans) and high-value animal fodder that helps increase milk production. 'Push-pull' systems are based on locally available crops, have low external input levels and fit within traditional, mixed cropping systems. Thus they are appropriate for resource-poor smallholders"[215].

2.13.5 <u>Integrated Pest Management (IPM)</u>

The Food and Agriculture Organization of the United Nations (FAO) defines IPM as "the careful consideration of all available pest control techniques and subsequent integration of appropriate measures that discourage the development of pest populations and keep pesticides and other interventions to levels that are economically justified and reduce or minimize risks to human health and the environment. IPM emphasizes the growth of a healthy crop with the least possible disruption to agro-ecosystems and encourages natural pest control mechanisms."

"FAO promotes IPM as the preferred approach to crop protection and regards it as a pillar of both sustainable intensification of crop production and pesticide risk reduction."

IPM has led to a great reduction, and in some cases the complete elimination of pesticide use.

There are many other examples where sustainable systems and traditional breeding practices have performed better than their chemically-intensive and genetically engineered counterparts. As discussed in chapter 2.5, a conventional breeding program in Uganda has produced a virus-resistant, high-yielding sweet potato which produced roughly 100% higher yields and at a fraction of the time and cost of Monsanto's GMO variety[164] and a new variety of cassava developed by the International Institute of Tropical Agriculture (IITA) has produced a virus and drought resistant variety that has 6 to 10 times higher yields[165] than other varieties grown in those regions. This high-yielding cassava has been successfully implemented across Africa.

2.13.6 <u>Organic Farming</u>

Besides the obvious benefit to human health in eliminating toxic insecticides, herbicides, fungicides, and chemical fertilizers, the benefits to the farmer, and to the environment are immense. A 30-year side-by-side Farming System Trial (FST); the longest-running trial of its kind, performed by the Rodale Institute[221] concluded that "Organic farming is far superior to conventional systems when it comes to building, maintaining and replenishing the health of the soil. For **soil health** alone, organic agriculture is more sustainable than conventional. When one also considers **yields, economic viability, energy usage, and human health**, it's clear that organic farming is sustainable, while current conventional practices are not."

The trial demonstrated that while conventional farming systems erode the soil, organic systems do the opposite by preventing erosion, increasing carbon content, increasing ground water recharge, reducing runoff, improving water retention and uptake by the crops, and regenerating the soil.

Organic methods also produced comparable, and even higher yields with less input and cost. Particularly in times of drought, organic methods produced 31% higher corn yields than conventional methods, while genetically engineered "drought tolerant" varieties produced only a 6.7% to 13.3% increase in yields over the conventional, non-drought resistant varieties, the report states, clearly demonstrating that GMOs are not necessary, and with rising temperatures, the need for a system that mitigates crop-losses, and increases water retention and soil health is essential to our survival.

From an economic perspective, the report concluded that "Even without a price premium, the organic systems are competitive with the conventional systems."

According to a report from the United Nations, agroecological farming methods could double global food production in just 10 years.

Furthermore, in looking at the human health impact from conventional and GMO farming, "Numerous studies have begun to capture the true extent of how our low-level exposure to pesticides [a general term which includes insecticides, herbicides, and fungicides] could be quietly causing serious health problems in our population. The toxins are nearly inescapable in the water we drink, the food we eat and the air we breathe ... More than 17,000 pesticide products for agricultural and non-agricultural use are currently on the market. Exposure to these chemicals has been linked to brain/central nervous system disruption, breast, colon, lung, ovarian, pancreatic, kidney, testicular, and stomach and other cancers ... The EPA has required testing of less than 1% of the chemicals currently in commerce."

"The groundwork established in the FST is now being replicated and validated in the wider academic and agricultural community."

2.14 GMOs IN A NUTSHELL

So let's once more review the industry's claims in light of the information presented in this chapter;

- **GMOs are an extension of natural breeding and do not pose different risks**

As I've outlined all throughout this chapter, the process in which GMOs are produced, and the outcomes of those genetic alterations cannot be compared with natural breeding. For starters, natural breeding cannot violate natural species boundaries, while cross-species DNA commingling is the basis of the genetic engineering technology. Since nature does not allow for this type of commingling, genetic engineers have to go to great lengths to fool nature and force the foreign DNA into the plant cells, but of course, always at a cost. Additionally, natural breeding cannot produce novel toxins – toxins which are not already present in the parental lines of the plants being bred, or even toxins which are entirely unknown to science. In GMOs however, the production of novel toxins, and especially toxins novel to plants are 1) part of the design – such as the bacterial Bt toxin incorporated into the DNA of Bt crops, which is not natural to plants and is not present in the produce derived from conventional and organic plants under natural circumstances, and 2) are unintentionally and unpredictably, and in many cases unknowingly produced in genetically modified organisms, as was the case with Showa Denko's genetically modified bacteria which led to the EMS epidemic.

- **GMOs increase yields**

As was shown in the "Failure to yield" report, GMOs have not increased yields, and in many cases, have reduced yields. This is due to disturbances in energy distribution in the plant's physiology, and the disruption of natural mechanisms caused by the genetic alteration. In India and other parts of the world, many farmers have had complete crop failures due to unintended consequences of the genetic modification.

While GMO manufacturers have been promising yield increases, and have been failing at every attempt, as was demonstrated in the Rodale Institute trial, and several other reports, organic practices and conventional breeding have been steadily delivering two and three-fold, and even ten-fold increases in yields, at a fraction of the cost and time that it takes to develop a GE crop, and at a lower cost to the farmer.

- **GMOs reduce herbicide and insecticide use**

Not only have GMOs not decreased herbicide and insecticide use, but they have actually increased both. While GMOs have initially reduced insecticide spraying, they simply moved the insecticide from the outside of the plant to the inside of the plant. This reduced the need for farmers to spray insecticides onto the plant, but it actually increased the amount of insecticide that is in and on the plant, and in the environment exponentially, since spraying is done periodically, whereas the Bt insecticidal toxin within the GE plant is produced 24/7 throughout the life cycle of the plant. Additionally, and ironically, many pests have developed resistance to the crop's Bt toxin which forced farmers to return to spraying greater amounts of more toxic chemicals to combat the resistant pests. So, not only are the Bt crops producing a much greater amount of insecticide within the plant than were ever used in sprays, farmers are now spraying additional chemicals on top of the plants.

Furthermore, with the advent of Roundup Ready crops, the usage of Roundup herbicide has also increased greatly, and with the development of herbicide-resistant superweeds, farmers are once again resorting to using higher amounts of Roundup, as well as more toxic herbicides, such as 2,4-D.

- **GMOs make farmers' lives easier**

While initially GMOs have reduced the work-load required by the farmer by making weeding and pest control simpler, through the development of herbicide resistant weeds and insecticide resistant pests, farmers are much worse off than they were before the advent of GMOs. The problem of resistance is so severe in some places, that many farmers had to abandon their lands.

- **GMOs are safe to eat**

While industry and industry-funded studies tend to paint a rosy picture, their studies are always heavily doctored to remove inconvenient truths, and their testing methods routinely violate scientific protocols. Even then, upon close inspection of the data, most studies report significant adverse effects on tissues and organs, which are downplayed and written off by the industry as biologically insignificant. Additionally, industry studies almost never go beyond short term. Long term studies are the only way to determine chronic toxicity. Chronic toxicity is the cause of almost all diseases and disorders. Additionally, industry studies are rarely published. The fact that the industry has not produced a single peer reviewed long-term toxicological study that shows that GMOs are safe suggest that in reality they have performed many long-term studies that were not publicized due to findings of many toxic effects. The reason I say this is because the biotech industry would jump at the opportunity to show that their products are safe. But that clearly has not happened.

On the other hand, nearly all studies performed by independent scientists show disturbing signs of tissue and organ damage, carcinogenicity, immune response, endocrine disruption, fertility problems and harm to reproductive organs, and other effects. The FDA's own scientific experts, as well as scientific experts from other organizations and agencies worldwide have warned about those effects for decades and have been ignored and suppressed.

- **GMOs can be more nutritious than naturally bred crops**

While the GMO industry have been promising crops with increased nutritional values for years, they have yet to produce any. Their much-anticipated Golden Rice, which is intended to alleviate vitamin A deficiency in developing countries has been in development for over two decades, and racked up billions of dollars in development costs, yet, it is still not market-ready due a disappointing vitamin A content and low yields in field trials. Besides, vitamin A is already abundant in sweet potatoes, carrots, dark leafy greens, winter squashes, lettuce, dried apricots, cantaloupe, liver, and tropical fruits, so clearly there are plenty of natural sources of vitamin A and other vitamins, minerals, and other nutrients in presently available crops. The graph on the following page demonstrates this well:

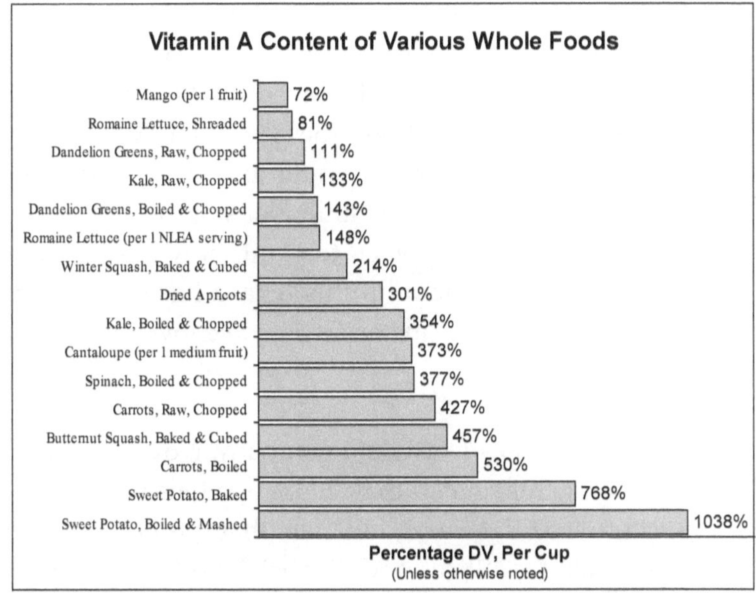

Although liver is also fairly high in vitamin A (126% DV per 1 chicken liver), I did not include it in the chart for three reasons; 1) most of the foods shown above contain a much higher concentration of vitamin A than does liver, 2) the liver is a detoxifying organ, and as such, if often times contains many toxins which accumulate in it, and 3) there is only 1 liver per animal, so it cannot be considered as a sustainable form of food for people of poor demographics. Additionally, it takes much more resources to produce a pound of animal product than it does to produce a pound of plant food.

- **GMOs are the solution to world hunger and increasing population**

Current food production is sufficient for feeding 11 billion people. Genetic engineering has not contributed one iota to increased yields, and the minor yield increases in GMOs where they are present, are not due to the genetic engineering, but to the parental stock that was used to create the genetically engineered line. As was discussed previously, conventional breeding techniques have resulted in almost all of the yield increases thus far. Additionally, the main reason for low yields in developing countries is not due to the limitations of the crop itself, but rather to education – when to plant, how to plant, how to irrigate, etc. Education in this regard has been attributed with the remaining increases in yield over the past few decades.

Steve Smith, head of GMO company Novartis Seeds UK (now Syngenta) stated that "if anyone tells you that GM is going to feed the world, tell them that it is not. To feed the world takes political and financial will - it's not about production and distribution."[222]

Likewise, a report by the United Nations Environment Programme (UNEP) and the International Fund for Agricultural Development (IFAD) stated that "Getting more (and more nutritious) food to the hungry has more to do with governance, distribution, food prices and protecting local food production than it does with raising global levels of farming output"[215]. More important than large corporations increasing their yields and their profits, which will do nothing to combat starvation and malnutrition in poor regions, the poor can gain more with proper education in sustainable farming. "Smallholdings can address one specific aspect of well-being very effectively: nutrition ... Smallholder farming can potentially impact human nutrition by providing a variety of foods in sufficient quantities to enable all household members to eat a nutritionally adequate diet. Greater and more-sustained yields may increase access of households to a larger food supply. The availability of a greater variety of nutritious foods at community and household levels can be increased through the introduction of new crops, the promotion of underexploited traditional food crops, and home gardens"[215].

- **GMOs are strictly regulated for safety**

GMOs are self-regulated by the industry that stands to gain from their sale in a fox guarding the hen-house manner. The FDA, USDA, EPA or any other agency do not in any way, shape or form regulate GMOs. The FDA conducts a voluntary consultation with the GMO developer, and is at the mercy of the GMO developer as to whether or not they get any scientific data to support the safety of the GMO to be marketed. The developer sends the FDA a statement claiming that the GMO strain intended for market has been tested and concluded to be safe for humans, animals and the environment, and in return the FDA sends the developer a letter back, in essence stating that they read their conclusion. This in actuality is not an approval process, but merely serves to give the appearance of regulation, without any actual regulation.

- **GMOs benefit the environment**

GMOs and their associated chemicals have damaged the environment in many ways. Beside the weed and insect resistance problems indicated above, GMOs and their associated chemicals have destroyed rhizomes in the soil, making nutrients less available to the plants, and reducing a crop's ability to get water from deeper soil, requiring more water to be used. They have also destroyed beneficial soil organisms and emboldened harmful soil organisms. Furthermore, Bt crops and herbicides are responsible for pollution of waterways, pollution of the air in and around farming communities, colony collapse disorder in bees, and the devastation to the population of Monarch butterflies through the killing-off of milkweed; their predominant food source.

- **GMOs are economically beneficial**

GMOs only benefit the GMO and chemical companies. Cross-contamination of conventional and organic plants alone has caused tremendous loss to farmers, and to the state. On several occasions, contamination of conventional and organic crops by GMOs has led to the rejection and subsequent destruction of those crops, and caused farmers to lose their organic certification. GMO seeds also cost more to the farmer than conventional seeds[223], and farmers are prevented by contractual obligation from saving their seeds for subsequent planting. "Over the past century, about 75 per cent of plant genetic resources have been lost and a third of today's diversity could disappear by 2050 ... Policies should help link formal and farmer-saved seed systems, and foster the emergence of local seed enterprises[215]. GMO companies reduce diversity just by the mere fact that development of GE seeds is an expensive process.

Whatever farmers have gained in the initial reduction in labor and pesticide costs, they have more than paid for in weed and pest resistance. Many farmers whom are now suffering financially do not switch back to conventional for the fear that GMOs from prior years' crops will unintentionally grow in their fields and they will be sued by the GMO company for growing their product without a contract. Many farmers have been bankrupted, especially by Monsanto because their fields were contaminated without their knowledge, and Monsanto had sued them, and won. Even so, many farmers are abandoning GMOs for non-GMO alternatives[223].

As you can see, the supposed benefits of GMOs are nothing but unfounded, over inflated hype, that might have been a good goal for the industry, but have fallen short in every respect. The driving force behind the industry's continued push forward is less influenced by their prior successes, and more influenced by their prior investments. Investments for which they intend to get a healthy return on, regardless of the consequences to individuals, or the entire world's ecosystem. What they fail to recognize is, when they have destroyed the world, their money will have no value.

Science is good, and using science to improve our food is a noble effort, but it needs to be an open and honest process, and in the case of biotechnology it has been neither. Monsanto especially has done a whole lot to destroy science by demonizing scientists who came out with findings which did not agree with their business ambitions, regardless of their own scientific findings or the consequences to human, animal, and environmental health. Unless this changes, there will never be trust between consumers and the GMO industry, and I (and others) will always be on the side of those who find ill effects, because when it comes to my health and the health of my family, my pets and the environment, I do not wish to take chances. Although I do not support open-air GMO farming, or using GMOs in the food supply at this time, I do support the continuation and furthering of the science, in a controlled, environmentally contained setting. It's only with the responsible continued exploration of the science that we will learn everything that needs to be learned about DNA and its control mechanisms, sufficiently, so that one day we might be able to alter nature to our benefit and the benefit of the planet as a whole; although I believe that working with nature, rather than modifying it is a better endeavor. As much as some genetic engineers have a big ego, and they like to think that they know a lot about genetics, the entire science of genetics is in its infancy and there is still much to be learned. There are discoveries made regularly in genetics and epigenetics that turn our existing knowledge on its head, so to think that we know enough to alter those enormously complex systems without repercussions is extremely egotistical.

With the current state of knowledge no genetically modified crop line can be proven to be safe unless each insertional event is thoroughly tested individually, by growing the crop in every possible condition, exposed to cross-pollination with every other GE and non-GE crop, grown with every pesticide and chemical fertilizer it is intended to be grown with, and evaluated for toxicological, allergenic, carcinogenic, and other deleterious effects in feeding studies on human volunteers, and then only the product of that specific insertional event can be deemed to be safe, and not the genetic "recipe" as a whole. This is due to the fact that the genetic insertion process, as well as the culture process are completely random and each insertional event results in a completely different set of genetic alterations, and cross-pollination leads to further genetic alterations, and of course, pesticides and chemical fertilizers effect soil health, nutrient uptake, and human and animal health. For this reason, it is also not possible to replicate a safety study by generating a new genetically engineered plant, even if it is done with the identical genetic cassette and process. Replication of results is a hallmark of the scientific process and is essential for demonstrating a scientific truth. Therefore, the genetic engineering process itself can never be assumed to be safe when performed using current techniques of genetic alteration and culturing.

For all those reasons, and many more, genetically engineered plants can never be considered financially beneficial, both from the financial burden of sufficiently testing them, and because of all that is already known about the deleterious effects caused by every step of the way, leading to an enormous economic burden from diseases and disorders brought on by GMOs and their associated chemicals.

- **GMOs are rigorously tested and proven safe**

Although the Biotech industry holds independent researchers who show evidence of harm to the highest standards, they do not do the same for themselves. Practically all industry tests are substandard, and most would not qualify for publication - missing data, inappropriate controls, using rats with widely varying starting weights, using bacterially-produced proteins and toxins in place of the plant-produced ones, replacing dead animals after the test has started, removing tumors prior to autopsy. And even then, when their studies still show adverse effects, they write them off as non-biologically significant, when in most cases they are extremely significant, especially considering that practically all industry studies are short to medium term. Contrary to the industry hard-line, GMOs have never been proven safe, and have never been approved by the FDA.

All that being said, when one day we have sufficient knowledge to ensure that GMOs are absolutely safe, labeling should still be mandatory for many reasons. As was aptly stated by the authors of the citizen response to the SLO Health Commission GMO Task Force report, "If the GMO food industry can't survive consumer choice, then those foods should not be sitting on the shelves of American grocery stores, and no scientist, corporation, political entity or university should stand in the way of that democratic process."[60]

2.15 RECOMMENDED DOCUMENTARIES AND INTERVIEWS:

- Documentary: Seeds of Death: Unveiling The Lies of GMO's - Full Movie
    - https://www.youtube.com/watch?v=a6OxbpLwEjQ

- Documentary: Genetic Roulette, The Gamble of Our Lives
    - http://geneticroulettemovie.com/

- Documentary: David Vs. Monsanto
    - https://www.youtube.com/watch?v=rf0BBDYl6bo

- Documentary: The World According to Monsanto (Full Length) HD
    - https://www.youtube.com/watch?v=6nNFmzAOtJI

- Documentary: GMO Trilogy - Hidden Dangers in Kids' Meals: Genetically Engineered Foods
    - (1 of 3): https://www.youtube.com/watch?v=oqc9-6dGWOw
    - (2 of 3): https://www.youtube.com/watch?v=B5ydsjKyBZA
    - (3 of 3): https://www.youtube.com/watch?v=SH6rStYRm_M

- Lecture: Dr Michael Antoniou : Sources & Mechanisms of health risks - GMO foods & glyphosate
    - https://www.youtube.com/watch?v=mckTJUXVbJM&feature=youtu.be

- Interview: Dr. Mercola Interviews Dr. Huber about GMOs
    - https://www.youtube.com/watch?v=yx4UVhJcnpo&feature=youtu.be

- Interview: The Health Dangers of Roundup (glyphosate) Herbicide. Jeffrey Smith & Stephanie Seneff
    - https://www.youtube.com/watch?v=h_AHLDXF5aw

2.16 COUNTRIES WITH MANDATORY LABELING OF GE FOODS[224]:

1. Australia
2. Austria
3. Belarus
4. Belgium
5. Bolivia
6. Bosnia and Herzegovina
7. Brazil
8. Bulgaria
9. Cameroon
10. China
11. Croatia
12. Cyprus
13. Czech Republic
14. Denmark
15. Ecuador
16. El Salvador
17. Estonia
18. Ethiopia
19. Finland
20. France
21. Germany
22. Greece
23. Hungary
24. Iceland
25. India
26. Indonesia
27. Ireland
28. Italy
29. Japan
30. Jordan
31. Kazakhstan
32. Kenya
33. Latvia
34. Lithuania
35. Luxembourg
36. Malaysia
37. Mali
38. Malta
39. Mauritius
40. Netherlands
41. New Zealand
42. Norway
43. Peru
44. Poland
45. Portugal
46. Romania
47. Russia
48. Saudi Arabia
49. Senegal
50. Slovakia
51. Slovenia
52. South Africa
53. South Korea
54. Spain
55. Sri Lanka
56. Sweden
57. Switzerland
58. Taiwan
59. Thailand
60. Tunisia
61. Turkey
62. Ukraine
63. United Kingdom
64. Vietnam

Chapter 3

CANCER
THE RACE FOR NO CURE

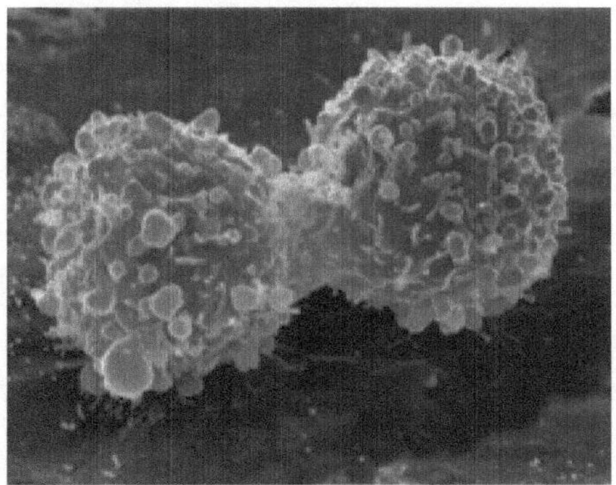

Image source: WikiMedia Commons

The person who takes medicine must recover twice, once from the disease and once from the medicine.

William Osler, MD was a Canadian physician and one of the four founding professors of Johns Hopkins Hospital.

The doctor of the future will give no medication, but will interest his patients in the care of the human frame, diet and in the cause and prevention of disease

Thomas Edison

I talked a lot about cancer in previous chapters, but in this chapter, I want to talk specifically about why cancer research has been going on for 250 years and why I believe that a true cancer cure, as opposed to life-long treatments, will never come from pharmaceutical cancer research organizations, and why cancer charities have no desire to find a cure. I will also discuss the many scientific studies that have been conducted for the past nearly 100 years that reveal what cancer is, what causes it, and the various natural substances that have been evaluated and have been shown to be extremely efficacious, despite the fact that the pharmaceutical and healthcare industries continue to deny that there are any effective alternatives to their current, approved "gold standard" therapies, which are themselves toxic, and have an abysmal success rate. Finally, I will talk about what the true heroes in the industry, many of which were blackballed, exiled, and even murdered, have to offer in the way of cancer treatments.

First off, I would like to say that as you read this chapter you might be thinking to yourself that it is not possible that there are so many effective and simple ways to eliminate cancer from your body. You might be saying that it is impossible that so many herbs, fruits and vegetables, and simple substances that are available for a few dollars in most grocery stores and supermarkets can have such a profound effect against cancer – that the public would have surely known about it by now. Let me offer you this thought in trying to make you understand why that is not only possible, but absolutely factual. Before the advent of ships, cars, and airplanes, people were largely confined to their little corner of the earth. They had no international commerce and no way of getting some special medicinal plant that only grows in some faraway corner of the globe. Differing regional climates meant and still means that certain plants grow in certain regions and certain other plants grow in other regions. Nature is smart though, and it thought it necessary to provide nutrition and healing to all people (and animals) regardless of where they are, so it placed those nutrients, enzymes, phytochemicals and so on in many plants, across most of the world. It also helps to think of cures or true medicine as nutrition, and as long as you are getting the proper nutrition, you are healthy. It goes a little bit deeper than that, but that's the basic gist of it. As I mentioned earlier in the book, the ancient Greek physician Hippocrates said, nearly two and a half millennia ago "Let food be thy medicine". The reason that this fact is not well known is due to the enormous power of corporations to shape and control public discourse, and to suppress knowledge that is seen as detrimental to their continued profits and dominance.

Cancer is very complicated and I don't want you to get the idea from reading this chapter that curing cancer is always simple, or that you can take one herb and your cancer will be gone. For many types of cancer, if you catch it at an early stage you can typically cure yourself on your own by cleaning up your diet and eliminating the likely cause (which might come from the food that you eat, environmental or workplace exposure to toxins, or possibly a toxic relationship or fears), and applying certain protocols that will target your specific type of cancer. Some types of cancer are more aggressive. For those types, and for more advanced stages of cancer it would be a good idea to find an alternative physician with experience in alternative cancer treatments to guide you and perhaps perform the necessary treatments. Since there are so many types of cancer, and each type responds to treatment differently, it would ideally be the job of an oncologist who has studied the different types and the corresponding natural, non-toxic treatment options. However, traditional oncologists generally know nothing about cancer beyond what pharmaceutical companies want them to know. They only know the approved modes of treatment (radiation, chemo, and surgery predominantly), and how to administer them, and even then, their success rates are abysmal, while at the same time they worsen the general health of the patient, which in most cases, ultimately leads to the patient's death.

Because of this, and because there are so many toxins in our foods, our water, and the air we breathe, and because so many of the devices we use on a daily basis, such as cell phones, microwave ovens, and other personal electronic devices, and even the electric meter found on the outside of your house, which emit electromagnetic radiation, damages our bodies on a cellular level, it is incumbent upon us to learn as much as we can about those causes, and about proper nutrition and the environment in which we live, and about the alternatives that we have at our disposal, if nothing else, so that if we are in a situation where we need medical help, that we know the right questions to ask.

The remedies discussed in this section are intended to be examples of several of many remedies that are known to be effective against cancer. Not all cancers respond to the same treatment, and treatments need to be multifaceted rather than taking a single herb for instance and expecting it to work. Cancer will try to evolve and spread, so it is critical for the assault to be from every direction and relentless. You must however do more research on your specific type of cancer and which combinations to use. Some combinations will work synergistically and some will not, or might even interfere with one another, so research the proper protocols and follow them.

There are many posts on social media about cancer cures, and although not all of them are right, there are many that are. I would recommend that when you come across a claim that a certain substance cures cancer, that you do some additional research to learn more about it. A good place to start is PubMed, which is a service of the U.S. National Library of Medicine, which provides free access to scientific publications.

There are more than 100 types of cancer, which might make you think that curing cancer is a losing battle, however, there are several common threads to all cancers, and knowing that means that there can be a common plan of attack. All cancers require an anaerobic (without air) or hypoxic (without oxygen) and by extension, an acidic environment to survive and thrive. Furthermore, all cancers get their energy from glucose (sugar), while healthy cells can thrive on a wider variety of energy sources, such as ketones, while cancer cannot. Thirdly, cancer cells are very wasteful in their metabolism of glucose and only use about 5% of the energy from the glucose, as compared to healthy cells[225]. There are other commonalities among all types of cancer, however, that does not mean that all cancers can be cured by one method or with one substance, because, for instance, there are certain substances that cannot cross the blood-brain barrier, and therefore might not work on brain cancers through oral administration or injection. The good news is that there are many natural substances, present in many foods and herbs that have fantastic cancer-killing properties. The other good news is that oxygen will penetrate all tissues of the body, including the brain, so blood oxygenation therapies of varying forms, in combination with other treatments will work against most, if not all types of cancer.

The cancer industry is worth hundreds of billions of dollars per year, and I would even argue that if you take other factors into account, such as illness caused by the fear mongering perpetuated by the cancer industry, and the propaganda campaigns (plastering everything in pink to appeal to consumers to drive up sales, etc., etc.), you will find that the true worth of the cancer industry is in the trillions of dollars per year.

> *"As a retired physician, I can honestly say that unless you are in a serious accident, your best chance of living to a ripe old age is to avoid doctors and hospitals and learn nutrition, herbal medicine and other forms of natural medicine. Almost all drugs are toxic and are designed only to treat symptoms and not to cure anyone. Most surgery is unnecessary. In short, our mainstream medical system is hopelessly inept and/or corrupt. The treatment of cancer and degenerative diseases is a national scandal. The sooner you learn this, the better off you will be."*
>
> Dr. Allan Greenberg, MD, 12/24/2002[226]

When you are a corporation, whether for-profit or not, money is a big driver. Don't get me wrong, there are genuine charities out there that seek out to do good, but usually the people at the top who run them are more interested in their big paychecks and bonuses. When you have a multimillion dollar salary and bonus package, the idea that one day, when you find what your organization is supposedly looking for, your job will come to an abrupt end, doesn't sound too good.

I would like to begin this chapter by discussing the cancer treatments sanctioned by the pharmaceutical industry, whom dictate the direction of medical treatment, and perhaps more importantly, dictate what treatment options doctors – especially in the U.S. and other world powers are forbidden from prescribing, or even discussing with their patients. In discussing the so-called "gold standard" treatments, I'll outline their effects on the body, and why those treatments are ineffective in curtailing cancer, and actually cause recurrences of the same cancer, as well as new, unrelated cancers, and other debilitating disorders.

3.1   THE BIG THREE

The main three allopathic methods of combating cancer are surgery, chemotherapy and radiation. To a lesser degree, hormone therapy, immunotherapy, targeted therapy, and bone marrow transplantation are also used, but are typically not the first choice provided by the treating physician.

Out of the three big modes of conventional treatment, chemotherapy is the most widely used, followed by radiation and then surgery.

Fig.1 gives an overall picture of "the big three", taken from data for treatments of all forms of cancers discussed in the American Cancer Society's 2012-2013 "Cancer Treatment & Survivorship Facts & Figures" report.[227]

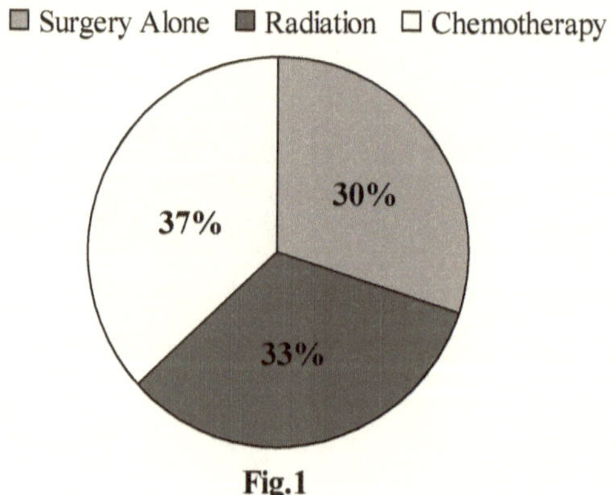

Fig.1

The birth of chemotherapy drugs came from a discovery resulting from a German bombing raid in Bari, Italy in December 1943. "German air raid in Bari, Italy led to the exposure of more than one thousand people to the SS John Harvey's secret cargo composed of mustard gas bombs. Dr. Stewart Francis Alexander, a Lieutenant Colonel who was an expert in chemical warfare, was subsequently deployed to investigate the aftermath. Autopsies of the victims suggested that profound lymphoid [a type of white blood cell associated with the adaptive immune system] and myeloid [a type of blood cell associated with the innate immune system] suppression had occurred after exposure. In his report Dr. Alexander theorized that since mustard gas all but ceased the division of certain types of somatic cells whose nature was to divide fast, it could also potentially be put to use in helping to suppress the division of certain types of cancerous cells."[228]

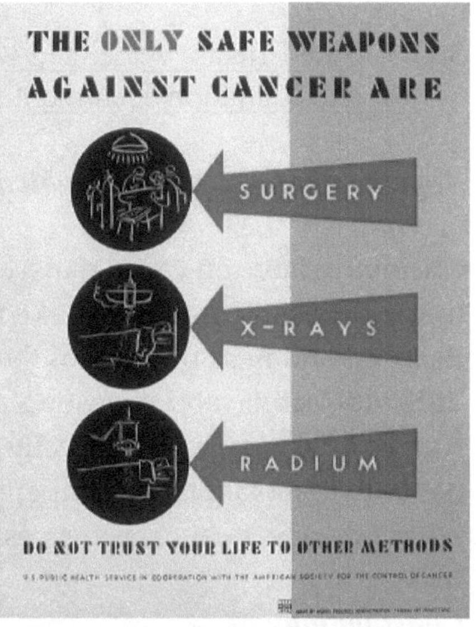

1938 poster by the United States Department of Health and Human Services, identifying surgery, x-rays and radium as the only treatments for cancer.
Image source: Wikimedia Commons

"Traditional chemotherapeutic agents are cytotoxic, that is to say they act by killing cells that divide rapidly – one of the main properties of most cancer cells. This means that chemotherapy also harms cells that divide rapidly under normal circumstances: cells in the bone marrow, digestive tract, and hair follicles. This results in the most common side-effects of chemotherapy: myelosuppression (decreased production of blood cells, hence also immunosuppression), mucositis (inflammation of the lining of the digestive tract), and alopecia (hair loss)."[229]

Radiation treatments likewise are harmful to soft tissue and causes a variety of deleterious effects. According to the

American Cancer Society report[227], the following are side effects of chemotherapy and radiation:

3.1.1 Side Effects Associated with Chemotherapy and Radiation Treatment

Appetite changes, eating problems, and weight loss

Chemotherapy can cause nausea, taste changes, or mouth and throat problems that may make it difficult to eat. Radiation to the head and neck or parts of the digestive system may lead to difficulty eating and digesting. Loss of appetite, as well as weight loss, may result directly from effects of the cancer on the body's metabolism. Appetite loss may also be related to other side effects, such as depression or fatigue.

Constipation

Some chemotherapy drugs and pain medications can cause constipation. Constipation may also result from changes in diet and/or activity level.

Diarrhea

Chemotherapy can cause diarrhea by affecting the cells lining the intestine. Radiation to the stomach, abdomen, or pelvis can also cause diarrhea. Diarrhea is usually defined as 2 or more loose stools in 4 hours.

Fatigue

Ranging from mild lethargy to feeling completely exhausted, fatigue is one of the most common side effects of cancer treatment. It is different from feeling tired after a long day and does not get better with rest or sleep. Fatigue tends to be the worst at the end of a treatment cycle.

Hair changes

Chemotherapy can cause hair loss (alopecia) on all parts of the body, not just the scalp, whereas hair loss resulting from radiation is limited to the specific area of treatment. Not all chemotherapy drugs cause hair loss. For most patients hair grows back after treatment, but it may be thinner or a different texture than it was before treatment. Some targeted therapies may cause facial hair to grow faster than usual, including longer, thicker eyelashes (don't get any ideas ladies…).

Immune suppression

Chemotherapy and radiation therapy can suppress or weaken the immune system by lowering the number of white blood cells (especially neutrophils) and other immune system cells or cause them not to work the way they should. A weakened immune system results in an increased risk of infection.

Infertility

For men, chemotherapy can reduce the number and quality of sperm, which may result in short- or long-term infertility. Chemotherapy can also cause infertility in women. Whether this happens and how long it lasts depends on many factors, including the type of drug, the doses given, and the age of the patient. Radiation to the pelvis can also affect fertility.

Memory and thinking problems

Chemotherapy and radiation to the brain can impact the cognitive (thinking) functions of the brain, including concentration, memory, comprehension, and reasoning. The changes that are found in patients are often very subtle.

Mouth, gum, and throat problems

Chemotherapy and radiation to the head and neck can cause sores in the mouth and throat. It can make these areas dry and irritated or cause them to bleed. This can interfere with the intake of food and even liquids, leading to malnutrition and dehydration. Mouth sores are not only painful, but there is also concern of infection that may spread to other parts of the body.

Nausea and vomiting

These symptoms may start during chemotherapy treatment and last a few hours. Less often, severe nausea and vomiting can last for a few days. Some people getting chemotherapy feel queasy even before treatment begins; this is called anticipatory nausea. Radiation to certain regions of the body can also cause nausea or vomiting.

Sexual problems

Chemotherapy and radiation to the pelvis can result in loss of libido, erectile dysfunction, and vaginal dryness and infections. Some sexual side effects of chemotherapy can remain after treatment.

Shortness of breath (dyspnea)

Radiation to the chest can cause shortness of breath. It may also occur as a result of chemotherapy-induced anemia.

Skin changes

Chemotherapy may cause minor skin problems, including color changes, redness, itching, peeling, dryness, rashes, and acne. When these symptoms occur on the palms of the hand and soles of the feet it is known as hand-foot syndrome. Some drugs may make skin more sensitive to the sun. Most chemotherapy-related skin problems go away, but a few require immediate attention. Certain drugs can cause long-term tissue damage if they leak out of an IV. Symptoms of an allergic reaction, including sudden or severe itching, rash, or hives, should be reported right away [note that there is no such thing as an allergic reaction to chemotherapy. Chemotherapy drugs are potent toxins, and a reaction to it is a reaction to toxicity, not allergenicity]. Radiation may make skin look red, irritated, swollen, blistered, sunburned, or tanned in treatment areas. After a few weeks, skin may become dry, flaky, itchy, or peel. Most skin reactions to radiation slowly go away after treatment; however, skin in the treatment area may remain darker than it was before.

Urine changes, bladder, and kidney problems

Some chemotherapy drugs can irritate the bladder or cause kidney damage. They may also cause the urine to change color (orange, red, green, or yellow) or have a strong or medicine-like odor. Radiation to the pelvis can also irritate the bladder and lead to painful or frequent urination.

3.1.2 <u>Side Effects Associated Primarily with Chemotherapy Treatment</u>

Anemia

A common side effect of chemotherapy, anemia is a condition where the body has too little hemoglobin contained in red blood cells to carry oxygen to the rest of the body. It can cause the following symptoms: fatigue, dizziness, paleness, a tendency to feel cold, shortness of breath, weakness, and racing heart.

Bleeding or clotting problems

Chemotherapy can affect the bone marrow's ability to make platelets that help stop bleeding. Patients without enough platelets may bleed or bruise more easily than usual, even from a minor injury. Some chemotherapy drugs also increase the risk of the formation of serious blood clots that form in the veins of the legs (deep vein thrombosis).

Nerve and muscle problems

Certain chemotherapy drugs can cause peripheral neuropathy, a potentially serious nerve problem that causes tingling, pins and needles, burning sensations, weakness, and/or numbness in the hands and feet. Some chemotherapy drugs can also cause short-term problems with the nerves in the throat, which can lead to pain with swallowing, especially food or liquids of extreme temperature.

Weight gain

Chemotherapy can cause some people to gain weight, which may be due to inactivity, electrolyte imbalances, fluid retention, or steroids contained in the drug regimen.

Through all this misery, the efficacy of the current allopathic methods of cancer treatment is abysmally insignificant, as demonstrated by Fig.2. It's noteworthy that the industry defines "cure" as 5-year survival. That is because a large number of cancer survivors do not live much past 5 years. That is because chemotherapy and radiation treatments themselves are toxic. Chemo and radiation are responsible for the premature deaths of millions of people every year. In their 2012-2013 "Cancer Treatment & Survivorship Facts & Figures" report, the American Cancer Society themselves admit to the fact that many survivors get "second primary cancers" due to "the carcinogenic effects of cancer treatment."[227] In what way does it make sense to treat cancer with methods that cause cancer?

552   CLINICAL ONCOLOGY

Table 2 — Impact of cytotoxic chemotherapy on 5-year survival in American adults

Malignancy	ICD-9	Number of cancers in people aged >20 years*	Absolute number of 5-year survivors due to chemotherapy†	Percentage 5-year survivors due to chemotherapy‡
Head and neck	140–149, 160, 161	5139	97	1.9
Oesophagus	150	1521	82	4.9
Stomach	151	3001	20	0.7
Colon	153	13 936	146	1.0
Rectum	154	5533	189	3.4
Pancreas	157	3567	–	–
Lung	162	20 741	410	2.0
Soft tissue sarcoma	171	858	–	–
Melanoma	172	8646	–	–
Breast	174	31 133	446	1.4
Uterus	179–182	4611	–	–
Cervix	180	1825	219	12
Ovary	183	3032	269	8.9
Prostate	185	23 242	–	–
Testis	186	989	373	37.7
Bladder	188	6667	–	–
Kidney	189	3722	–	–
Brain	191	1824	68	3.7
Unknown primary site	195–199	6200	–	–
Non-Hodgkin's lymphoma	200 + 202	6217	653	10.5
Hodgkin's disease	201	846	341	40.3
Multiple myeloma	203	1721	–	–
Total		154 971	3306	2.1%

*Numbers from Ref. [22].
†Absolute numbers (see text).
‡% for individual malignancy.

Fig. 2 [230]

"After treatment is completed, cancer survivors are at risk for a wide range of ongoing symptoms that are often referred to as long-term and late effects. Specifically, long-term effects are those symptoms that arise during treatment and remain problematic, while late effects tend to have a later onset, typically surfacing months or even years after cancer treatment has ended. Long-term and late effects may be emotional (e.g., anxiety, depression) and/or physical (e.g., heart, lung and kidney damage, mental impairment, and infertility). Cancer survivors are also at risk for recurrence of the original cancer or the development of a new, biologically distinct, second primary cancer"[227].

An earlier meta-analysis of 1,178 patients evaluated the effectiveness of two chemotherapeutic drugs against metastatic colorectal cancer[231]. The data revealed that when the chemotherapeutic drug fluorouracil (the first-choice chemotherapy drug for colorectal cancer) was used alone, the curative rate was only 2%. When combined with a second chemotherapeutic drug - methotrexate, the curative rate increased to 3%. Placebos have a better cure rate than that, yet these drugs are FDA approved and used extensively.

Other major long-term and late effects cancer survivors may experience as a result of the toxic therapies include: chronic pain as a result of nerve cell damage, cognitive problems such as problems with attention, concentration, memory, and delayed thought process, damage to the heart that may be permanent, decreased bone density (osteoporosis) and thinning of the bone mass (osteopenia), and decreased lung function, not only from surgical resection, but from progressive damage caused by chemotherapy and radiation.

Additional effects include fatigue, infertility, lymphedema (swelling of the arms and legs), sexual problems, and fear of cancer recurrence. It's interesting to note that people who cure themselves using natural treatments, either on their own or with the assistance of a naturopath generally do not have a fear of recurrence, and certainly do not have any negative side-effects. Quite opposite - they gain quite a bit of knowledge into proper nutrition and natural healing methodologies so that they generally lead much healthier lives after their treatment than they had beforehand.

Any reasonable person who reads this long list of horrendous side-effects caused by those allopathic treatments should ask him or herself why the industry would be so feverishly pushing for those types of treatments. You should know that it's not for lack of safe, effective and side-effects-free alternatives, as you will discover from reading the remainder of this chapter, but rather, it's because the alternatives are often inexpensive and highly effective, whereas surgery, chemo and radiation are extremely expensive and keep you coming back for more.

When their treatments inevitably fail, the National Coalition for Cancer Survivorship will give you a lecture about "Dying Well – The Final Stage of Survivorship"[232]. Apparently, dying well means being pumped full of palliative drugs, and making peace with dying. The following are their recommendations:

- Communicate with the members of your cancer care team, as well as family, friends, employers, and coworkers
- Manage hopes and expectations
- Deal with any anxiety or depression that may arise
- Make decisions about symptom management (including controlling pain) and continuing or stopping treatment
- Recognize what is happening during the dying process
- Make informed decisions about hospice/palliative care
- Manage grief

Absolutely despicable. There is nothing wrong with making peace with dying, but taking people's hope away, and squeezing every last cent out of them before their death is unconscionable.

3.2 WHAT IS CANCER AND WHAT CAUSES IT?

Cancer is merely a symptom of a much broader, systemic problem. As with everything else, the pharmaceutical industry aims to treat the symptom rather than eliminate the underlying problem because it is much more profitable – to the tune of over \$1 trillion in worldwide revenues[233]. It is impossible to truly cure cancer by only attacking the cancer. Likewise, it is impossible to prevent cancer through genetic interventions or vaccinations, because cancer is a systemic problem that arises from years of abuse. Even if scientists are able to prevent cancer from manifesting in a particular way, it will simply manifest itself in a different, and potentially worse way.

When I talk about abuse, it does not necessarily have to begin with you – the abuse could have started with your parents or even your grandparents, which led to your physiology being what it is at present time. You might have been born with gastroschisis, cleft palate, congenital heart disease, or another disorder. The medical industry claim that some of those are genetic defects that are passed down, but in actuality, they are epigenetic (environmentally mediated) phenomenon which are caused by your parents' poor eating habits, drinking habits, smoking habits, mental habits or even the environment that they live in, as through exposure to environmental toxins such as pesticides and industrial pollutants, or physical, verbal, and/or mental abuse, stress, and other influencers which induce negative emotional effects. Not to say that you are a victim of your physiology... There are still things you can do to live healthfully and prevent cancer from occurring. I'll expand on these points further in a bit.

Chemotherapy and radiation, besides being toxic and carcinogenic themselves, only kill mature cancer cells, but leave cancer progenitor cells (cancer stem cells) intact[234,235,236]. This ensures; especially with the immune system destroyed by the chemotherapy and/or radiation that the cancer will return if no other natural interventions are undertaken. To make things worse, the cancer progenitor cells develop resistance to those treatments, so when the cancer does return, it returns much more aggressively.

Surgery likewise, only removes the tumor and not the cancer progenitor cells. Surgery alone can often do more harm than good because while in the instance that a tumor is localized and perhaps easier to target, once it is incised, cancer cells are released into the bloodstream and induce metastasis. Don't get me wrong – sometimes surgery is necessary, such as when a tumor is pressing on an artery or organ and causes an immediate, life-threatening condition or severe pain, but tumors can and have been eliminated using natural methods that have no side effects or long-lasting damage to the immune system. Chemotherapy and radiation on the other hand is never necessary, under any condition. At the very least, chemo and radiation should be the absolute last resort. Interestingly enough, the pharmaceutical and cancer research industry are aware of most, if not all of the alternative treatments that are claimed by other physicians and researchers, and have done their own tests which confirm their efficacy in treating and eliminating cancer, but they will not let the public know, and they will not abandon their "cash cow".

So, going back to the statement I made before – cancer is merely a symptom of a much broader problem. To eradicate the cancer therefore, it is necessary to get to the root of the problem and address it. Once the root problem is addressed, the body will take care of the cancer on its own.

Nature is fantastically designed, and under normal circumstances, nature can defend against many assaults. The problem arises when we force substances and energies into our biology that do not belong there. Just as you wouldn't put sand in your car's gas tank, many substances that are present in our modern day "food", radiation from wireless devices or high voltage overhead power lines, toxic air and water pollutants and additives such as chlorine and fluoride, do not belong in our bodies and do great harm by direct assault on organs and tissues or by attacking or fooling our body's natural defense systems. Likewise, to continue with the car analogy, you wouldn't rev your engine past the red line, because doing so would overstress your engine and cause it to fail. Along the same line, overstressing the body over an extended period of time will cause its systems to fail, leading to diseases and disorders, and even death.

Cancer cells are cells that through a mutation have lost the natural ability to commit suicide – a process called apoptosis. Cells constantly multiply (mitosis) and so old cells need to die. Apoptosis is the mechanism that tells cells when to die. All healthy cells have this apoptotic mechanism, but in cancer cells it has been disabled. Cancer cells also multiply, but since they have effectively become immortal, the result is uncontrolled growth which in many cases lead to tumors.

Macrophages are part of the innate immune system and are effectively scavengers within our bodies. In addition to gobbling up cellular debris and dead cells, they are also the first line of defense against bacteria and viruses. Once a macrophage envelopes a bacteria or virus, it releases a protein from its surface which alerts the acquired immune system to the presence of

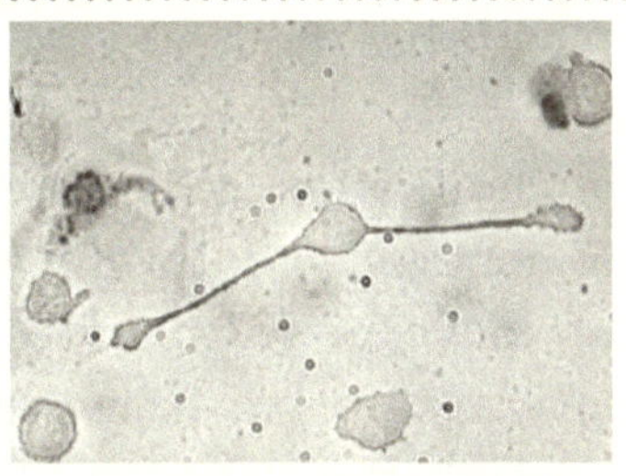

Image Source: Wikipedia
Macrophage of a mouse
spreads its "arms" to engulf
two particles

the invader. The acquired immune system then takes over and sets out to eliminate those invaders.

Cancer cells downregulate MHC class I molecules which effectively makes them invisible to macrophages and the immune system.

So what causes cancer and how can we cure and prevent it? In truth, there are many, many causes of cancer. It is impossible to list all of the things that cause cancer, but it can be said that anything that causes an imbalance, a disorder, or a dysfunction in cellular activity, or prevents it from carrying out its functions, could potentially lead to cancer. Once you realize this, the next question should be, what promotes health? That question is a little bit easier to answer, but not so simple to fully put into practice. The answer is, everything that the cells require to carry out their functions, in the quantities, forms and combinations that are needed, and at the time that they are needed, will bring about health. Everything else is unnecessary and undesirable for a healthy body. There are two problems with that... 1) as consumers, we don't know everything that is in our foods, even if we read labels, and 2) no one on earth can answer the question of what are all the things that cells need, at any moment in time, throughout the seasons, in all geographical locations, and at what quantities and in which combinations, and on top of that, which foods provide those nutrients and none or little of those that do not promote health.

For clarification, cells respond to signals (vitamins, minerals, hormones, etc.) in their environment in one of three ways - 1) they move towards the "signal" in order to assimilate it, 2) they move away from it and shut themselves down in order to protect themselves from a toxic "signal", or 3) they do not react to it at all.

So let's simplify things a bit... What *can* science tell us, and what can history teach us?

You sort of have to get yourself in the mindset of what is natural and what is not. If it is not natural, it will cause disease and disorder in the body. Not to say that there aren't natural toxins - there are many…

Additionally, there are certain foods that we have been told are healthy for us, but in reality, are not. For instance, soy is being pushed as a health food, but soy is very high in phytoestrogens, which "have the ability to cause estrogenic or/and antiestrogenic effects, by sitting in and blocking receptor sites against estrogen"[237], or breakfast cereals which are supposedly "a part of a balanced breakfast", but are full with sugars, artificial flavors, dies, and other industrial chemicals such as bleach and glyphosate[238].

Additionally, processing certain foods in certain ways, such as heating may lead to toxic effects. For example, oils containing polyunsaturated fats produce a toxic chemical called lipid peroxide when heated to high temperatures.[239]   Lipid peroxide toxicity can lead to cell membrane damage, damage and mutations to DNA as well as cause the formation of cancer (oncogenesis).[240]

Many years back, people knew how to eat and what to eat, and what foods to combine with other foods and what not to. This information has for the most part been lost, other than in certain pockets of indigenous populations. Fortunately, there is an effort under way to preserve a lot of that information.

For example, "The [Matsés Traditional Medicine Encyclopedia] "marks the first time shamans of an Amazonian tribe have created a full and complete transcription of their medicinal knowledge written in their own language and words". This 500-page encyclopedia "compiled by five shamans with assistance from conservation group Acaté, details every plant used by Matsés medicine to cure a massive variety of ailments."[241]

So let's talk about some specifics:

3.2.1   <u>A Historical Approach</u>

We can look back at what our ancestors ate and what diseases they developed, which will give us an idea of which foods are compatible with our genome and which are not. One such example is dairy products. Most of the world's population are actually lactose intolerant. Only about 35% of the world's population have a Lactase Persistence mutation that keeps the lactase gene turned on past the age of 7 to 8.

"During the most recent ice age, milk was essentially a toxin to adults because — unlike children — they could not produce the lactase enzyme required to break down lactose, the main sugar in milk ... around 11,000 years ago, cattle herders learned how to reduce lactose in dairy products to tolerable levels by fermenting milk to make cheese or yogurt. Several thousand years later, a genetic mutation spread through

Europe that gave people the ability to produce lactase — and drink milk — throughout their lives."[242]

Lactose intolerance might not present itself with immediate, severe symptoms, but rather, might cause long-term, chronic inflammation that will manifest itself years down the road as other diseases.   Regardless of lactose, animal proteins, including those from milk, have been linked to every chronic disease known to man, including type 1 diabetes in children, so consuming milk is not advisable. Milk is also acidifying to the body, which brings me to the next point:

3.2.2   Acidity, Alkalinity, and Blood Oxygen

If you are a gardener or a farmer, you know that each type of plant in your garden or farm has its unique biological needs. Some plants need more sun, some need less sun. Some require an acidic soil at a certain range, and some require a more alkaline soil. If you expose a plant to an environment that it was not designed for, the plant will be stressed, develop disease, and possibly die. Every living organism on the face of the earth works in this way.

The colorful hot springs in Yellowstone are a great example. Each band of color in these rainbow-colored pools is a different temperature range. The water in the center is the hottest, and as it gets farther away from the center and closer to the shoreline, the water cools down more and more. The different colors in those pools are caused by different microbes which are uniquely adapted to living within each temperature range. Each of those microbe colonies could not survive in the other rings, because the environment in the other rings would not serve their specific biological niche.

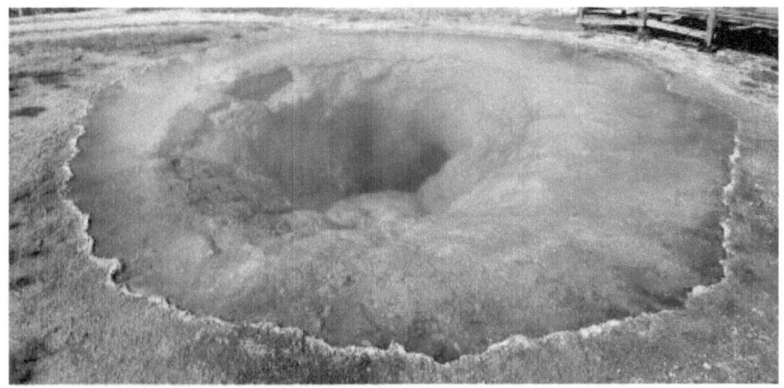

Morning Glory Pool, Yellowstone National Park

Likewise, as humans, we have an ideal pH that our bodies require (about 7.4 for blood) and any drastic departure from this pH is detrimental to our health. A pH of 7 is neutral. Anything above 7 is alkaline and anything below 7 is acidic. With all of the acidifying substances in western diets, it is very common for people to be too acidic. Over acidity in the body causes a reduction in blood oxygen, depletion of good bacteria, proliferation of harmful bacteria, such as Candida, and leads to almost every disease and disorder known to man, including cancer. As a matter of fact, most medications are acidifying to the body and only serve to perpetuate our diseased state. Of course, not all of the parts of our body require the same pH; for instance, the mouth and the stomach need to be acidic in order to break down food, while food is present. Blood pH on the other hand must remain at a fairly constant 7.4 ± 0.5. Urine pH will vary throughout the day, and from day to day with what you eat and drink, but urine pH, when measured on a regular basis is a good indication of your overall pH health. If your urine is alkaline more often than it is acidic (again, at around 7.4), then you are doing well, but if it is below 7 for long stretches of time, you might want to change your eating habits.

I mentioned blood oxygen above – it's interesting to note that cancer cannot propagate or survive in the presence of high levels of oxygen, so for cancer to start, blood oxygen needs to be low, and once a tumor forms, the tumor creates its own acidic microenvironment to ensure the displacement of oxygen and its continued survival and proliferation.

In 1931 Dr. Otto Heinrich Warburg was awarded The Noble Prize in Physiology or Medicine[243] for his discovery that cancer is caused by a lack of oxygen at the cellular level and proving that cancer thrives on anaerobic (without oxygen) or acidic conditions. It is interesting that nearly 100 years have passed since this discovery and yet doctors dismiss pH levels, and pharmaceutical companies have no interest in harnessing this knowledge.

In his 1925 paper on "The Metabolism of Carcinoma Cells"[244], Otto Warburg concluded the following:

"During our work we repeatedly asked ourselves what can the causative factors be, and just as often has the idea obtruded itself that the causative factor in the origin of tumors is nothing other than oxygen deficiency." Of course, scientific knowledge evolves over the years, and with new discoveries. However, these facts are as true today as the day that Dr. Warburg discovered them, yet the direction of the pharmaceutical and food industries have not improved, and have even become much worse.

Over-acidity leads to a reduction of blood oxygenation as explained by the Bohr Effect (see Fig. 3).

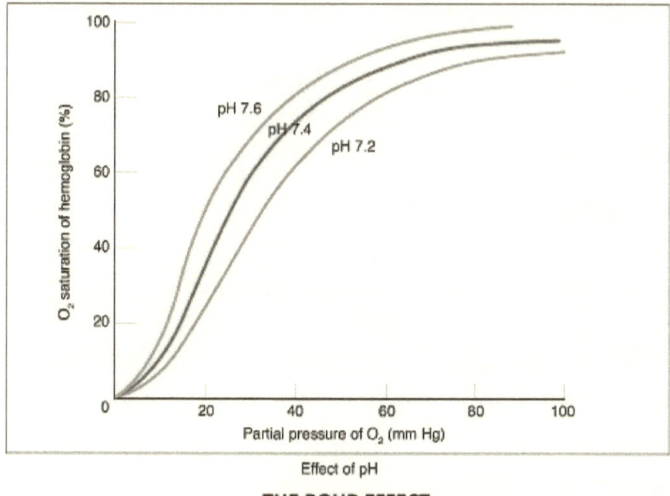

THE BOHR EFFECT

Fig. 3

Of course, acidity and lack of oxygen is not a root cause, but a symptom or effect of a broader problem.

The following is a list of some alkalizing foods. Note that the food's initial pH is not necessarily an indication of its acidifying or alkalizing effect in the body. For example, citrus may be acidic, but the metabolism of the citric acid contained within citrus fruits has an alkalizing effect on the body.

Vegetables:

Beets, Broccoli, Cauliflower, Celery, Cucumber, Kale, Lettuce, Onions, Peas, Peppers, Spinach

Fruits:

Apple, Banana, Berries, Cantaloupe, Grapes, Melon, Lemon, Orange, Peach, Pear, Watermelon

Seeds and Nuts:

Chestnuts, Coconut, Macadamia Nuts, Pine Nuts, Pumpkin Seeds

Spices:

Cinnamon, Curry, Ginger, Mustard

The USDA developed the PRAL formula to calculate the acidifying / alkalizing effects of the foods you eat based on the amounts of Magnesium, Phosphorus, Protein, Calcium, and Potassium they contain.

The PRAL formula is as follows:

value per 100g serving =   0.49 x (g) protein +
0.037 x (mg) phosphorus -
0.021 x (mg) potassium -
0.026 x (mg) magnesium -
0.013 x (mg) calcium

Interpreting the results:
A negative number indicates an alkalizing effect whereas a positive number indicates an acidifying effect. The lower the number the more alkalizing and the higher the number the more acidifying.

You can obtain nutritional data for various foods from www.nutritiondata.com.

3.2.3   DNA Damage and the Immune System

In addition to acidity and lack of oxygen, there are many substances that cause our immune system to be suppressed (immunosuppressants) and cause genetic damage (genotoxins) and mutations (mutagens).

With regards to the immune system, keep in mind that there are cancer cells and cancer progenitor cells floating around everyone's bodies at all times, but when we are healthy, our immune system keeps them in check. Same with Candida and other harmful fungi and bacteria, or collectively: opportunistic organisms. They are called opportunistic organisms because, given the opportunity, they will take over.

Manifestations of mutagenic and genotoxic substances are not so easily detectable in the population, because they typically take a long time to cause a significant effect. I've heard people tell me "I've been eating this my entire life and I haven't grown a second head yet". While they may be right in that extreme example, they may not realize that certain ailments that they've carried with them for many years, or increased susceptibility for developing cancer due to adverse mutations of genes, or development of allergies are directly cause by those substances. For example, glyphosate, a popular herbicide has been shown to negatively affect Cytochrome P450 enzymes[127], which are abundant in the liver, thereby greatly reducing the liver's ability to eliminate toxins. By doing so, every day substances which would not normally cause an allergic or toxic reaction due to the liver's ability to detoxify them, now would be rendered more toxic.

Additionally, if you pass your genes along to your children, they may be born with genetic abnormalities, and even physical deformities or birth defects such as anencephaly, cleft palate and gastroschisis to name just a few.

There was a study done recently of poor and low-income whites, blacks and Hispanics where it was discovered that there was significant genetic damage and mutations occurring in those groups in comparison with the general population. The authors of the study did not consider food intake or environmental toxins as a cause, but if you look at the results and varying levels of genetic damage, it is easily correlated with the types of diets that those particular groups consume. For example, it was shown that first generation Mexican immigrants had less genetic damage than Mexican descendants who were born in the United States and less genetic damage than white and black populations of the same economic class. If you consider that Mexican immigrants tend to eat more home-cooked meals and more vegetables, grains and legumes than low income whites and blacks, and low-income whites, blacks, and integrated Mexicans tend to eat more fast food and junk food, it is no surprise that the study's results were what they were.

Another review of the scientific literature summates that immigrants to the U.S. are healthier than U.S. born individual, and the longer those immigrants live in the U.S., the more their health deteriorates[245].

The presence of toxins in foods is ubiquitous. The so-called advancement in modern food science in the past 100 or so years is more of a significant step backwards in nutrition and promotion of health. Food and health scientists like to point out that advancements in vaccines, medicine and nutrition has led to an increased life expectancy, but in reality, people are living longer mostly due to personal hygiene and cleanliness practices in the medical field (washing of hands, sterilization of surfaces and instruments, etc.) particularly in delivery room settings, as well as in the home, and due to antibiotics, which unfortunately have been overused to the point where nearly all antibiotics today are ineffective.

Aspartame, sucralose, acesulfame potassium, saccharin, propylene glycol, etc. are all artificial sweeteners that are nothing more than a combination of toxic chemicals that cause anything from suppression of the immune system to cancer.

Potassium sorbate, sodium benzoate, Calcium Sorbate, Butylated Hydroxytoluene (BHT), etc. are food preservatives which are known to cause suppression of the immune system, gene mutations and damage, gene toxicity, endocrine (hormone) disruption and cancer. [246-252]

Red 2, Red 3, Red 40, Yellow 5, Yellow 6, Blue 1, Citrus Red 2 and Orange B are all food colorings that have been shown to cause cancer, hypersensitivity reactions, and genotoxicity[253].

Many of these substances, when combined with other substances common in the diet, such as sodium benzoate in combination with ascorbic acid (vitamin C) cause the formation of other toxic compounds (benzene in this example)[254], which is genotoxic, mutagenic, clastogenic and carcinogenic.

Nearly all processed foods, organic or otherwise, but especially non-organic, contain many of those additives, and some, as with the example of the "water enhancer" I've given earlier in the book are comprised of almost nothing but artificial chemicals. As a matter of fact, if they didn't need to add water to liquefy and thin out their concoction, it would be exclusively artificial chemicals.

This truly highlights the importance of reading labels and being selective in what you purchase and what you put in and on your body. Keep in mind that cosmetics, lotions, sunscreens and other products you put on your body contain many chemicals that can and do get absorbed through the skin and cause cancer, endocrine disruption and other conditions. Many deodorants for example contain aluminum, which is a neurotoxin. In today's age, where almost everyone carries a smart phone with internet connection, it is easier than ever to research things that you don't know, so if you see a chemical name on the label that you do not recognize or know what it is, Google it.

Keep in mind that if you see, especially on Wikipedia, information that states that there is no evidence of carcinogenicity or no evidence that a certain natural substance or treatment is effective against cancer, that in many cases those entries are made by industry shills, and I have personally found dozens of instances where those Wikipedia statements were explicitly false and contradicted by hundreds of published scientific studies. If you want to get a better idea, search the scientific literature on sites such as PubMed - which is a service of the U.S. National Library of Medicine - or others, and make sure that the authors of the study do not have conflicts of interest. Also keep in mind that if you see a statement that says "Generally Recognized as Safe" or "GRAS" – this is an FDA designation and it means absolutely nothing. Look at what independent research scientists have to say about it. The FDA gets its revenue from industry, and it is also run by a revolving door of industry executives. The FDA and CDC have had a long history of suppression of information when it comes to public safety, as is becoming more and more evident in recent days with several whistleblowers coming out[255], as well as with cases going back decades, which are now in the public domain. The FDA also does not test anything. As part of the certification and consultation programs, they require the manufacturer of the additive, drug, chemical, etc. to do their own testing, and most times the reports that come out of those tests are highly biased and doctored.

Let's consider for a moment that nature is not a fool. Everything in nature has a purpose and nature has a mechanism to address every deviation from a balanced state. Again, looking at the case of GMOs and overuse of herbicides, insecticides, and in general, monoculture. Nature loves diversity, so when a farmer grows acres upon acres of a single crop, nature says – that doesn't feel right... I'm going to send pests to get rid of this crop, because it's taking over... On the other hand, when you have a variety of different plants growing together or side by side, insects don't get numerous enough to cause a problem for any particular plant species. But it's easier to grow and cultivate just one crops, so humans, thinking they're smart, poison the insects with insecticides, and poison the weeds with herbicide. But nature is smarter – it develops resistance to those chemicals and just keeps on pushing towards diversity and balance.

Humans, as much as some would like to think that we are above nature, are part of nature, and as such, nature has a plan for us as well. So when we get sick because we deviate from the plan, nature has the mechanisms to heal us. This is the case with a simple cold, as well as stage 4 cancer.

If you are like me and you pay attention to developments in alternative medicine and research being conducted on natural substances, you may think to yourself that it sounds a bit odd that so many plants have anti-cancer properties, especially with the cancer industry claiming that there are no known cancer cures besides chemo, radiation and surgery (neither of which is a cure). But remember, nature had a plan well before humans were around, and nature had a plan well before boats and airplanes allowed humans to have global trade of foodstuffs, so nature decided that it would be a good idea to put those anti-carcinogenic (and other health promoting) substances into many plants; different plants that grow in every corner of the earth. That way, all humans and animals would have access to those substances. When looking at it from this perspective, it is no surprise that everywhere you look there are anti-cancer, anti-inflammatory, anti-oxidant, health promoting, disease-fighting substances. You just have to use them as nature intended – in a whole food, plant-based diet.

3.3   NATURAL CANCER CURES

Like humans, animals in nature also get sick from time to time, and with so much pollution of soils, air and water, animals get cancer as well. It has been observed and documented on many occasions that when animals get sick, or even when they get cancer, they intuitively find a particular herb, bush or tree, which they either consume or rub themselves on. Shortly thereafter, their cancer, or disease, goes away.

So let's look at some of those plants and their benefits:

3.3.1   <u>Coriolus Versicolor</u>

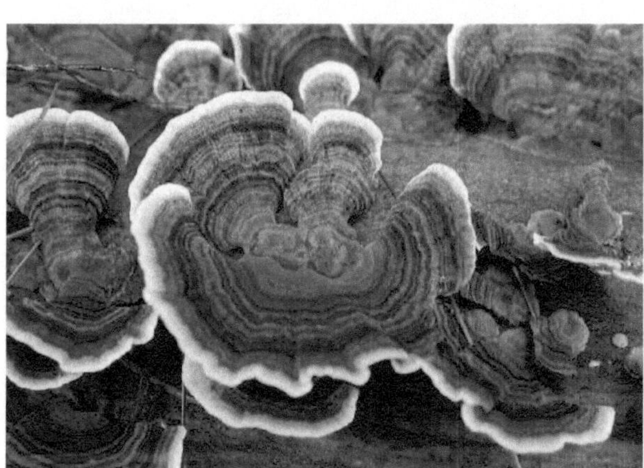

Coriolus Versicolor (Turkey Tail Mushroom): Picture source: WikiVisually

Coriolus Versicolor is a mushroom, also known as Turkey Tail mushroom for its bands of color resembling a turkey's tail. It is found around the world and has been used in Chinese and Japanese medicine, mainly to treat cancer. It has been shown in lab tests and clinical trials to be very effective at curing several types of cancer, and preventing cancer from recurring[256-259]. Unfortunately, the influence of the pharmaceutical industry is so great that even when such findings are reported, there is still an insistence on using chemotherapy, radiation and other toxic treatments, and only using the natural options as adjuvant treatments to reduce the symptoms from the main course of treatment, and to keep the cancer from returning. In this way, they can credit the success of the treatment with the chemo, etc. and continue to greatly benefit from its use.

Some studies show that hot water extract of Coriolus Versicolor cause an increase in large intestinal tumors. This may be due to chemical changes mediated by the hot water extraction process, as it is known that certain beneficial substances undergo chemical changes when heated which renders them toxic, such as pasteurization or roasting of almonds and other nuts, which creates harmful levels of Acrylamide – a known human carcinogen. Other extraction methods using solvents produce larger yields, but often they tend to degrade the quality of the extract, and in some cases residues of the solvents can be harmful. Cold, solvent-free extraction methods are always preferred, and of course, whole-plant forms are ideal.

3.3.2   <u>Reishi Mushroom</u>

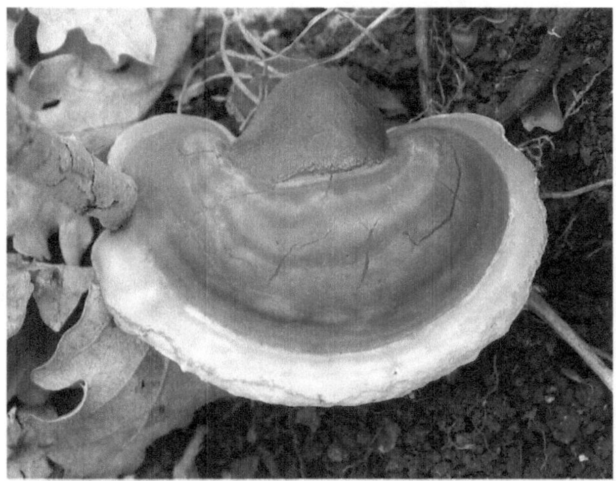

Ganoderma lucidum: Picture source: Wikimedia Commons

Reishi mushroom, also known as lingzhi mushroom is a mushroom of the genus Ganoderma. Like Coriolus Versicolor, Reishi mushrooms have been used extensively in Asian medicine for the treatment of cancer. In vitro and in vivo tests have been demonstrating the mushroom's tremendous effects against various cancer types[260,261,262].

3.3.3 <u>Moringa Oleifera</u>

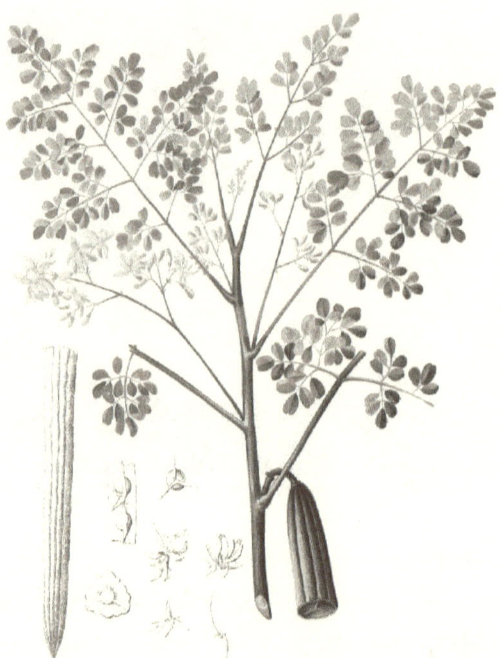

Moringa Oleifera: Picture source: Wikimedia Commons

Moringa Oleifera, also known as drumstick tree, horseradish tree, ben oil tree, or benzoil tree "is a fast-growing, drought-resistant tree, native to the southern foothills of the Himalayas in northwestern India, and widely cultivated in tropical and subtropical areas where its young seed pods and leaves are used as vegetables. It can also be used for water purification and hand washing, and is sometimes used in herbal medicine."[263] Nearly all parts of this tree can be consumed, and it is one of the most widely studied plants for its immense nutritional value, and its wide array of medicinal uses, including treatment of cancer. It has been shown in many studies to cause cancer cell death lin breast cancer[264,265,266], colorectal cancers[264,265,267], hepatocellular carcinoma/liver cancer[265,267,268], lymphoma[269], leukemia[270], lung cancer[266], adenocarcinoma[266],   epidermoid   carcinoma[266], fibrosarcoma[266], multiple myeloma[271], neuroblastoma[272], and many other cancers, while leaving normal, healthy cells untouched. Additional benefits of Moringa Oleifera include antimicrobial, anti-inflammatory, antidiabetic, and antioxidant effects.

In a 2014 mini-review of scientific studies performed on moringa[273], the authors found that the list of health benefits offered by the use of moringa is extensive, and includes the effective non-toxic treatment of cancer, along with its chemopreventive (cancer-preventing), protective effect against toxic chemicals, as well as protective effects against liver fibrosis and other hepatocellular damage. Moringa also induces a reduction in medication and disease-induced gastric ulcers. It possesses anti-inflammatory, anti-hyperlipidemia, and anti-hyperglycemia properties (hyperglycemia - high blood sugar, is associated with diabetes). It was also found to have anti-bacterial, anti-microbial, anti-tumor, anti-oxidative, and anti-clastogenic properties. Moringa has also been shown to promote the proliferation of beneficial liver enzymes, such as cytochrome b5 and cytochrome P450 (which was discussed in the chapter on GMOs and pesticides), which are responsible for detoxifying the body of cancer and disease-causing toxic chemicals. It also reduces free-radical formation.

Other reviews of the scientific literature reached the same conclusions[274,275].

3.3.4 <u>Ginger, Turmeric, Galangal & Cardamom</u>

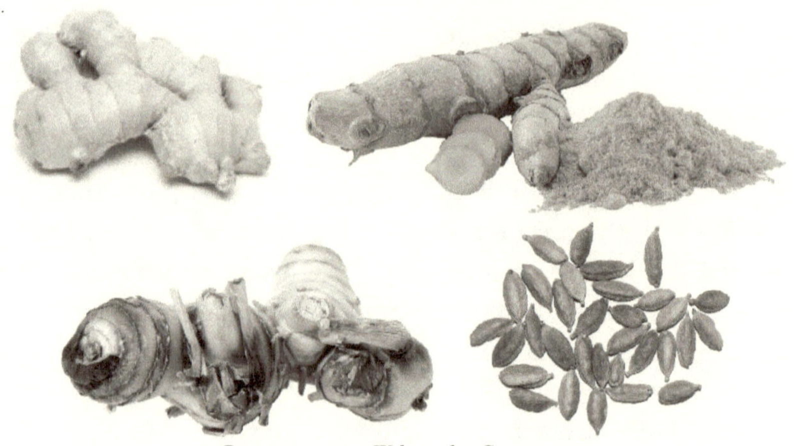

Picture source: Wikimedia Commons

Ginger, turmeric, galangal, and cardamom all belong to the zingiberaceae family. Ginger, turmeric, and galangal are rhizomes (creeping rootstalks), and cardamom is a seed. All four have been used for thousands of years as spices, as well as for medicinal purposes. Ginger has anti-inflammatory, antioxidant and antiproliferative activities[276]. It has also been shown in countless medical studies to prevent nausea, dizziness, and vomiting, and stimulate digestion[277] and is used for that purpose in allopathic medicine, as well as in traditional medicine. Many studies have demonstrated ginger's anti-cancer activity in combating prostate cancer[277], ovarian cancer[278], liver cancer[279], cervical cancer[280], pancreatic cancer[281], and many others, while being non-toxic to healthy cells. Ginger has also been demonstrated to have anti-angiogenic properties, which is "useful in the treatment of tumors and other angiogenesis-dependent diseases"[282]. Angiogenesis is the formation of new blood vessels from existing ones. Angiogenesis in tumors go into overdrive due to the tumor's inefficient energy metabolism, which means that tumors require more blood than normal tissue. Cutting off the ability of a tumor to create more blood vessels prevents it from growing.

Ginger has also been shown to have radioprotective effects. In a 2016 study[283], ginger essential oil extract (GEO) was shown to protect against the effects of whole body gamma-irradiation. Doses of "100 and 500 mg/kg [body weight] (orally) significantly ameliorated decreased hematological and immunological parameters. Radiation induced reduction in intestinal tissue antioxidant enzyme levels such as superoxide dismutase, catalase, glutathione peroxidase and glutathione was also reversed following administration of GEO. Tissue architecture of small intestine which was damaged following irradiation was improved upon administration of GEO". Additionally, "GEO significantly decreased the formation of micronuclei, increased the P/N ratio, inhibited the formation of chromosomal aberrations and protected against cellular DNA damage in bone marrow cells." In other words, ginger not only protected against radiation, but also repaired tissue, chromosomal, and DNA damage caused by radiation when administered after exposure. Ginger has been shown to be safe when taken at very high doses. Turmeric (Curcumin), galangal and cardamom likewise have shown great efficacy against many forms of cancer, against inflammation, as well as at generally promoting good health[284,285,286].

3.3.5   <u>Graviola (left) & Paw Paw (right)</u>

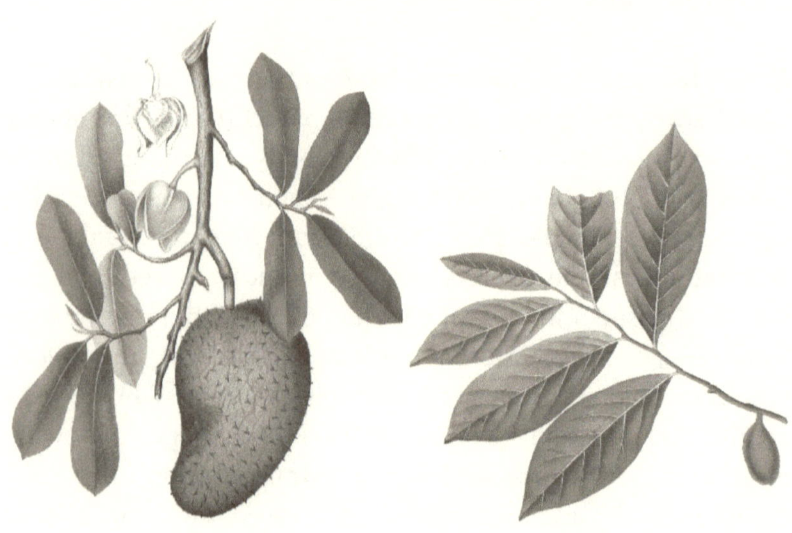

Picture source: Wikipedia

Graviola (Annona Muricata) and Paw Paw (Asimina triloba) are both from the same plant family - Annonaceae. Both have an extensive list of health benefits, and both have been shown in studies to have highly effective anti-cancer/anti-tumor properties. They were shown to be effective against multidrug resistant mammary adenocarcinoma[287,288], pancreatic cancer[289,290], breast cancer[291,292,293], leukemia[294,295,296], prostate cancer[297,298,299], lung cancer[300], colon cancer[301], liver cancer[302], skin cancer[303], and ovarian cancer[296]. Paw Paw has been shown to cause neurotoxicity and liver toxicity with prolonged exposure, so it is not recommended as a cancer preventive measure, or for people with liver disease. Aside from their anti-cancer properties, Graviola and Paw Paw also possess antimalarial, antiviral, antimicrobial, antiparasitic, and pesticidal activities.

Those are only a few of the many natural foods and substances that have amazing anti-cancer and other health-promoting properties, and I will discuss a few more as we get further along.

As living beings, we have certain nutritional needs, such as vitamins, minerals, protein, etc., and so nature has deemed it important enough to provide those nutrients in many sources throughout the world, so that regardless of where you are, you will be able to obtain the nutrition you need. Since cancer is a systemic problem that arises from an imbalance or toxicity, it is therefore logical to not look at cancer cures as cures or medicine, but as nutrients and substances that are necessary for elimination of toxins, imbalance and disarray, and for proper functioning of the body's systems, which leads to good health. When contemplated from this perspective therefore it is easy to see why there are so many cancer "cures" in every corner of the earth. It is however less of a cure and more of a nutrient.

Furthermore, it is then clear to see why some natural treatments work for some people, but not for others. It is important to examine your habits and your environment to determine the cause of your deficiency or toxicity and tailor your treatment accordingly. If it is not so easily discernible however, then a multifaceted approach might be called for, and will be a good idea regardless of the reason. It is never a bad idea to get more and better nutrition from a greater variety of fruits, vegetables, nuts, and other natural, wholesome sources, and to improve our mental health, while at the same time eliminating those foods, thoughts and environmental factors which do not serve us. Consulting with a physician who specializes in natural medicine and nutrition, such as an orthomolecular medicine practitioner will be helpful in determining what is lacking in your body, what needs to be flushed out, what to avoid, and what course of treatment to implement for your particular type of cancer.

Keep in mind that aside from vitamin B12, which cannot be obtained from cleansed plant-based foods, and vitamin D, which comes from sun exposure, but can be difficult to obtain in winter months or in high latitude zones, obtaining nutrition from organic, whole-food, plant-based sources is always superior to isolated supplements.

Once you eliminate the toxicity from your body, your mind, and your environment, and provide a balanced nutrition for your cells to do their job, then your body can and will heal itself. It is absolutely beyond belief how amazingly intelligent our biology is, and all of the systems within our bodies that are designed for self-maintenance; repair, cleanup, disposal, defense, and many other functions, that given the opportunity, will fight and win against any disorder or disease, including end-stage cancer.

Note: Many supplements, and foods, especially ones that are sourced from China, but also many other places around the world, are contaminated with high amounts of lead, cadmium, arsenic, and many other toxic substances. Remember that I said that many plants bioaccumulate toxins which are present in the soil? This attribute is what makes them efficient at scavenging and eliminating toxins within the body as well, but you want to make sure that they are not already contaminated. Make sure that the products that you purchase are tested for, and are free of those contaminants.

The problem arises when we stop listening to the signals that our bodies are giving us, like acne, oily skin, bloatedness, headaches, bad breath, and on and on, and continue to consume and slather ourselves with substances that are bad for our biology. Drinking one glass of soda might not kill you, but drinking soda every day for 30 years will lead to all sorts of diseases and disorder that you might not think are related, including cancer. When combined with all the other junk you eat and drink, the assault is compounded, to the point where you're taking a pill for fatty liver, and another one for high blood pressure, and a third for diabetes, and a few more to manage the side effects from the first three, and surprise, surprise, all those pills are actually destroying your liver, your kidneys and your digestive tract, suppressing your immune system, leaving you susceptible to other diseases, and you end up worse than when you started.

According to a 2013 study published in the journal Mayo Clinic Proceedings, nearly 70% of Americans take at least one prescription drug[304]. That is the equivalent of every man and woman in the United States, ages 20 and over, or 223 million people[305]. According to a 2015 report by the U.S. Department of Health and Human Services[306], in 2014, Americans spent $297.7 billion on prescription drugs, and $3.03 trillion (with a "t") total in healthcare costs. Houston, we certainly have a problem... Is it starting to make sense now why the healthcare industry has no interest in making you healthy?

In today's age of profits over morality and decency, it is your job to do the research and implement some common sense when it comes to your health. Doctors will not help you, because they are trained by a system that wants you sick, and the pharmaceutical industry will certainly not help, because they are a major stakeholder in that industry, and the main architect of the way that the industry operates today.

When reading research papers, you need to read between the lines. While the researcher may be testing a natural substance, such as ginger, in hopes of developing drugs from it, the fact is, it's the ginger that does the healing, and the whole ginger or whole ginger extract will work a lot better than an isolate of ginger, because that is how nature works... In nature nothing is in isolation, because nature works by synergy. Yes, it might be difficult to get the concentrations that are present in medications from food, but if you maintain a healthy lifestyle, you will not need to treat disease with high concentrations, and if you are in reaction mode, and you are treating a disease that was caused by years of abuse, getting those high concentrations are still possible with juicing and whole-plant extracts. It might not be as easy as popping a pill, but it will be more effective, and will make you healthier overall, rather than making you sicker overall.

According to research by Chunhua Yang et al. on the effects of Graviola (Annona Muricata) on prostate cancer, "Isolation of 'most-active fraction' [active ingredient] or single constituents from whole extracts may not only compromise the therapeutic efficacy but also render toxicity, thus emphasizing the importance of preserving the natural composition of whole extracts."[298]

Let's get back to a few other offending substances that are responsible for so much disease in the world, and then we'll get back to some more solutions:

3.4   WHAT IS CANCER AND WHAT CAUSES IT? (CONT.)

3.4.1   Pharmaceutical Drugs

The first fact that you need to understand is that the doctors that prescribe those drugs are almost always ignorant of what is in the drug, and how it affects your body, aside from the symptom it claims to treat. If you are currently on medication, research the side-effects of the medications you are taking, and the next time you visit your doctor, ask him or her what the side-effects of those medications are on your liver, or your digestive tract, or your heart, acidity, gut biome, etc. You will be surprised when the doctor either gives you rosy information that contradicts the published data on the drug, or they tell you that they don't know and need to check. They certainly didn't check when they pulled out that prescription pad...

Likewise, if you are planning on taking a vaccine, ask your doctor what's in it. Most doctors would not be able to answer that question, and most doctors will not know that almost all vaccines, besides being completely unnecessary, contain aluminum and mercury[307] which are both neurotoxic and carcinogenic, formaldehyde[307] which is genotoxic, mutagenic, clastogenic, and carcinogenic, and some vaccines have even been found to contain a cancer-causing virus. Additionally, some vaccines contain human DNA, human albumin (a constituent of human blood), and genetically engineered human albumin[308], which have been linked to autism.

Here are a few of the many adverse reactions of MMR vaccine as reported by the vaccine manufacturer[309]:

- Atypical <u>Measles</u>
    - o   the measles vaccine will give you measles

- Vasculitis
  - inflammation of blood vessels
- Pancreatitis
  - inflammation of the pancreas
- Parotitis
  - inflammation of the parotid gland, or <u>Mumps</u>
- Diabetes
- Arthritis, Arthralgia, Myalgia and Polyneuritis
  - features of infection with wild-type <u>Rubella</u>
- Subacute sclerosing panencephalitis
  - a progressive, debilitating, and deadly brain disorder related to <u>Measles</u> infection
- Guillain-Barré Syndrome
  - a condition in which the immune system attacks the nerves

So, in summation, the MMR (Measles, Mumps, and Rubella) vaccine can give you measles, mumps, and rubella, in addition to other, extremely severe conditions, of which some may lead to death. Additionally, because vaccines contain inactivated viruses, the body still reacts to them as if the live virus is present and it puts the immune system in overdrive. This is not really immunity, it is more like persistent immune response, and the problem with that is that it will eventually lead to adrenal fatigue and degradation of the immune system. When you get multiple immunizations, the effect is compounded, while the intended protection is diminished[310].

A recent peer-reviewed and published study – the first of its kind in the United States has compared vaccinated to unvaccinated children, ages 6 to 12. The researchers had found that "Vaccinated children were significantly less likely than the unvaccinated to have been diagnosed with chickenpox and pertussis, but significantly more likely to have been diagnosed with pneumonia, otitis media, allergies and

NDDs (defined as Autism Spectrum Disorder, Attention Deficit Hyperactivity Disorder, and/or a learning disability)". As expected, almost immediately after this study was published, it was retracted. What's worse is that typically when a study is retracted, the text is still accessible, but with the word "RETRACTED" at the top of the paper. In this case, they simply wiped it out of existence, and in its place, a barrage of pro-vaccine articles mocking and attacking the study. Luckily it was republished in another journal early this year.[311]

Many drugs are metabolized in the liver, and cause serious liver damage. Most drugs are also extremely harmful to the digestive tract. Furthermore, most drugs are acidifying, leading to a host of diseases and infections, and ultimately to cancer. Now, don't get me wrong – there are many herbs that can have negatives effects on the liver when taken at inappropriate doses, or cause hormonal disturbances, or other issues, but as a rule, most herbs which have been in use for thousands of years have that track record of safety, while most pharmaceuticals have very short track records, and in that short time have been shown to cause more harm than good. Not to say that all medications are bad at all times. In some extreme situations pharmaceuticals might be necessary, but in most cases, they are not, and certainly not for any extended period of time.

Here are some alarming statistics from IMS Health about prescribed drug use among children in the United States[312]:

- 227,132 children 0 to 1 year of age are on anti-anxiety medications. When you look at children up to 5 years of age, that number jumps to 757,645, and over 2 million children ages 0 to 17.

- 26,406 children 0 to 1 year of age are on anti-depressants. That number jumps up to 118,330 children ages 0 to 5 and again, over 2 million children in the 0 to 17 age group.

- 274,804 children ages 0 to 1 are on psychiatric drugs in general. That number jumps up to 1,146,530 children ages 0 to 5 and nearly 8.4 million children ages 0 to 17. That is more than 10% of all children ages 0 to 17 in the United States in 2013[313] - the same years this data was collected.

What is making American infants and children so anxious, depressed, and psychotic?

3.4.2   Carnivore Vs. Omnivore Vs. Herbivore

By now it's fairly common knowledge that consumption of animal products causes cancer, heart disease, diabetes, and many other diseases and disorders in humans.   But less known is why...   Contrary to what some may say, while humans can survive on consuming animal products, the human body is not designed to process it, and consuming it over the long run causes disease.

Let me try to explain this using an analogy of anaerobic microbes.   Anaerobes are organisms which grow in the absence of air or require an oxygen-free environment to live. Under the anaerobic umbrella, there are two main types - facultative anaerobes and obligate anaerobes.   Facultative anaerobes prefer an environment free of oxygen, but they can survive in the presence of some oxygen.   In an oxygen-containing environment, facultative anaerobes will continue living, but will expend more energy, and will strain to do so.

In an environment high in oxygen, facultative anaerobes will die off.

Obligate anaerobes on the other hand can only live in an oxygen-free environment and will die if exposed to even a minute levels of oxygen.

Humans are physiologically-speaking *facultative herbivores*. That is to say that by nature, humans are herbivores, but we can survive by consuming meat. Consuming meat and other animal products will not kill us immediately, but it will strain our organs, release toxins into our blood which we are not equipped to handle as the meat putrefies in our digestive tracts, and cause diseases and disorders. Over the long run, meat consumption will degrade out health and shorten our lives.

Let's look at those physiological factors which separates us from carnivores and omnivores:

- Humans have teeth designed for grinding. Yes, we have canines, but our canines are short, and herbivores have canines as well. Cattle, sheep, goats, llamas, alpacas, deer, and other herbivores all have canines. While chimps and gorillas have huge canines, their diet consists of almost entirely vegetation, and a small portion consisting of ants. While chimps occasionally kill other animals, and eat them, it is not part of their normal diet. Carnivores, likewise, have carnassial teeth, designed for slicing flesh, while herbivores, like humans, do not.

- Our jaws move side-to-side and front-to-back for grinding, while carnivores' jaws move in an open-and-shut, and shearing fashion with very minimal side-to-side movement. There are many other physiological differences in the jaws and facial musculature between herbivores, omnivores and carnivores.

- Carnivores and omnivores do not chew their food, and therefore they do not have salivary enzymes. Humans on the other hand, like other herbivores chew their food. Human/herbivore saliva is full of carbohydrate digestive enzymes to help with breaking down plant food.

- The length of the intestines of carnivores and omnivores is between 3 and 6 times the length of their torso, while the length of the intestines of humans and herbivores is between 10 and 12 times their torso. The reason for this is, meat putrefies very quickly, so it is necessary to move it through the system rapidly. For that reason, carnivores' intestines are also smooth to facilitate rapid elimination. When humans eat animal products, it sits in the intestines for a long time, rotting and releasing toxins. Plant matter on the other hand take much longer to break down in an anaerobic environment, which the intestines are, so human/herbivore intestines are designed to extract as much nutrition out of the plant food over a longer period of time. Human and herbivore intestines are also sacculated for this purpose.

- Carnivores and omnivores have sharp claws for holding onto prey and ripping flesh. Humans on the other hand have flattened, thin nails that would not do much good in ripping much of anything.

- Meat and other animal products are very acidifying to the body, leading to metabolic acidosis. "It is well established that diet and certain food components have a clear impact on acid-base balance."[314] According to a study published in the European Journal of Nutrition, "We know that clinically-recognized chronic metabolic acidosis has deleterious effects on the body, including growth retardation in children, decreased muscle and bone mass in adults, and kidney stone formation, and that correction of acidosis can ameliorate those conditions ... Our group has shown that contemporary net acid-producing diets do indeed characteristically produce a low-grade systemic metabolic acidosis in otherwise healthy adult subjects, and that the degree of acidosis increases with age, in relation to the normally occurring age-related decline in renal functional capacity."[315] When your blood becomes acidic from consuming animal proteins, the body has to correct for this acidity. If your blood is too acidic for an extended length of time, you will slip into a coma and die if not corrected. The body has several mechanisms for correcting acidosis - one of them is an increase in breathing to eliminate carbon dioxide from the blood. Another way is an increase in acid secretion into the urine by the kidneys. Finally, the body will rob calcium carbonate and calcium phosphate out of the bones, and use the carbonates and phosphates to increase the blood pH (alkalinity). In response to the increased free calcium in the blood, your body will excrete the calcium through the urine, leading to bone-loss. Meat consumption will therefore lead to chronic metabolic acidosis, which will lead to osteoporosis, cancer, and a whole multitude of other health conditions.

- Carnivores and omnivores have a stomach volume of 60% to 70% of their entire digestive tract, while the stomach size of herbivores is less than 30%, and humans 21% to 27% of the total volume of their digestive tract.

- The livers of carnivores and omnivores are able to detoxify vitamin A, while the livers of herbivores and humans cannot. Toxicity of vitamin A, which can come about from chronic consumption of as little as two times the recommended daily limit, can lead to various health issues. Now, here's a fascinating fact about vitamin A toxicity in humans… There are two types of vitamin A – preformed vitamin A, which comes from meat, poultry, fish and milk, and provitamin A which comes from fruits, vegetables, and other plant-based products. Too much preformed vitamin A (from animal products) can cause vision problems, bone disease, digestive issues, liver damage, coma, and even death. Provitamin A (from plants) on the other hand is entirely safe and does not cause any toxicity in humans at any level. Although our ancestors have been eating meat for millions of years, the archeological record supports the fact that humans are not designed to eat meat. "Fossilized skeletal remains of early humans suggest that bone abnormalities may have been caused by hypervitaminosis A. From these and other reports, vitamin A toxicity is known to be an ancient phenomenon."[316]

- Carnivores and omnivores produce their own vitamin C. Herbivores (and humans) get their vitamin C from their diet (from fruits and vegetables).

- Lastly, according to William C. Roberts, MD – an authority on cardiac pathology, and an editor for both the American Journal of Cardiology and the Baylor University Medical Center Proceedings, "Atherosclerosis [the build-up of fats, cholesterol, and other substances in and on the artery walls] affects only herbivores. Dogs, cats, tigers, and lions can be saturated with fat and cholesterol, and atherosclerotic plaques do not develop."[317] He further states that "Although most of us conduct our lives as omnivores, in that we eat flesh as well as vegetables and fruits, human beings have characteristics of herbivores, not carnivores."[317]

The China-Cornell-Oxford Project, which was the largest and most thorough study on nutrition and its effect on disease ever conducted, demonstrated beyond a shadow of a doubt that animal proteins in the diet are responsible for nearly all chronic diseases. The book "The China Study" by T. Colin Campbell, who lead the China project, chronicled its results, and many other studies in making the case that humans are herbivores. I highly recommend reading this book.

All this being said, if you grew up eating meat and you become vegan, you might feel that you're having cravings for meat. This could be one of several things. It could be the memory of the taste of meat that you are craving, and not a biological need per-se. It could also be, if you quit meat in the recent past (and this is very common with sugar for instance) that your body is weaning off of it, and it's not craving it because it needs it, just like with weaning off of a drug. Lastly, it could be that because you do not get enough nutrition from your new vegan diet due to a lack in variety or proper food combinations, that your body will respond to this deficiency by sending out craving signals to your brain asking for the type of food that it knows will fulfill its immediate need. That does not mean that it's overall healthy for you, but if you are low in iron for instance, you might crave a steak, and in that instance, it is better to eat the steake than make yourself ill. Unless you have been vegan your entire life, or your meat consumption prior to becoming vegan was low, you might need to "supplement" with eggs or meat once in a while. It is always better to supplement with food than with synthetic supplements, although there are food-based supplements on the market that work well. Also keep in mind that the soil has become so depleted in recent decades that foods today don't have nearly the levels of nutrients they used to, and should have, so getting complete nutrition from food alone is becoming increasingly difficult. However, as was discussed previously, organic farming leads to more nutrition in the soil, and consequently, more nutrition in the crops. Yet another reason to eat organic.

Additionally, since we have become such a sterile society, it is difficult to get vitamin B12 from plant foods. While plants contain all of the amino acids, vitamins and minerals that our bodies need, the only way to get vitamin B12 is from animal products, or bacteria. In the past, humans got their share of vitamin B12 from soil-borne bacteria on their fruits and vegetables, but today, we wash our produce thoroughly. Additionally, there is some evidence to show that vitamin B12 degrades with cooking, so getting it exclusively from meat / fish, etc. does not guarantee that you are getting enough of it. However, many products, including vegetarian and vegan products, are fortified with bacterially-derived vitamin B12, so while proponents of meat-eating like to harp on this issue, it is not really an issue.

What it comes down to is, you have to learn to listen to your body's subtle signals and it will tell you what you need or should stay away from. Going to your doctor periodically for blood work would be a good idea, because it will tell you where you need to focus your efforts, but keep in mind that blood tests, in some instances are not good indicators, such as in body acidity/alkalinity, so you need to look at other indicators, such as spots, discoloration, grooves, etc. on your nails, spots on your iris, the appearance of your tongue, skin discoloration or acne, and other bodily signs that tell you about the state of your internal health. A holistic health practitioner will be able to diagnose you using those body signs.

3.4.3   Vaccines

I've already mentioned vaccines in the section on pharmaceuticals, and I don't want to get too deep into the topic of vaccines because it would literally take another book of equal length, but there are a few concepts to keep in mind when it comes to vaccines:

- The premise of vaccines is that it causes an immune response which leads the body to develop immunity to a particular pathogen. At face value, this seems to be a good thing, but when you receive dozens on vaccines over a lifetime, your immune system goes into overdrive and eventually fatigues.

- Vaccines contain adjuvants, such as Aluminum, and preservatives such as mercury, as well as formaldehyde, acetone, animal and human serum (blood product), polysorbate 80 and many more toxins and allergens
    - Aluminum is a neurotoxin and is also associated with the formation of certain cancers,

such as sarcoma, as well as brain and bone disease. According to the FDA, the safe limit of aluminum in drinking water is 0.2mg/L, and according to the CDC, it is 0.05 to 0.2mg/L, although the CDC makes a nonsense disclosure that states that their recommendation is based not on health, but on smell, taste and color, because the CDC cares about smell, taste and color... Aluminum that enters the body through food and water is not entirely absorbed and only a very small amount of it enters the bloodstream (about 1%). Now here's an interesting fact about vaccines - on the first day of life, infants are given a Hepatitis B vaccine (yes, for a sexually transmitted disease, because you know those babies nowadays), which contains 0.25mg of aluminum, injected directly into their vein. By its first birthday a baby can expect to get a total of 4.225mg of aluminum injected directly into their veins. For visual reference, this is what 0.25mg and 4.225mg of aluminum foil looks like (full size):

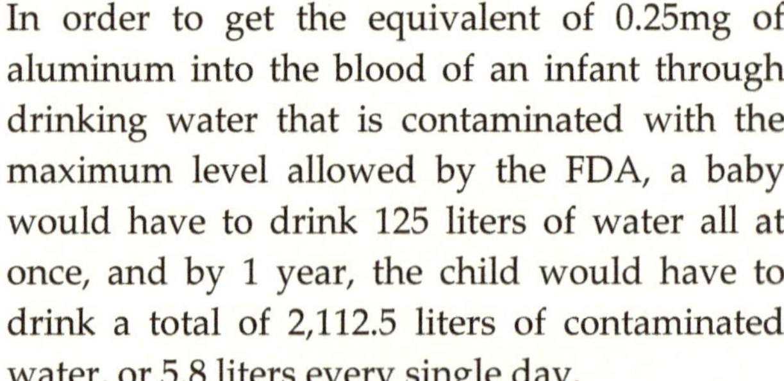

In order to get the equivalent of 0.25mg of aluminum into the blood of an infant through drinking water that is contaminated with the maximum level allowed by the FDA, a baby would have to drink 125 liters of water all at once, and by 1 year, the child would have to drink a total of 2,112.5 liters of contaminated water, or 5.8 liters every single day.

Paul Offit is a pediatrician specializing in infectious diseases, vaccines, immunology, and virology who is very outspoken in favor of vaccines. He is a member of the Centers for Disease Control (CDC) Advisory Committee on Immunization Practices, which means that he makes decisions on which vaccines get included in the vaccine schedule. He also holds patents on vaccines, which have made him tens of millions of Dollars, and is a clear conflict of interest. Offit constantly spews lies and misinformation in his attempt to discredit anti-vaccine or vaccine safety activists, and pushes his vaccine agenda.

In a paper co-authored by Paul Offit that aims to address parents' concerns regarding vaccinations, he makes the most absurd statement that an infant could theoretically take 10,000 vaccines all at once without any negative effects.[318]

His assumptions were deduced, as people like him like to do, by focusing on only one aspect of a system (antigens and epitopes in this case) and ignoring everything else. To illustrate what I mean by that, let's look at the aluminum example shown above. 10,000 Hepatitis B vaccines would contain 2,500mg of aluminum, which is equal to a 9.5 x 9.5 inch sheet of aluminum foil. In another example, 10,000 influenza vaccines equals to 245,000mcg of mercury. The EPA's safe limit of mercury in drinking water is 2mcg/L. If you drank the recommended 8 glasses of water per day, it would take you 177 years to accumulate that much mercury from water contaminated with 2mcg/L mercury (assuming that your body does not chelate any of it along the way).

Looking at only those two examples, it is easy to see how vaccine-pushers use misinformation – picking only the data that suits their agenda and discarding the rest, and are just plain lying.

In a report on the detection of glyphosate in vaccines, Dr. Toni Bark, MD, MHEM, LEED, AP stated: "Injection is a very different route of entry than oral route. Injected toxins, even in minute doses can have profound effects on the organs and the different systems of the body."[319]

3.5   NATURAL CANCER CURES (CONT.)

Let's look at a few more plants with amazing anti-cancer activity. The following plants are considered pests and dangerous drugs, but in reality, they are some of the most potent health-promoters. There is a reason why weeds are so prolific and resilient - they provide excellent nutrition for humans and animals, and they enrich the soil. Many of these "weeds" are found in disturbed areas, such as in the cracks of your driveway and roadsides, around railroad tracks, and on your lawn, if you don't use herbicides. I would not recommend eating them from those areas because they extract toxins from the soil by binding them in the plant tissue, so you need to be certain that the soil where they are grown is toxin-free. All of these are available for purchase as supplements, herbs, and even in some grocery stores. I would, as with everything else, suggest that you look for organically grown whole-plant extracts rather than isolated compounds:

3.5.1   Dandelion (Taraxacum)

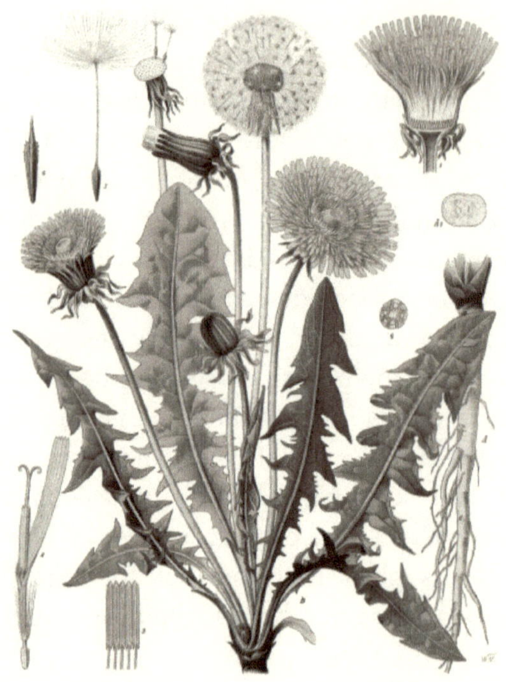

Picture source: Wikipedia

Dandelions are recognizable pretty much all over the world. They grow in disturbed areas as well as in lawns, and are considered a weed. However, dandelions are highly nutritious, and have been used for culinary and medicinal purposes for thousands of years. The leaves - dandelion greens which can be found in grocery stores, contain more iron and calcium than spinach. They are also high in vitamin K (741% daily value per 100g) and vitamin B_1, B_2, B_6, C, E, calcium, manganese, and protein. They also contain many other vitamins, minerals and health-promoting phytochemicals.

The flower buds and flowers can be eaten raw. The flowers are also used for making wine, soft drinks, jams, and honey substitutes, and the roots have been used as a non-caffeinated coffee substitute as well as medicinally in dandelion root tea.

Dandelion has been shown in scientific studies to have "diuretic, choleretic, anti-inflammatory, anti-oxidative, anti-carcinogenic, analgesic, anti-hyperglycemic, anti-coagulatory and prebiotic effects"[320]. For cancer specifically, it has been shown to be effective against hepatocellular carcinoma[321], drug-resistant/chemoresistant melanoma[322,323], breast cancer[324], prostate cancer[324,325], leukemia[326], skin tumors[327], and mammary tumors[328].

In a study showing the efficacy of dandelion root extract against Chronic Myelomonocytic Leukemia, the authors stated that "Chronic Myelomonocytic Leukemia (CMML) is a heterogeneous disease that is not only hard to diagnose and classify, but is also highly resistant to treatment. Available forms of therapy for this disease have not shown significant effects and patients rapidly develop resistance early on in therapy. These factors lead to the very poor prognosis observed with CMML patients, with median survival duration between 12 and 24 months after diagnosis."[329]. Yet, DRE was demonstrated to effectively kill this aggressive cancer. "In this study, we demonstrate the selective efficacy of dandelion root extract in inducing apoptosis and autophagy in highly aggressive and resistant CMML cell lines. We observed the induction of apoptosis in three of the CMML cell lines used for this study. More importantly, this effect was selective, as non-cancerous PBMCs and NHFs remained unsusceptible to DRE-induced apoptosis"[329].

In another study, the authors commented that "Pancreatic cancer has a 100% mortality rate ... DRE [Dandelion Root Extract] has the potential to induce apoptosis and autophagy in human pancreatic cancer cells with no significant effect on noncancerous cells"[330].

While dandelion has many health benefits, including cancer-fighting properties, it has been shown to be particularly non-toxic to normal cells.

As I mentioned before, whole plant extracts, especially from those plants that are non-toxic, as dandelion is, is always better than isolates[331].

3.5.2   <u>Milk Thistle (Silybum Marianum)</u>

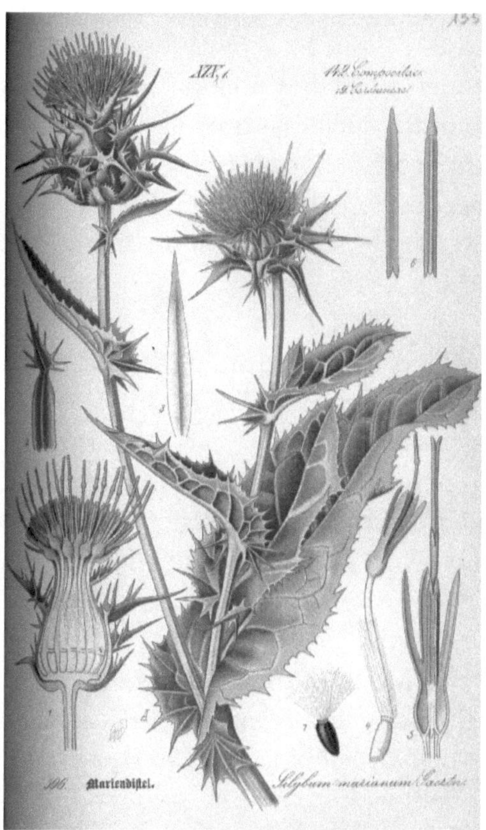

Picture source: Wikipedia

Milk thistle is another one of those "weeds" that grows in disturbed areas. It has been used extensively in herbal medicine to treat liver diseases and has been shown in in vitro and in vivo studies to have hepatoprotective properties[332,333,334] which contributes to its overall protection against chemically-induced cancers.

In [334] the authors describe how "The anticancer effects of most naturally occurring plant extracts can often be attributed to one compound ... or few compounds ... The current studies were initiated to determine which compounds are responsible for documented antiproliferative effects of milk thistle extracts. Interestingly, none of the four most closely related milk thistle compounds was devoid of activity on any of the end points tested [in Human Prostate Carcinoma Cells] thus far. Several other compounds, such as taxifolin and silychristin, also possessed antiproliferative activity when used at higher exposure concentrations." This plant is very remarkable in the sense that it possesses so many cancer-fighting compounds in one small package.

"Untreated patients with BM [brain metastases] have a median survival of about 1 month"[335]. A study of the response of brain metastasis from lung cancer patients to an oral nutraceutical product containing silibinin from milk thistle seeds showed a "suppressive effects of silibinin on progressive BM, which involved a marked reduction of the peritumoral brain edema"[336].

A 2016 study in Molecular Carcinogenesis demonstrated the efficacy of Silibinin from milk thistle, and its oxidation product 2,3-dehydrosilibinin (DHS) against basal cell carcinoma in both in vitro and in vivo models[336]. "Basal cell carcinoma (BCC) is the most common cancer worldwide, and its current treatment options are insufficient and toxic." The results of the study indicated that "Both silibinin and DHS significantly inhibited cell growth and clonogenicity while inducing apoptosis in a dose - and time-dependent manner, with DHS showing higher activity at lower concentrations ... these results provide the first evidence for the efficacy and usefulness of silibinin and its derivative DHS against BCC".

In yet another published study on liver cancer[337], the authors write that "Current therapeutic options for [Hepatocellular Carcinoma], including surgical resection and liver transplantation, have limited benefits and are essentially ineffective ... On the basis of numerous studies conducted using various liver cancer cells, chemically induced xenograft, orthotopic, and transgenic animal models, and human participants, as summarized in this review, silymarin and its principal phytoconstituent silibinin were found to play an important role in the prevention and treatment of HCC [hepatocellular carcinoma]. From the results of various preclinical in-vitro and in-vivo studies, it is evident that the constituents of silymarin could inhibit all stages of hepatocarcinogenesis, namely, **initiation, promotion, and progression** [emphasis added] ... It is tempting to speculate that several bioactive phytochemicals present in silymarin could act through coordinated regulation of multiple discrete pathways to prevent the occurrence of liver tumors and kill established hepatic carcinoma cells. This is in line with emerging evidence that plant phytochemicals manifest chemopreventive and antitumor effects when they are used in combination rather than individually ... On the basis of an impressive body of evidence presented in this review, milk thistle-derived products, especially silymarin and silibinin, have been found to show significant promise for the prevention and treatment of liver cancer without any adverse effects."

Additional studies have shown great efficacy in treating and preventing colorectal cancer[338], prostate cancer[339], breast cancer[340,341], renal cell carcinoma[342], and ovarian cancer[343].

3.5.3   <u>Artichoke (Cynara L.)</u>

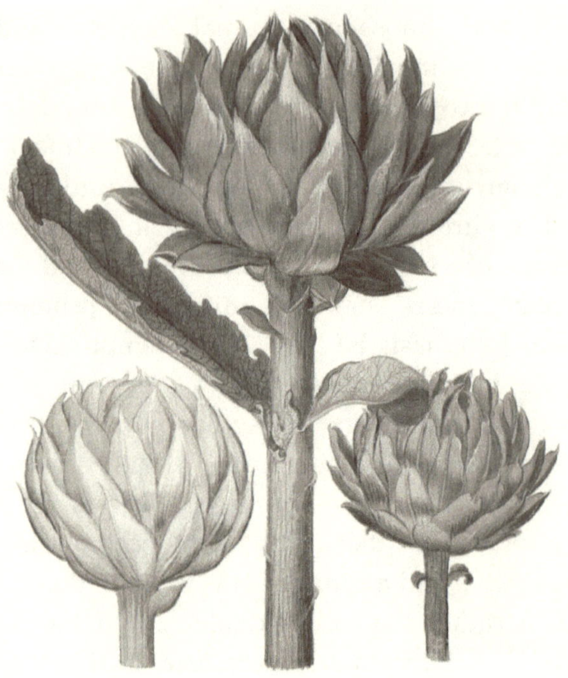

Artichoke is in the thistle family, just like milk thistle and has many of the same biological activities as milk thistle does. Artichoke leaf extract has been studied extensively for its liver protective and liver healing properties, as well as for its effects on various types of cancer. It has been shown to be very effective at killing cancer cells by various mechanisms, such as cell cycle arrest, apoptosis, and other routes[344 - 347]. It has also been shown to be entirely non-toxic to healthy cells in all tested concentrations.

In one study, artichoke, borututu, and milk thistle were tested alone and in combination with each other, in varying ratios. It was discovered that all three had liver-protective, and liver cancer killing activity, and that the various combinations, without exception, had synergistic effects on anti-oxidant activity, while at the same time being non-toxic to healthy cells[348].

Lastly, the next plant is a controversial one, but for no good reasons. Although it is illegal to grow, use or sell in most parts of the world, I suspect that it has nothing to do with anything other than its tremendous health-promoting effects, as well as its disease-fighting effects. It is likely the most studied plant in all of human history and poses a great risk to the pharmaceutical industry if it becomes legal globally.

3.5.4   Cannabis / Hemp

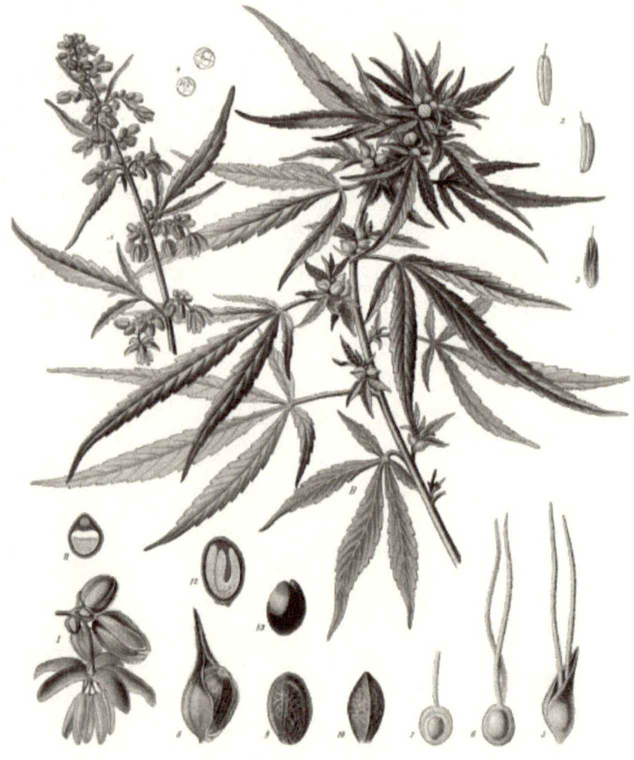

Picture source: Wikimedia Commons

While I personally do not condone smoking of any kind, including cannabis, cannabis does have some well-known therapeutic properties even when smoked. However, I see the greatest benefits in its extracts and whole-plant use (such as in juicing or eating the leaves and/or buds). Cannabis has been used medically for nearly 5,000 years, and for its fibers and as building materials for at least 10,000 years.

The two main constituents of cannabis are THC (tetrahydrocannabinol), which is responsible for the mind-altering effects that recreational use of cannabis is known for, but also has many medical/therapeutic applications – and CBD (cannabidiol) which actually has an anti-psychotropic effect. As a matter of fact, CBD moderates the effects of THC when the two are taken together.

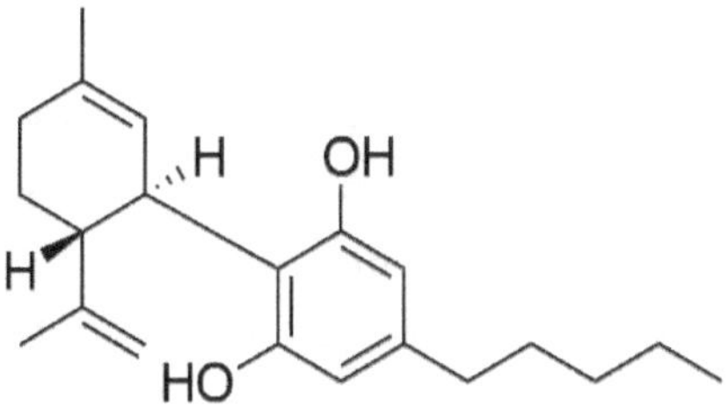

2D structure of cannabidiol (CBD)

There are hundreds of other phytochemicals – cannabinoids, terpenes, flavonoids, etc., with medicinal benefits in cannabis that are being discovered and studied on a daily basis, such as cannabigerol, cannabinol, cannabichromene, β-myrcene, linalool, luteolin, kaempferol, and many others. CBD and THC, and many of the terpenes and flavonoids in cannabis and other plants, have repeatedly been shown to be exceedingly effective in the fight against cancer, as well as many other ailments.

Cannabis' effectiveness against cancer has been recognized in the scientific community since 1975 when it was discovered that cannabinoids suppress lung cancer cell growth[349].

In the early 1990's scientists had discovered that humans and all mammals have what is called an endocannabinoid system (endo meaning endogenous – originating inside of an organism, tissue or cell). The system is comprised of cannabinoid receptors; a class of cell membrane receptors which are located throughout the body, and are responsible for a variety of physiological processes including mood, memory, pain-sensation, and appetite. Cell membrane receptors are a type of Integral Membrane Proteins (IMPs), as discussed earlier, and are responsible for sensing chemicals in the cellular environment and initiating a cellular function in response to those chemical signals. The mammalian brain produces an endocannabinoid called anandamide, which is nearly identical to THC (interestingly, the name anandamide is taken from the Sanskrit & Pāli word ananda, which means "joy, bliss, delight", and amide.), and another, called 2-AG, which is nearly identical to CBD. Both anandamide and 2-AG produce effects which mirror THC and CBD, respectively, from plant sources, such as cannabis.

While everyone knows what cannabis, marijuana, pot, or weed is, and many know their therapeutic effects for glaucoma for instance, not many people know their effects on calming or eliminating seizures[350,351], Tourette's symptoms[352], and symptoms of many other neurological conditions[353], and even fewer know how effective they are at ameliorating or curing an impressive variety of cancers. The following impressive list of nearly 100 studies illustrate the consensus in the scientific community as to the efficacy of cannabis at killing cancer cells. This list is by no means the extent of the scientific studies that have been performed on cannabis which show its amazing cancer-killing abilities, such as its effects on tumors[354-375], colorectal cancers[376-379], brain cancers[380-398], breast cancer[399-405], lung cancer[406,407], prostate cancer[408,409], blood cancer / leukemia[410-413], liver cancer[414], and other cancers[415-422].

Clinical trials on cannabis are very limited due to its classification as a schedule 1 drug, and the subsequent governmental control and oversight, but one such pilot clinical trial on incurable glioblastoma multiforme; a fast-growing brain cancer showed excellent results[423].

If you read all of the referenced studies on cannabis you will notice an impressive trend. Not only does cannabis repeatedly kill cancer cells via multiple routes, but in all of the studies, it "selectively" kills cancer cells, and only cancer cells. In other words, it specifically targets cancer cells and not their normal, healthy counterparts. As you have read previously, chemo, radiation, and gene therapies kill indiscriminately and cause massive collateral damage that can last a lifetime, and more often kills the patient.

Schedule 1 drugs are defined as having a high abuse potential, no medical use, and severe safety concerns, and include narcotics such as Heroin, LSD, and cocaine. However, cannabis has many medical uses, and not a single person has ever died as a direct result of cannabis use, especially its non-psychoactive components. Not only does the U.S. government know this to be fact – but there are several FDA-approved synthetic-cannabinoid prescription medications that have been in use for over three decades, such as Marinol. Additionally, the U.S. government holds a patent for "Cannabinoids as antioxidants and neuroprotectants" (U.S. patent No. 6,630,507). Their patent abstract states:

"Cannabinoids have been found to have antioxidant properties, unrelated to NMDA receptor antagonism. This new found property makes cannabinoids useful in the treatment and prophylaxis of wide variety of oxidation associated diseases, such as ischemic, age-related, inflammatory and autoimmune diseases. The cannabinoids are found to have particular application as neuroprotectants, for example in limiting neurological damage following ischemic insults, such as stroke and trauma, or in the treatment of neurodegenerative diseases, such as Alzheimer's disease, Parkinson's disease and HIV dementia. Nonpsychoactive cannabinoids, such as cannabidiol, are particularly advantageous to use because they avoid toxicity that is encountered

with psychoactive cannabinoids at high doses useful in the method of the present invention."

The patent further states:

"As used herein, a "cannabinoid" is a chemical compound (such as cannabinol, THC or cannabidiol) that is found in the plant species Cannabis saliva [sic] (marijuana)"

While cannabis is illegal in much of the U.S., the good news is that hemp is legal in all 50 states. There are three strains of cannabis – cannabis sativa, cannabis indica, and cannabis ruderalis. Hemp is actually a breed of cannabis sativa. The legal distinction between what qualifies as cannabis and what qualifies as hemp is, a cannabis plant that contains more than 0.3% THC is considered illegal cannabis, while a cannabis sativa strain containing less than 0.3% THC is considered hemp, and is perfectly legal.

There are other distinctions between the illegal cannabis sativa and hemp. Unlike the illegal kind, hemp grows taller and faster, and can be planted much closer together. However, CBD from hemp and CBD from other cannabis strains and breeds, is the same.

Hemp CBD oil is available for purchase all over the U.S., in stores and online. However, keep in mind that all strains of cannabis are bioaccumulators, which means that when grown with herbicides, insecticides, and chemical fertilizers, they will accumulate those toxins into their tissues. For this reason, it is important that you do your research and find a company that grows their hemp organically. You will also want to make sure that they do not extract the oil using high heat methods because high heat will degrade the oil. The best extraction method used at this time is supercritical CO_2 extraction.

When you find the right company, call them and ask which concentration is right for your condition.

Lastly, get involved politically to make sure hemp CBD oil maintains its supplement status. There are steps currently being taken by the FDA to halt the sale of hemp CBD in favor of pharmaceutical company GW Pharmaceuticals, which petitioned for Investigational New Drug (IND) status for its drug Epidiolex, which is intended for use in rare, treatment-resistant epilepsy conditions. These are the very conditions that Charlotte's Web CBD was developed for and is currently being used for, and is more effective at alleviating than Epidiolex has been shown to be in all its clinical trials to date.

There are many documented cases of the efficacy of CBD at treating all forms of seizures, and I would suggest that you watch the following videos and share them far and wide, to open the eyes of as many people as possible and alleviate the ignorance surrounding cannabis:

- The surprising story of medical marijuana and pediatric epilepsy | Josh Stanley | TEDxBoulder
    - https://www.youtube.com/watch?v=ciQ4ErmhO7g

- Why I changed my mind about medicinal cannabis | Hugh Hempel | TEDxUniversityofNevada
    - https://www.youtube.com/watch?v=3N8QMeIsX2c

- Making peace with cannabis | Zachary Walsh | TEDxPenticton
    - https://www.youtube.com/watch?v=Jv2GG_csUc8

Note: The above links have been verified at the time this book was written. In the event that they do not work, search the video title.

Speaking from personal experience with my dog, Hemp CBD also works extremely effectively for seizures in animals.

In addition to the fantastic disease-fighting properties of cannabis/hemp, its nutritional profile is impressive in its own right. Hemp seed contains more protein than beef. 100g of beef contains 28g of protein, while 100g of hemp seed contains 33g of protein. Hemp also has an excellent ratio of Omega-6 to Omega-3. It contains all 9 essential amino acids. It is also high in iron, phosphorus, magnesium, zinc, and dietary fiber.

Although more human clinical trials need to be conducted on the cancer-fighting properties of many of the plants and natural substances discussed, it is undeniable that a great number of studies on cells and animals, as well as human cancer cells implanted into animals, and in some human trials have shown exceptional cancer-fighting efficacy, while at the same time being completely safe for healthy cells. The same cannot be said for pharmaceutical anti-cancer drugs and radiation therapy, or most pharmaceuticals for that matter. It is also undeniable that the efficacy of these plants and natural substances against cancer has been known for thousands of years and that now science is catching up and confirming those results.

Epidemiologists studying the effects of self-administered alternative treatments, such as special diets or protocols carry their own challenges. For one, scientists need to control the test environment, otherwise they have no way of knowing if the results were attributable to the treatment alone, or to a combination of treatment and diet, exercise, environmental exposures, etc., etc. However, clinicians don't always control all of those aspects, and many times they don't even look for them in the first place, because most medical professionals have been trained with the idea in mind that diet has no effect on curing disease. This may explain the reason why so often different studies result in different outcomes, and even why there is such wide variability within a single study. However, Epidemiologists nevertheless can detect patterns and draw conclusions more effectively based on trends and time scales when it comes to the safety or toxicity of substances, and in this regard, many natural substances that have been in use for thousands of years and have been shown to be effective in treating disease through generations and across a diverse range of cultures.

Although preclinical predictive analysis remains mostly ineffective – for example, results from animal testing translate to similar outcomes in clinical studies less than 8% of the time[424] – when a very large number of in vitro and in vivo studies of natural substances present the same outcomes, coupled with historical records showing successful treatment of disease with the use of those substances, it should be given more credence, rather than being dismissed offhand.

It is furthermore unrealistic to control for every aspect in a test and then expect a treatment to be effective in the population at large. Whole, natural substances tend to have a greater success in treating disease over a wide range of circumstances than synthetic or isolated compounds do, because our genetics were designed, and have evolved alongside those substances, and so it would make sense that nature would offer a much wider range of medicinal and therapeutic remedies than humans could through their manipulations.

3.6 WHAT IS CANCER AND WHAT CAUSES IT? (CONT.)

Although cancer has been around for thousands of years, it used to be extremely rare. 100 years ago, cancer was extremely rare. Today cancer is on an epidemic scale, and it can be attributed to a great many things. Some of those things are:

- the rise in industrialization and the stresses, pollutants and increase in radiation from electronics and other sources that came along with it. I am not against advancement and industrialization, but it is no secret that much disease and ecological damage has resulted from those advancements. Microwave ovens are known to cause cancer, both directly and by degrading and altering the food that is cooked within them. Overhead high voltage power lines create electromagnetic radiation which is known to cause cancer at distances of hundreds of meters when exposure is sustained, such as in people who live or work nearby to those power lines. Buried powerlines are much less of a concern. A recent two year study conducted by the U.S. National Toxicology Program (NTP) has concluded that exposure to cell phone radiation, and devices which emit the same or similar type of radiation, such as electric Smart Meters, boosts rates of brain and heart cancers[425,426], which really is no surprise, since both the heart and the brain are electromagnetic in nature. These findings confirm previous tests which prompted the International Agency for Research on Cancer (IARC) to classify radiofrequency electromagnetic fields including those from cell phone use as a possible human carcinogen (Group 2B)[427]. Smart Meters, and even their predecessors which transmit shorter distances, are of particular concern, because they transmit at a much higher signal strength, and they transmit continuously. 5G technology is another major concern. 5G is a military technology and is actually being used as a weapon to inflict severe pain on enemy combatants. 5G is now being installed all over the United States, with many individuals and groups fighting their proliferation. The same resistance is transpiring against Smart Meters and the "Smart Grid", which is also a major violation of privacy rights due to the fact that Smart Meters will be collecting personal information on every household, which utility companies will sell without consumer consent.

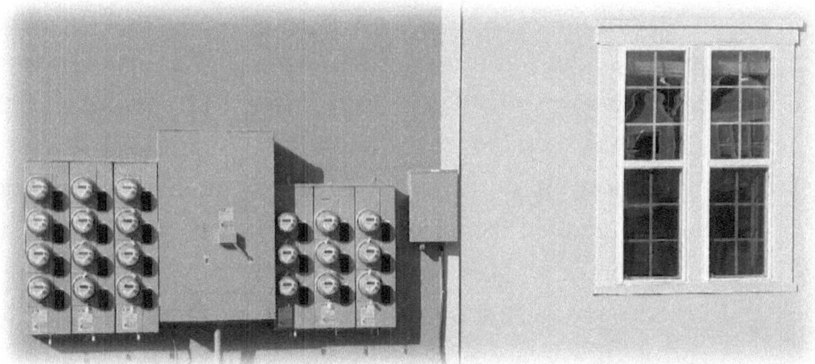

A bank of 21 Smart Meters next to a bedroom window. These Smart Meters are continually, wirelessly sending and receiving information from appliances and other meters in the area, and wirelessly transmitting this information long distances to the utility company. Does this look safe?

- the industrialization of our food, and the prevalence of toxic chemicals that are applied to our foods and soil. As discussed extensively in the chapter on GMOs, toxic agrochemicals have been killing the diversity of life within our soil and above-ground, therefore depleting it of its nutrients. Those same chemicals have also made their way into our bodies through residues on the food, which is used for human consumption and animal feed – which in turn, is present in the meat and dairy which humans consume.   Those chemicals are also present in the air and water supply.   As also discussed, many toxic chemicals are being used in food preparation and as food additives that are causing much disease and disorder.

- the increase in the consumption of animal products (meat, dairy, etc.) and the reduction in the consumption of plant foods.   This has caused a widespread epidemic of chronic metabolic acidosis in the population, which leads to premature aging, wasting away of muscle and bone mass, and a whole host of diseases. In an article in the European Journal of Nutrition on the pathophysiologic effect of modern diets[428], the author states that "We know that clinically-recognized chronic metabolic acidosis has deleterious effects on the body, including growth retardation in children, decreased muscle and bone mass in adults, and kidney stone formation, and that correction of acidosis can ameliorate those conditions ... Our group has shown that contemporary net acid-producing diets do indeed characteristically produce a low-grade systemic metabolic acidosis in otherwise healthy adult subjects, and that the degree of acidosis increases with age, in relation to the normally occurring age-related decline in renal functional capacity", and that many health problems arise from this "mismatch between our genetically determined nutritional requirements and our current diet".   Yet another study on the consumption of milk states that "Although we talk about lactose intolerance as if it is a disorder or a disease, in fact it is the norm. In most human populations, as in nonhuman mammals, lactase activity decreases by mid-childhood (age 5 years in humans) such that lactase nonpersistence is the rule, not the exception ... dairy protein consumption has been positively associated with elevated levels of insulin-like growth factor-I [IGF-1] which has been implicated with increased risk of colorectal carcinomas. Not to mention the ongoing concern that dairy consumption and calcium may lead to an increased risk of other malignancies, particularly prostate cancer."[429]   IGF-1 has also been linked to breast cancers and melanoma[430,431].

- the intentional acidification of processed foods during the manufacturing process in order to increase shelf life, and generally, the destruction of the food during its processing. For instance, Potassium Sorbate, which is a common food preservative, as well as a mutagen and genotoxin[432,433], has to be in an acidic environment in order to be effective[434], so the pH of the food item is intentionally lowered in order to make the already toxic preservative effective.

- the bastardization of our foods through genetic engineering, as already discussed extensively, and

- Processed sugars are added to everything nowadays, including raw meat. Processed and artificial sugars have been linked to many diseases, including cancer. The consumption of sugar of the average American has gone up by 1,600% over the past 190 years, from 9g per day in 1822 to 153g per day in 2012[435].   153g is equivalent to over 38 teaspoons of sugar **per day!**

"Tumors have a greater reliance on anaerobic glycolysis for energy production than normal tissues, a phenomenon that is known as the Warburg effect."[436]

In other words, tumors process glucose (sugar) at a much higher rate than normal cells do. Over consumption of sugars cause tumors to grow rapidly. While it is entirely possible, though very unlikely, that cancer was just as prevalent back in the 1800's as it is today, since it is well known that cancer progenitor cells / cancer stem cells circulate in everyone's blood; with the low consumption of sugar at that time, cancer would have progressed so slowly that people would have died of old age before tumors would cause any health effects. Again, with the explosion of carcinogenic environmental toxins, acidifying chemicals in foods, acidifying and toxic meat consumption, and all the other food-like substances that humans consume on a daily basis in the modern era, it is extremely unlikely that sugar alone would be responsible for the explosion in cancer rates, but it certainly compounds the problem.

- the conversion of human and animal life to currency by the healthcare industry - creating disease in order to sell drugs, which create more disease in order to sell more drugs, and the cycle goes on. This one may shock you, but the number one tool that doctors promote for the early detection of breast cancer - mammography, not only has been shown to be useless at doing so, but actually causes cancer and metastasis[437].

3.6.1   <u>Candida</u>

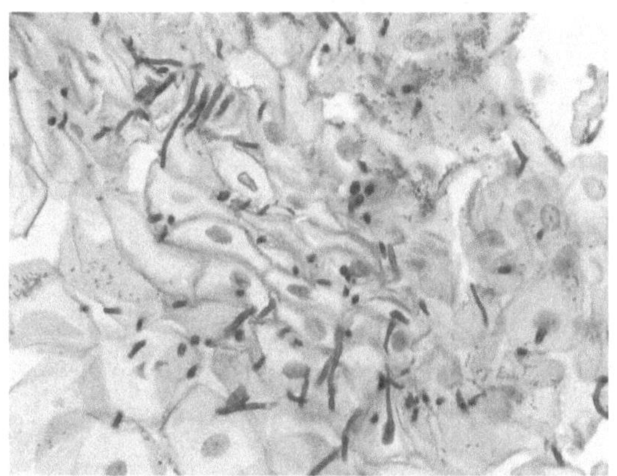

Image source: WikiMedia Commons

Candida is a fungus, which is a part of the many microorganisms in our gut flora. It is typically a symbiotic organism when kept in balance. It only becomes pathogenic when the conditions are right for its over-proliferation, such as when the immune system is compromised through illness, such as HIV, or through immunosuppressive medical interventions, such as chemotherapy, radiation therapy and organ transplantation, or through the use of many pharmaceutical medications, including antibiotics. Candida overgrowth, known as candidiasis is responsible for the majority of hospital-acquired infections. Common forms of Candida infections are thrush when it is present in the mouth and yeast infection, but presents itself in many other forms and spreads all over the body, inside and out.

A poor diet consisting of refined sugars, simple carbohydrates (which are actually sugar), and other foods with a high-glycemic index, and lack of fiber-rich foods, have been implicated in the overgrowth of Candida[438].

Candida has long been associated with cancer. Many studies are now surfacing which support this hypothesis and demonstrate the mechanisms by which Candida, and other fungi and pathogens lead to cancer. According to a review of the scientific literature, "the most recent findings demonstrate that [Candida] albicans is capable of promoting cancer by several mechanisms, as described in the review: production of carcinogenic byproducts, triggering of inflammation, induction of Th17 response and molecular mimicry"[439].

Candida proliferates in an overly acidic environment that is consequently low in oxygen. Ironically, as will be discussed below, Candida waste products lead to a further reduction of blood and tissue oxygenation, which worsens the acidic state of the body. Whether Candida leads to cancer or simply feeds its proliferation, the fact is, the same environment that leads to Candida overgrowth also leads to the formation and proliferation of cancer.

In an article on yeast and inflammation by Dr. Carolyn Dean MD ND[440], she states that "Candida albicans is a fungus living in our intestines that produces 180 chemical toxins capable of making you feel dizzy and fatigued, shutting down your thyroid, throwing your hormones off balance, and causing you to crave sugar and alcohol, and gain weight. It's associated with PMS, loss of libido, painful intercourse, infertility, numbness, tingling, MS, Crohn's, colitis, IBS, acne, Lupus, insomnia, drowsiness, white tongue, breath bad [sic], body odor, sinusitis, bruising, sore throat, bronchitis, shortness of breath, heart palpitations, spots in front of eyes, and dozens more symptoms ... [it is] the culmination of the side effects of drug and food technology and the disservices of our stressful way of life. The miracle of antibiotics has its downside as an underlying cause of yeast overgrowth. The refining of sugar and wheat has its downside by creating a simple food source for yeast. The tremendous levels of stress hormones that flood our bodies daily, hourly, and every minute in our sped up world also make us prey to yeast".

She goes on to say that among the many toxins that Candida produces through its metabolism of sugars, acetaldehyde, a potent toxin, "readily combines with red blood cells, proteins, and enzymes; travels to all parts of the body; and even passes through the blood brain barrier. It damages the structure of red blood cells making them unable to squeeze through tiny capillaries to convey oxygen to needy tissues. Acetaldehyde also blocks the attachment of oxygen to red blood cells." This effect of acetaldehyde contributes to the acidification of the body and the formation and proliferation of cancer. I highly recommend reading the rest of Dr. Dean's article, which includes recommendations for eliminating Candida overgrowth.

IARC has classified acetaldehyde as a Group 1 carcinogen[441], meaning that it is a known carcinogen in humans and animals. It is in the same group with arsenic, benzene, asbestos, and many other known carcinogens.

3.6.2   Sugar

Sugar is a general term used to describe sweet, short-chain, soluble carbohydrates, such as table sugar (sucrose). When consumed, sucrose is converted to glucose and fructose. Glucose and fructose, as well as galactose, are "simple sugars", or monosaccharides. Galactose is also known as milk sugar, which combined with glucose make the disaccharide lactose, which most of the world's population cannot digest.

Monosaccharides are the most basic units of carbohydrates. Glucose and galactose are absorbed rapidly, while fructose is absorbed slowly. However, it is now well documented in the scientific literature that cancers' main fuel sources are simple sugars, such as glucose and fructose. Cancer cells metabolize sugar at a rate 15 times higher than normal cells due to their inefficient metabolism. Various animal and human studies have shown that the mortality rate from cancer is directly proportional to sugar intake[442]. Those results have also shown that a lowering of sugar intake resulting in hypoglycemia reduces mortality.

Normal cells can use glucose as an energy source, but they also have other options, like ketones, which cancer cells cannot use. Coconut oil is a medium chain triglyceride, which is metabolized to ketones in the liver. The added benefit of ketones is that, unlike sugars, they do not get stored as fat, and do not require insulin[443]. In light of this information, it is important to keep sugar consumption (especially processed and artificial sugars) to a minimum in daily life. If you are battling cancer, it is recommended that you eliminate all sugars, with the exception of small amounts of sugars from vegetables, such as carrots, and increase the amount of healthy saturated fats, such as those in organic extra virgin coconut oil, or avocado, which contains health-promoting monounsaturated oils. Healthy cells will use those oils for energy, while cancer cells will be unable to do so.

3.7   NATURAL CANCER CURES (CONT.)

3.7.1   <u>Frankincense</u>

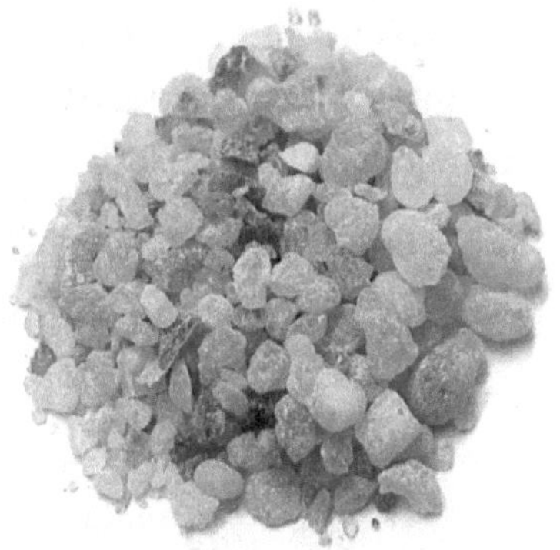

Image source: WikiMedia Commons

Frankincense is a resin obtained from the Boswellia tree. It has been in use for over 5,000 years and has been mentioned multiple times in both the old and new testaments.

The component of frankincense which has been reported to have the highest anti-cancer activity is boswellic acid, although other compounds have been shown to have anti-cancer effects as well. Note that steam and hydro distilled frankincense oils contain only trace amounts to no amount at all of boswellic acids. Boswellic acid concentrations in frankincense extracts are much higher (40% to 60%).

Studies on frankincense oils and extracts have been shown to cause selective cancer cell death by multiple routs. A 2009 study on bladder cancer cells demonstrated that "Frankincense oil can discriminate bladder cancer cells and normal urothelial cells in culture. The oil suppresses cell survival and induces apoptosis in cultured bladder cancer cells."[444] A 2014 study reported the same results, on the same cell-lines as the 2009 study, stating that "frankincense essential oil elicited selective cancer cell death via NRF-2-mediated oxidative stress"[445]. Frankincense has been reported to be effective against other cancer lines as well, such as colon cancer[446], chemoresistant prostate cancer[447], and many others[448]. In addition to being effective against cancer, frankincense also has neuroprotective properties and improves cognition. It also has anti-inflammatory, antiseptic, expectorant, tissue / wound healing, and many other properties.

3.7.2   <u>Myrrh</u>

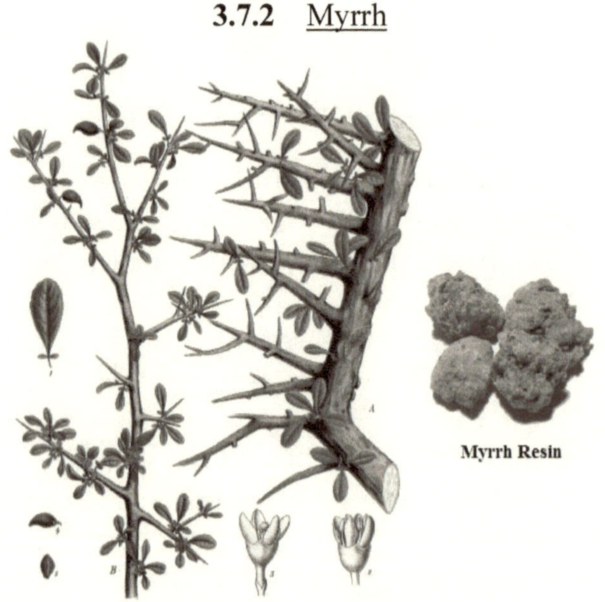

Image source: Wikipedia

Although myrrh, like frankincense has been in use for thousands of years, it has been conjectured that the source of myrrh from ancient times was derived from a different species of tree than today's myrrh. The research presented will be in regard to the myrrh being used in the modern era.

Myrrh and its active ingredient Guggulsterone (GS) has been shown to kill cancer cells through multiple routes. One review of the scientific literature notes that "There is a growing evidence now that GS is capable of preventing tumor growth and proliferation through activation of pro-apoptotic and inhibition of anti-apoptotic signaling pathways ... GS has been shown to cause effects on the biological function of cells including cell proliferation, angiogenesis, inflammatory response and apoptotic cells death in cancers cells"[449].

The authors site many studies that demonstrate myrrh's effectiveness against multiple types of aggressive and drug-resistant cancers, including pancreatic cancer, head and neck squamous cell carcinoma, esophageal adenocarcinoma, colon cancer, breast cancer, prostate cancer, and liver cancer.

A limited number of studies into lung cancer, ovarian cancer, leukemia, lymphoma, and multiple myeloma using Guggulsterone have also shown promising results.

3.7.3   <u>GcMAF</u>

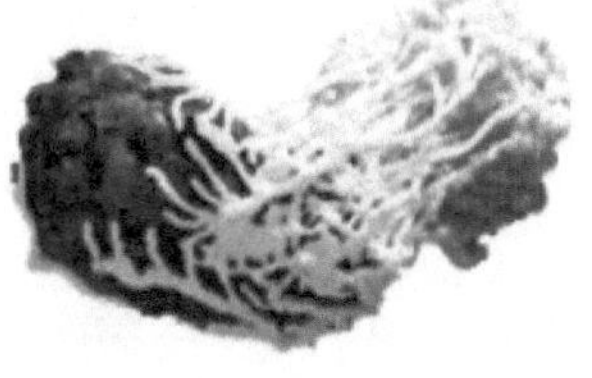

In the process of tumor invasion, cancerous cells secrete nagalase - an extracellular matrix-degrading enzyme. Nagalase is also secreted by viral-infected cells. In other words, nagalase breaks down the scaffolding surrounding cells, thereby allowing the cancerous or infected cell to invade surrounding tissue. Elevated nagalase in the blood therefore points to either an active viral load or cancer. Likewise, if you are undergoing cancer treatments and the level of nagalase in your blood decrease, it is a good indication that the treatments are having a positive effect.

In addition to facilitating tumor invasion, nagalase also degrades the immune system by deglycosylating the vitamin D3-binding Gc-protein, which is the precursor for the major macrophage-activating factor (MAF). "Macrophage activation for phagocytosis and antigen presentation is the first step in the immune development cascade. Lost precursor activity, therefore, leads to immune suppression."[450]

Most, if not all cancers secrete nagalase, and elevated nagalase blood levels are a good indication of cancer (of course when viral infection is ruled out) even before tumors can be detected through imaging technologies.

Treatment with GcMAF, or Gc protein-derived macrophage activating factor, has been shown to lower blood concentrations of nagalase and have a positive effect against cancer. There is much controversy surrounding GcMAF as a treatment for cancer, HIV and many other diseases and infections, but all of the pushback seems to be from organizations that are not interested in alternatives to the current status quo.

GcMAF is available in various forms, including injection, nebulization, suppositories, as well as oral preparations.

3.7.4   <u>COX-2 Inhibition</u>

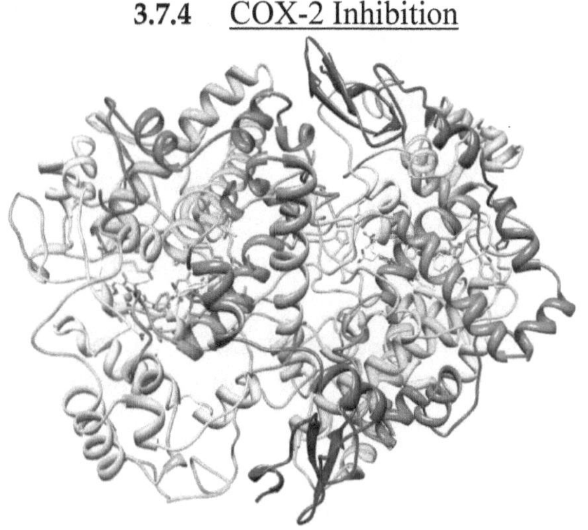

Image source: Wikipedia

Cyclooxygenase-2 (COX-2) is an induced isoform of the cyclooxygenase family of enzymes. It is upregulated during both inflammation and cancer. It has been reported that COX-2 plays a role in cell proliferation, cancer progression, and tumor invasion. Inhibition of COX-2 has been shown to reduce the incidence of many types of cancer, however, synthetic drugs which downregulate COX-2, such as NSAIDs, while having a positive effect on cancer, have had a negative effect on cardiovascular health.

Natural COX-2 inhibitors however have been shown to be much safer, and include bromalain (present in pineapples), curcumin (present in turmeric), coumarin (found in numerous plants and spices), fisetin (a plant flavonoid), sulforaphane (found in cruciferous vegetables), apigenin (a flavone found in many plants), EGCG (from green tea), butein (a chalconoid found in various flowering plants), and willow bark extract[451], all of which can be found in whole foods and concentrated supplement form, and all of which have been shown to have many additional health benefits.

COX-2 inhibition has also been shown to inhibit cancer cell proliferation as well as to sensitize cancer cells to other treatments, making other treatments more effective[452].

"Growth factors such as IGF-I increase cox-2 expression by several complementary mechanisms; hence, decreased cox-2 activity may play a role in the remarkably low mortality from 'Western' cancers enjoyed by Third World cultures in which systemic growth factor activity was minimized by quasi-vegan diets complemented by leanness and excellent muscle insulin sensitivity."[453]

Salicylic acid (SA) is the active ingredient in Aspirin – an NSAID drug. It has been shown to reduce the risk of cancer by a third when taken daily over many years. As mentioned before, NSAID drugs have their own issues. Luckily, salicylic acid is ubiquitous in natural foods:

"SA is ubiquitously present in fruits and vegetables, and herbs and spices contain the highest concentrations."[454] "Red chilli powder, paprika, and turmeric contained total salicylates in excess of 0.1% (by weight), and cumin, an ingredient used in very large amounts in Indian cookery, had a content of >1.5% (by weight), most of which was the phenolic acid itself."[455]

"Consequently, populations that incorporate substantial amounts of spices in foods may have markedly higher daily intakes of salicylates. Indeed, it has been suggested that the low incidence of colorectal cancer among Indian populations may be ascribed in part to high exposure to dietary salicylates throughout life from spice consumption".[456]

3.8   ALTERNATIVE CANCER THERAPIES AND PROTOCOLS

First, let me address the stance of the allopathic medical community on natural, alternative cancer treatments. Although our history is full with snake oil salesmen, the therapies and protocols outlined below are backed by scientific research. Additionally, as I've stated before, the medical industry – especially the pharmaceutical industry – do not like competition, and they go to extraordinary lengths to suppress competition – especially natural substances which cannot be patented, and therefore cannot make them a profit. Towards the goal of eliminating competition, they fabricate phony studies, suppress scientists with threats and bribery, and even resort to murder.

In August 1987, a U.S. federal court found the American Medical Association guilty of conspiracy to destroy the chiropractic profession[457].

A 1953 Fitzgerald report commissioned by congress found the American Medical Association, the American Cancer Society and other orthodox medical organizations guilty of conspiracy to suppress alternative cancer treatments which have been shown to be effective, and were worthy of further studies. The report stated the following in regard to the orthodox medical community:

"Behind and over all this Is the weirdest conglomeration of corrupt motives, intrigue, selfishness, jealousy, obstruction, and conspiracy that I have ever seen."[458,459]

World cancer expert Dr. Samuel S. Epstein, M.D., a recipient of the Right Livelihood Award for his contributions on avoidable causes of cancer stated:

"That the NCI (National Cancer Institute), with enthusiastic support from the ACS (American Cancer Society) – the tail that wags the NCI dog – has effectively blocked funding for research and clinical trials on promising non-toxic alternative cancer drugs for decades, in favor of highly toxic and largely ineffective patented drugs developed by the multibillion dollar global cancer drug industry. Additionally, the cancer establishment has systematically harassed the proponents of non-toxic alternative cancer drugs"

Keep in mind that most of the protocols outlined below, on their own, might not do enough to combat cancer. In order to effectively eliminate cancer, it must be attacked from every direction, with each protocol having its own unique effect, with some overlap between protocols. You should do research on your type of cancer to learn what its weaknesses are in order to come up with a treatment plan that will most effectively exploit those weaknesses. Consult alternative practitioners to help you along. Also consult a qualified physician, who is open to alternative and traditional therapies, to make sure that you do not have contraindications that would prevent you from conforming to your treatment, such as a condition, sickness, or a medication that you are taking that might negatively interact with a substance that you plan on taking. There is no substitute for research.

3.8.1 Sodium Bicarbonate (Baking Soda) Protocol

Sodium bicarbonate, more commonly known as baking soda, is an amazing, versatile, and essential substance for health. Bicarbonates are present in soils, plants, and in the human body, and play an essential role in the physiological pH buffering system.

Sodium bicarbonate has been used medically for over 100 years, and has been in use over 1,000 years ago in Hindu medicine for various health issues, including cancer[460]. It is used in hospital settings intravenously to combat acidosis, and it is also used orally for acid reflux. Additionally, it is used as a treatment of hyperkalemia – a condition resulting from elevated levels of potassium in blood serum, in aspirin and tricyclic antidepressant overdoses, bone loss, and various other conditions.

As mentioned previously, in acidic conditions, the body will leach calcium carbonate and calcium phosphate out of the bones and muscles, leading to bone loss. Administration of sodium bicarbonate and potassium bicarbonate are used to raise the pH of the body, increasing absorption of calcium in bones and increasing bone strength.

There is much debate in the scientific community as to whether sodium bicarbonate directly kills cancer, and research is continuing. However, here is what we know:

Cancer is not a cause – it's a result of dysregulation and dysfunction caused by years of exposures to toxins from food, the environment and the mind. Truly curing cancer therefore cannot be done by solely attacking the cancer, and any therapy that addresses the underlying dysregulations and dysfunctions is therefore worthwhile, especially when there are minimal to no adverse side effects.

Sodium bicarbonate very quickly and safely raises body pH (alkalinity). Alkalinity facilitates blood and cell oxygenation, while the opposite is true for acidic conditions. Cell oxygenation is absolutely crucial to all body function and the lack thereof leads to disease. Oxygen is also toxic to cancer cells.

It is well known that acidic conditions cause inflammation, and the reverse effect is true of alkaline conditions. Inflammation is a major contributor to cancer development, growth and proliferation.

Most of the enzymes responsible for cancer cell invasion and proliferation require an acidic microenvironment and will be denatured in an alkaline environment. Administration of sodium bicarbonate in drinking water has been shown to greatly reduce circulating tumor cells in the blood, thereby reducing metastasis, as well as reducing various cancer biomarkers[461,462], showing that it does have a direct effect on cancer's ability to carry out its functions. Maintaining stress on the cancer, preventing its proliferation and functions, and decreasing its growth and viability, "essential glycolytic ATP production [in the cancer cells] will be exhausted to the point of collapsing energy utilization."[463] Doing so, while at the same time attacking it with other cancer-fighting phytochemicals and natural substances is therefore a winning strategy.

For solid cancers, the most effective way of treating with sodium bicarbonate is to bring it in contact with the cancer/tumor. For example, in digestive tract cancers, the best means of administration is orally (drinking sodium bicarbonate in water). For skin cancers, making a paste with sodium bicarbonate and a little bit of water and applying directly to the affected area is most effective. Enemas for rectal cancers, douches for vaginal/uterus cancers, and nebulized/aerosolized sodium bicarbonate for upper respiratory and lung cancers

With oral administration, you want to raise your urine pH to a higher level than normal body pH in order to have a positive effect. In this instance, you will want to raise your urine pH to 8 – 8.5 and maintain it there for no longer than 5 days in a row. Thereafter you should discontinue using sodium bicarbonate and let your pH stabilize at 7 – 7.5. Periodically (especially if you are having a hard time maintaining normal pH) you can repeat the protocol.

Caution!

Raising your pH too high for an extended period of time can lead to adverse health conditions, so while taking sodium bicarbonate, you will want to monitor your urine pH daily using litmus paper (pH strips).

Dr. Tullio Simoncini – an Italian Oncologist – after researching the commonalities between the various types of cancer had concluded that cancer is a result of fungal infection by Candida Albicans – an opportunistic organism that under normal conditions lives symbiotically in the body, but proliferates under acidic conditions. While there is no scientific consensus that Simoncini's hypothesis is correct, it is well known that candida and cancer go hand-in-hand. At the same time, Dr. Simoncini has a great track record in curing many cancer patients using sodium bicarbonate. On his website (www.curenaturalicancro.com), he gives protocols for nearly every type of cancer.

For more information on Dr. Simoncini's research and the waves it made in the scientific community, watch the documentary "Cancer – the forbidden cures"[464] (time: 1:11:59).

With that being said, acidity is also not a cause, but rather a symptom of bad eating habits, which brings us to the next protocol:

3.8.2   The Gerson Diet
(The Gerson Institute / CHIPSA Hospital)

The Gerson diet was developed by German Dr. Max Gerson M.D.   Dr. Gerson's journey began when a diet he was developing for himself to treat his migraines had also cured one of his patients of skin tuberculosis, leading to the establishment of a special skin tuberculosis treatment program at the Munich University Hospital. "In a carefully monitored clinical trial, 446 out of 450 skin tuberculosis patients treated with the Gerson diet recovered completely".[465]   As time progressed, the Gerson diet was successfully applied to every other form of tuberculosis, type II diabetes, heart disease, kidney failure, cancer, and many other chronic diseases, many of which are incurable by modern medicine's standards.

After moving to the United States, in 1938 Dr. Gerson was licensed to practice medicine in New York. For the next twenty years, Dr. Gerson proceeded to successfully treat cancer patients whose conventional treatments had failed and were told they were going to die.

The Gerson therapy hinges on two principles:

1) that cancer is caused by a toxic load, and therefore toxins need to be removed from the body through proper nutrition and chelation therapies, and

2) that the body's inability to defend itself against the cancer and other conditions is due to deficiencies in vitamins, minerals, enzymes, beneficial bacteria, and other biologically necessary constituents.

The Gerson therapy aims to treat the whole body, mind and spirit, rather than the cancer. In other words, the Gerson therapy does not treat cancer – it treats the underlying problems in the body, and once the body is healed, it will eliminate the cancer on its own. Participants in the Gerson therapy are expected to change their lifestyles in support of this goal. For this reason, the Gerson therapy has been very successful, not just at eliminating cancer, but eliminating many other chronic diseases at the same time – many of which the allopathic medical community has labeled "incurable", such as arthritis, multiple sclerosis, diabetes, digestive disorders, heart disease, and many others.

Caution!

The diet and supplementation portion of the therapy rapidly releases toxins from the organs and tissues of the body. The toxins are released into the bloodstream to be disposed of and if not combined with the proper chelation protocols will end up back in the liver and could cause complications. For this reason, it is important to consult with a certified Gerson Therapy practitioner prior to beginning the protocol.

Although the American Cancer Society, the National Cancer Institute, and other "cancer authorities" claim that there is no merit to the Gerson therapy, the scientific literature begs to differ. A very large number of studies have shown that the kind of diet that the Gerson therapy utilizes is associated with decreased cancer rates, decreased heart disease, decreased diabetes, and every other chronic disease, and an increase in general health. On the other hand, the gold standard therapies that those cancer organizations promote are carcinogenic in themselves, they destroy the immune system, and they cause more death and disease than any other treatment in the history of medicine, which spans thousands of years. Even the up-and-coming targeted genetic and hormonal cancer therapies that the cancer cartel is currently pushing, have been shown to have devastating effects in most of their patients, such as autoimmune diseases, where the immune system attacks healthy cells, causing extreme pain and permanent damage to tissues and organs. Clearly, the authority which they've bestowed upon themselves is misplaced and unwarranted.

Opponents of the Gerson therapy like to point out the few cases where the therapy did not cure patients of their cancers. However, keep in mind that the death rate from the "gold standard in cancer therapy" – chemotherapy and radiation – is 97%, and nearly all of those patients die as a result of the treatment, not the cancer, and of those that survive, their quality of life is seriously degraded. With the Gerson therapy, quality of life is not only improved, but full health is usually restored.

"It is not necessary for healthy persons to care so much about enough or too many carbohydrates and proteins, and their caloric value should be ignored. However, one cannot ignore the absolutely necessary minerals, vitamins and enzymes in their most natural composition and in sufficient amounts for a relatively long term and remain unpunished."

Dr. Gerson; Book - "The Gerson Therapy: The Proven Nutritional Program for Cancer and Other Illnesses"

I find it laughable that opponents of cancer diets keep on saying that cancer diets can be dangerous. Have they looked at pharmaceuticals lately? Drinking water in excess can kill you. Generally speaking, cancer diets are not in themselves dangerous – the danger stems from inappropriate application of the diet, or not getting sufficient nutrition due to lack of diversity in the foods consumed, which could be alleviated with supplementation if necessary. If there is ever doubt, periodic bloodwork can put those concerns to rest, rather than demonizing the method. How many pharmaceutical drugs require periodic bloodwork to ensure liver toxicity does not go out of control? I don't see the industry demonizing those drugs.

Back in 2004, Prince Charles was speaking in front of a group of doctors, when he recalled the experience of a friend of his, whom had cancer, and was treated for it using all of the conventional methods. At the conclusion of her treatment, her doctors told her that there is nothing more they can do and that she will die of her cancer. He then said that after receiving that news, she had changed her diet and did the Gerson therapy, and that it is now seven years later, and she's alive and well. He did not claim to have any understanding as to what the therapy entails or even how it works, but nevertheless, the scientific community and the pharmaceutical industry put words in his mouth and attacked him – calling him crazy, and a criminal that should be hung. The controversy had encircled the world. It only stopped when they realized that they were giving free publicity to the Gerson therapy.

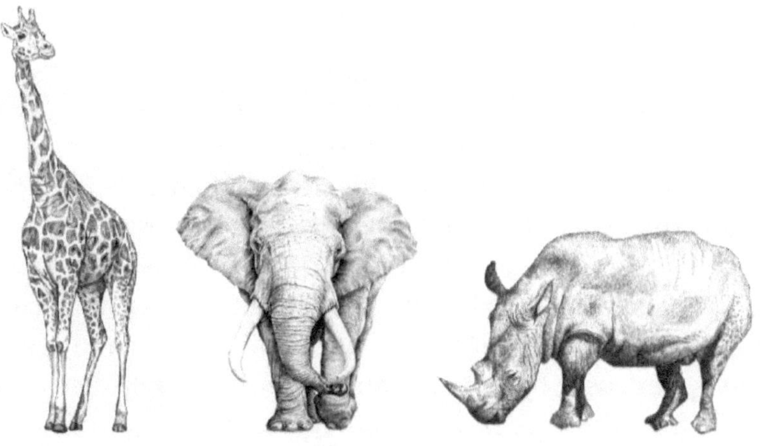

Another nonsense argument that the medical community uses in opposition to the Gerson therapy, and other vegan diets is "protein deficiency".

The largest land animals in the world are all herbivores. You might ask yourself – where are they getting their protein? The answer, of course, is from plant food. Grasses, leaves, barks, etc. Looking at those huge, amazingly strong, magnificent animals should bring into question the decades of indoctrination leading us to believe that we need to consume large amounts of protein from animal flesh and milk to support our growth and health. As a matter of fact, there are many vegan athletes, such as world-record holder Patrik Baboumian; strongman, and world-record holder Fiona Oakes; marathon and ultradistance runner who compete alongside their meat-eating counterparts.

Charlotte Gerson who runs The Gerson Institute has been a vegan for decades. She is now 95 years old, and she does not have osteoporosis, arthritis, cardiovascular disease or any other chronic condition. She is sharper than most people a fraction of her age, and she regularly gives hour-long lectures. Many of her lectures and interviews are on YouTube, and you should certainly watch them.

Protein deficiency is very rare in people eating sufficient calories. Still there are those who claim that there are millions of people all over the world who are protein deficient. While that is true, what they fail to mention is that those are mainly people in poor demographics who do not consume enough food / calories. So really, the issue is not protein sufficiency, but food sufficiency, or caloric sufficiency. Yes, some vegans or vegetarians who do not eat a diverse enough diet could suffer from protein deficiency, but it is rare.

On the other hand, most Americans get too much protein. Bacon and eggs for breakfast, chicken for lunch, steak for dinner, day after day. Excess protein has its own problems, especially when not getting sufficient fiber as well. Proteolytic enzymes – the ones responsible for breaking down protein, can only break down a certain amount of protein per day. Undigested or partially digested proteins lead to kidney damage, leaky guy syndrome, brain fog, and other health issues.

A recent study[466] of 71,751 subjects, the largest of its kind, evaluated the diets of non-vegetarians, semi vegetarians, pesco vegetarians, lacto-ovo vegetarians and strict vegetarians, and they had found that everyone in the study group had consumed more protein than the average dietary protein requirement of 42g per day, including the strict vegetarians (Fig. 4). They had found that only about 3% of the population do not get the minimum requirement, most likely due to calorie restriction diets or economic reasons. The study also found that more than 97% of the population do not get enough fiber in their diets, with an average consumption of less than half the minimum daily requirement for dietary fiber.

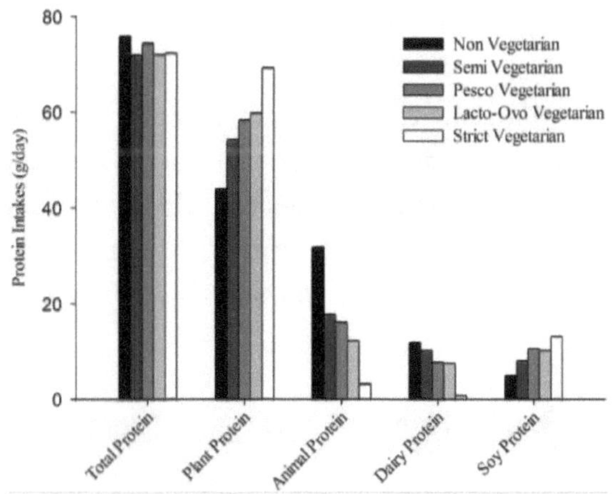

Dietary mean protein intakes by dietary pattern in the AHS-2. Adjustments were made for age, sex and race.

Fig. 4 [466]

According to Charlotte Gerson, most cancer patients also have other chronic diseases. In following the Gerson therapy, it is impossible to cure cancer and not also cure all other chronic diseases. The Gerson Therapy brings the body into homeostasis, and a body in homeostasis cannot support the existence of disease.

3.8.3 High Dose Vitamin C

Just like with sugar, cancer cells love vitamin C (ascorbate). The problem is, vitamin C is oxidized to hydrogen peroxide within the cell, and cancer cells are much less efficient than normal cells at disposing of it. This makes cancer cells much more prone to damage and death from the increased tide of hydrogen peroxide.

It is hypothesized that the reason for this is that some cancer cells have a lower level of catalase than normal cells. Catalase is an enzyme that catalyzes the reduction of hydrogen peroxide to water and oxygen.

Oral intake of vitamin C however is typically insufficient, due to gut metabolism and excretion pathways, which lessens the amount of vitamin C that reaches the blood by a factor of 100 to 500. For this reason, high-dose intravenous vitamin C (IVC) has been utilized successfully in the fight against cancer.

3.8.4 Hyperbaric Oxygen Therapy

Oxygen is essential for higher life forms, and cells require oxygen in order to operate properly. When the level of oxygen goes down, acidity increases, leading to the proliferation of anaerobic bacteria, fungi/yeasts, inflammation, dysfunction and cancer. Likewise, as discussed before, chronic acidifying diets lead to the displacement/reduction of blood oxygen, and therefore cellular oxygen, which leads to all of the aforementioned conditions.

Hyperbaric oxygen therapy (HBOT) is used for many conditions, including serious infections, wounds that will not heal as a result of diabetes or radiation therapy, decompression sickness and bubbles of air in the blood vessels. It is also used in cancer treatment to saturate the blood with oxygen, which cancer cells do not like.

In a hyperbaric chamber, pure oxygen is pressurized to 3 times normal atmospheric pressure, facilitating rapid absorption through the lungs, and saturation of the blood, tissues and organs. Increased blood oxygen promotes the production of therapeutic chemicals in the body.

Hyperbaric therapy along with a ketogenic diet has been shown to have significant anti-cancer benefits.

3.8.5   Ketogenic Diet

The ketogenic diet is a low-carb, high fat diet. Keep two things in mind: sugars are carbs, and not all fats are healthy fats. Coconut oil is an excellent choice. While it is a saturated fat, and saturated fats (for no good reason) have been demonized, it is not like other saturated fats from animal products. Coconut oil is a medium chain triglyceride, and unlike other fats, it is sent directly to the liver to be processed for energy and ketone bodies. Coconut oil, unlike saturated fats from animal products, also does not contain any cholesterol, not that cholesterol is bad for your health – it is absolutely essential for every cell in the body, and especially the brain, which contains 25% of all cholesterol in the body.

Coconut oil is also the easiest oil to use because it actually tastes good and can be eaten by itself, mixed into shakes, and cooked with. It is also one of the heathiest oils to cook with for the reason that, unlike most oils, it is very stable at high temperatures and does not break down into toxic byproducts. While olive oil is a very healthy oil, it is very sensitive to heat damage, and therefore should only be used cold – never for cooking. Avocados / avocado oil and hemp seed hearts / hemp seed oil are also excellent fat sources.

As a matter of fact, hemp seeds are one of the most nutritious foods on the planet. Hemp seeds have significant amounts of all 9 essential amino acids (the basic building blocks of protein), which is rare in plant foods. Also, unlike soy and beans, which are also high in amino acids, and even meat; hemp seeds do not contain trypsin inhibitors. Trypsin is an enzyme that is present in the digestive tract and is involved in the breakdown of proteins. For this reason, amino acids from hemp are assimilated in their entirety, while proteins from meat for example are not – due to the trypsin inhibitors. Additionally, hemp has 33g of protein per 100g serving, while beef has only 28g per 100g serving.

Hemp seeds also have a perfect balance of omega-3 to omega-6 essential fatty acids, and many vitamins and minerals that are critical for a healthy immune system.

Ketones, unlike sugar, do not turn into fat.

The goal of the ketogenic diet is to induce ketosis, whereby the body switches from burning sugar for energy to burning fat for energy. Fat is converted to ketones in the liver, providing energy for the brain, heart and kidneys.

Caution!

People with deficiencies in the enzymes responsible for ketone body synthesis and degradation should not follow ketogenic diets. Typically, people with this deficiency will get ill in periods of fasting.

Ketogenic diets have been shown to have numerous health benefits.

"The effects of ketone body metabolism suggests that mild ketosis may offer therapeutic potential in a variety of different common and rare disease states. These inferences follow directly from the metabolic effects of ketosis and the higher inherent energy present in d-beta-hydroxybutyrate relative to pyruvate, the normal mitochondrial fuel produced by glycolysis leading to an increase in the $\Delta G'$ of ATP hydrolysis. The large categories of disease for which ketones may have therapeutic effects are:

(1) diseases of substrate insufficiency or insulin resistance,
(2) diseases resulting from free radical damage,
(3) disease resulting from hypoxia."[467]

Ketogenic diets are associates with better weight-loss as compared with low-fat / caloric restriction diets. Again, be mindful of the source and type of fats. Ketogenic diets comprised of animal products, such as the Atkin's diet, are extremely toxic.

The biggest benefit from the ketogenic diet is the elimination of sugars, which as discussed before, is responsible for nearly every chronic disease, including cancer.

3.8.6   The Budwig Protocol

The Budwig protocol was developed by German scientist Dr. Johanna Budwig – a seven-time Nobel Prize nominee. Dr. Budwig was an expert in fats and oils.

The Budwig protocol hinges on the combination of flaxseed oil (a highly unsaturated fat) with low fat cottage cheese, or quark cheese (a sulfur protein-containing cheese).

"The mixing of the oil and cottage cheese allows for the chemical reaction to take place between the sulfur protein in the cottage cheese and the oil, which makes the oil water soluble for easy absorption into your cells."[468] Flaxseed oil by itself is not well absorbed, and therefore the combination of sulfur proteins is essential to making it water-soluble and absorbable.

The principle behind this therapy is that the mixture promotes cell oxygenation. As a matter of fact, flaxseed oil is used in oil-based paints to promote faster drying through oxygen permeation. Unlike other highly processed oils, flaxseed oil contains electron-rich fatty acids, which are critical for proper cell division and other cellular processes.

The protocol also heals the body's ability to absorb the energy from sunlight, which is highly deficient in people with cancer. Sunlight exposure is critical for proper functioning of the digestive system and detoxification systems of the body. Many cancer patients cannot tolerate the sun. The Budwig protocol restores the body's ability to tolerate sun exposure.

"electrons in our food serve as the resonance system for the sun's energy and are truly the element of life. Man acts as an antenna for the sun. The interplay between the photons in the sunbeams and the electrons in the seed oils and our foods governs all the vital functions of the body."[468]

Healthy, highly unsaturated, electron-rich fats are absolutely crucial to our health. Without healthy fats, internal organs dry out, the digestive system is more prone to acid erosion and disease, and the immune system is compromised. Fats/oils which have been processed to last longer on the shelf, have been stripped of their electrons, making them less susceptible to oxidation, but also making them highly toxic, leading to heart disease and other ailments.

The following video shows how to prepare the oil-protein mixture:

- Budwig Diet Flaxseed Oil & Cottage Cheese, available on:
    - https://www.youtube.com/watch?v=RSoddptWL0s
    - www.budwig-videos.com

- The protocol can also be found here:
    - https://www.cancertutor.com/budwig/

Caution!

People with liver, gallbladder, or pancreatic disease should start slowly and work themselves up. Also keep in mind that the Budwig protocol takes time to work, and should be combined with other clean, high-nutrient diets, such as the Gerson diet. Also, keep cottage cheese / quark cheese consumption to a minimum, and combine with lots of plant based foods for the reasons discussed previously regarding animal proteins, especially if you have a weak digestion.

In the scientific literature, flaxseed and flaxseed oil has been shown to have anti-cancer effects[469,470,471], as well as cardioprotective effects against arsenic poisoning from arsenic trioxide-based chemotherapeutic medications[472].

3.8.7   Vitamin B17 / Laetrile / Amygdalin

Vitamin B17, Laetrile, and Amygdalin are more-or-less different names for the same substance, however it is not actually a vitamin. Amygdalin (the natural form) is found in many plants, but in highest concentrations in the kernels of stone fruit, such as apricot, peach, bitter almond, and plum, as well as in apple seeds.

"The LD50 [lethal dose - the amount of an ingested substance that kills 50 percent of a test sample] for ingestion is 50-200 milligrams, or 1-3 milligrams per kilogram of body weight, calculated as hydrogen cyanide."[473]   Lower doses have caused adverse reactions requiring hospitalization.

The only reason I am mentioning Vitamin B17 / Laetrile / Amygdalin is because it is so widely cited by proponents of natural cures, and while I have read the science and believe that it is a viable cure, and in small quantities, critical for good health, I believe that the upper dosing limit is very critical and it is too risky for self-administration, and there are so many other, safe options. Certainly, the amount of cyanide that you would get from apple seeds is insignificant, and I regularly juice, or add apples to my shakes, seeds-and-all, with no adverse effect.

3.8.8   Colon Hydrotherapy

Colon cleansing is a process that has been practiced for millennia. The ancient Egyptian Edwin Smith Papyrus (from around 1,700 BCE) and Ebers Papyrus (from around 1,550 BCE) prescribe the use of enemas to cleans the bowels.

"Enemas were known in ancient Sumeria, Babylonia, India, Greece and China … there is hardly a region of the world where people did not discover or adapt the enema."[474]

The human colon (large intestines) is about five feet long. Over many years, lots of waste can accumulate in the colon and cause disease. You can have 20 pounds or more of waste in your colon that could remain there for weeks, months, or even years. Waste in the colon that has become stagnant is linked to leaky guy syndrome, diverticulosis, diverticulitis, polyps, cancer, compromised immune system, prostate issues, hernias (from pressure buildup), and even halitosis (bad breath), giving a whole new meaning to the colloquialism "your breath smells like sh…".

A buildup of toxins in the colon from layers of fecal matter and poisonous waste can cause toxic chemicals to leach into your bloodstream, causing fatigue, headaches, and even serious, chronic diseases.

"John Harvey Kellogg, M.D. reported in the 1917 Journal of American Medicine that in the treatment of gastrointestinal disease, in over 40,000 cases, he used surgery in only 20 cases. The rest were helped as a result of cleansing the bowels, diet, and exercise."[474]

According to Betsy Exton, MA[475] – an I-ACT Advanced Certified colon hydrotherapist who is one of only a very few therapists that work for the world-renowned Tony Robbins, colon hydrotherapy opens up the haustra (pockets) in the colon, releasing the buildup of stagnant waste, and hydrates the colon. According to Exton, stress, lack of fiber in the diet, lack of exercise, and depletion of nutrients prevents elimination, and colon hydrotherapy gently, safely, and effectively hydrates and dislodges waste from the colon and carries it out of the body. In her years of working with her patients she has seen people have increased clarity and focus, improved vision, a reduction in aches and inflammation, and a greatly improved immune system.

Colon cleanses can be done at home, but it is highly recommended that you go to an I-ACT (International Association for Colon Therapy) certified colon hydrotherapist, who will have the equipment to do a proper and safe cleanse. If your hydrotherapist is not using an FDA approved colonic irrigation system that is regularly maintained, look for another practitioner.

Note: Colon hydrotherapy should not be performed on people who have had part or all of their colon surgically resected, or people who have had radiation therapy or chemotherapy. Those therapies may weaken the integrity of the colon and there is a risk of tears occurring from the procedure. There are other contraindications to be aware of. Consult a qualified colon hydrotherapist to make sure you are eligible for the procedure.

3.8.9   Dietary Fiber

Nearly the entire population of the United States is deficient in dietary fiber. Meat contains no dietary fiber at all, while plant foods are high in fiber. Dietary fiber is not only necessary, but is critical in many ways. It maintains a healthy body by:

- Removing toxic waste products from our intestinal tract. Removing toxins from the intestines keeps our immune system functioning properly. Toxin buildup in the intestines due to lack of dietary fiber leads to diverticulosis and colon cancer.

- Slowing down the absorption of sugars into the bloodstream. Eating low-fiber, sugary foods causes a spike in blood-sugar. On the other hand, even with high sugar-content fruits and vegetables, the sugar is released into the bloodstream slowly and steadily, preventing blood-sugar spikes. For this reason, eating a diet high in fiber is crucial for diabetics.

- Promoting the growth of beneficial bacteria in the intestinal tract, which builds up and maintains the proper function of the immune system.

- Binding to excess hormones and pharmaceutical drugs in our bloods and carrying them out of the body. This helps detoxify, and eliminate or alleviate hormone related conditions, such as PMS, menopausal hot flashes, and reproductive organ cancers.

- Eliminating excess cholesterol, which lowers LDL ("bad" cholesterol) levels.

- Facilitating the proper flow of waste through the intestines, which prevents constipation and hemorrhoids.

3.8.10 Exercise

There is no doubt that exercise promotes healing in many ways. Sweating releases toxins through the skin. Exercise also helps with clearing out the bowels. Additionally, since the lymphatic system does not have a pump, like the cardiovascular system does, movement is essential for circulating the lymphatic fluids.

The lymphatic system is responsible for detoxification and fighting bacterial and viral infections. Ayurvedic medicine, thousands of years ago, had described the location, structure, and function of the lymphatic system, and the ailments associated with congested lymph, and how to bring health back to the lymphatic system. Modern science is only now starting to catch up, and not until very recently, modern science discovered that there are lymphatic channels in the brain and central nervous system, draining away toxins and beta-amyloid plaque, which Ayurveda had described all those thousands of years ago. A stagnant lymphatic system – one that does not properly drain away toxins and fight infections is linked to metastasis and tumors, among many other ailments.

Cardiovascular exercise has many benefits, including reduction of stress, strengthening of the heart and lungs, improved sleep, improved mood and mental clarity, and even a reduction in the risk of cancer. Exercise also increases blood oxygenation, which as discussed previously is a critical component in the fight against cancer.

Although exercise is very beneficial, for healthy and sick people alike, depending on your state of health, it might not be a good idea to do strenuous exercise. Consult your physician to determine how much you can do, but consider that some level of movement is essential for restoring your health.

3.8.11 Oral Health

Poor oral health is known to cause a whole host of diseases, including cardiovascular diseases, respiratory infections, dementia, and even cancer.

Dental fillings which contain mercury are known to leach small amounts of mercury into the bloodstream over a period of many years. Another rout of exposure from mercury-containing fillings is mercury vapor. Mercury bioaccumulates and is extremely destructive to the central nervous system and cardiovascular system. It is also carcinogenic.

Root canals can also lead to extensive health complications, including death. When a root canal is performed, the cavity is disinfected, but most times, the disinfection process is insufficient. When the cavity is sealed, it creates the perfect environment for anaerobic bacteria to proliferate. Those bacteria then release highly toxic byproducts into the bloodstream, which can lead to a weakened immune system, disease, cancer, and even death.

If you have amalgam fillings, it is very important that you replace them with biologically compatible fillings. However, you should go to a qualified holistic or biological dentist, because they are trained in proper amalgam removal, and if the amalgam fillings are not removed properly, large amounts of mercury and other toxins can be released into your body.

For qualified, accredited practitioners in your area, visit the websites of the International Academy of Oral Medicine and Toxicology (IAOMT), the International Academy of Biological Dentistry and Medicine (IABDM), and the Holistic Dental Association (HDA).

3.9   FOOD COMBINATIONS

The Proper combination of food items is a topic that is so important that it should be a part of standard school curriculum, starting early in life, yet you never hear of it. Which foods are okay to combine and which are not. There are some disagreements between nutritionists on some of those combinations - for example, some say that it is okay to combine cucumbers with tomatoes and some say it is not, but there are several basics that all nutritionists (or at least most) agree on. Just like there are food combinations that are favorable or synergistic, such as adding black pepper to turmeric, which enhances the turmeric's absorption in the body, or rice and beans, which together are considered a complete protein, there are combinations which when eaten together form toxins, or do not get properly digested. Proteins for example require an acidic stomach to break down - they require pepsinogen along with hydrochloric acid to form pepsin, which is an enzyme which breaks down the protein bonds. Carbohydrates (and starches, which are complex carbohydrates) on the other hand require an alkaline stomach because carbohydrate digestion does not occur in the stomach. Carbs begin their digestion in the mouth where enzymes in saliva called salivary amylase start the breakdown of polysaccharides - long chains of sugars in the carbohydrate food. The food is then swallowed and passes through the stomach, where it spends very little time, into the duodenum (the beginning of the small intestines). In the duodenum, the pancreas releases pancreatic amylase to further break down the polysaccharides into disaccharides; a chain of two sugars linked together. The small intestines then produce several other enzymes which further break down the disaccharides into monosaccharides (single sugar molecules), which are then absorbed into the blood through the small intestines. In the large intestines, bacteria break down any of the remaining sugars, and indigestible fiber is passed in the feces.

When for example you combine protein with starch (complex carbs), such as potatoes, or with simple carbs such as bread or pasta, the carbohydrates spend too long in the stomach and begin to ferment, whereby toxic fermentation products are formed and subsequently disturbs the balance of good and harmful bacteria in your gut flora. Those toxins also enter the bloodstream. Many of those toxins cause inflammation and cellular damage which leads to a diseased state over many years, including cancer.

Here are some simple rules to follow:

3.9.1   Fruits

Fruits should be eaten on their own. Give half an hour to an hour before eating protein or starches and at least three hours after. Fruits contain simple sugars and combining them with other foods that require a more complex digestive process will cause those sugars to ferment in the stomach. Melons should be eaten on their own because they do not combine well with other fruits.

3.9.2   Animal Protein & Carbs

Putting the debate as to whether consumption of animal products is healthy or necessary aside, eating steak and potatoes, or pasta with chicken, or chicken between two buns will cause the digestive juices required for the digestion of each of those items to nullify one another. As I mentioned before, animal protein requires an acidic digestion while carbs require an alkaline digestion. Eating those two items together will cause the meat to sit in your stomach for too long and putrefy, while the carbs will ferment. Both will cause the release of harmful toxins. Plant-based proteins are not an issue in this regard.

3.9.3   Soaking Seeds (Cereals, Legumes, Kernels, and Nuts)

Plant seeds are designed to "hibernate" for a long time until the right conditions are present for them to grow. What makes this possible is called "enzyme inhibitors". Enzymes inhibitors are also the reason why seeds are not well digested, because they also inhibit digestive enzymes. There is a way around that however – soaking the seeds overnight will neutralize those enzyme inhibitors and begin the germination process. Dehydrating the seeds after soaking will restore the crispiness of the seeds, if desired.

3.9.4   Cold Drinks with Meals

While there are good arguments for drinking with meals, the fact is, drinking warm liquids aids digestion, while drinking cold liquids hampers digestion. According to Ayurveda, which is a 5,000-year-old science (Ayurveda in Sanskrit means life knowledge) Agni, or "digestive fire", which is the enzymatic processes of digestion, is extinguished by cold temperatures, leading to ama – another Sanskrit word which refers to toxins that develop as the byproducts of poor digestion and metabolism, leading to other digestive and systemic disorders.

Temperature plays a critical role in biology, and enzymes are no exception. Enzymes have an optimal temperature range. At temperatures above and below their optimal range, enzymatic activity decreases, and at temperature extremes they become altogether inactive. For humans, the optimal range is 98.6°F to 107.6°F / 37°C to 42°C. Yes, the body will eventually regulate the temperature of the foods and drinks you consume, but digestion on its own is an energy-intensive process, and using up additional time and energy to warm up the stomach's contents will both strain the body and as mentioned before, will slow down digestion and lead to the creation of toxins.

Throughout the millions of years of human evolution, humans have always eaten in season. It is only in the modern era, with technological advancements and global trade that humans are eating out of season. A large number of scientific studies are showing that eating in season, in synch with the circadian rhythm, has enormous health benefits, and eating out of season causes many ailments.

3.10   THE POWER OF THE MIND

The mind, by far, is the most powerful epigenetic force over your physiology. The mind on its own is capable of creating disease, or curing disease. Emotional traumas, especially those from young age can program your mind for failure and disease. Have you even been called ugly, or useless, or told that you don't deserve certain things? Have you seen lots of people around you dying from cancer and were fearful that you will succumb to the same fate? Because your subconscious mind is literal, all of those emotions and fears generate programs in your subconscious that ensure that what you are focusing on will come to pass.

A 2008 study evaluated the genetic expression of 30 men with low-risk, early-stage prostate cancers who chose not undergo surgery, radiation, or chemotherapy treatments. The men had submitted prostate biopsies to evaluate gene expression at the beginning of the study, and three months later, after undergoing comprehensive lifestyle changes;

"The changes included a plant-based diet (predominant fruits, vegetables, legumes, soy products, and whole grains low in refined carbohydrates), moderate exercise (walking 30 minutes per day), stress management techniques (yoga-based stretching, breathing techniques, meditation, and guided imagery for one hour per day), and participating in a weekly one-hour support group. The diet was supplemented with soy, fish oil (three grams/day), vitamin E (100 units/day), selenium (200 mg/day), and vitamin C (2 grams/day)."[476]

The initial samples were compared to the samples obtained after three months, and the differences were astounding. "We found that many disease-promoting genes (including those associated with cancer, heart disease, and inflammation) were down-regulated or 'turned off', whereas protective, disease-preventing genes were up-regulated or 'turned on' ... These genes are the target of many new drugs that are being developed. Clearly, changing lifestyle is less expensive, and the only side-effects are good ones."[476]

All-in-all, 48 genes were up-regulated and 453 genes were down-regulated.[477]

Note: I do not recommend consuming soy and soy products for two main reasons; 1) soy is very high is phytoestrogens which over the long term can actually cause hormonal imbalances and reproductive organ cancers, and 2) because soy is one of the most prolific GMO crops in the world.

Although this study was not purely a mind exercise, another study that evaluated the effects of mindfulness meditation alone demonstrated the same effects;

"The study investigated the effects of a day of intensive mindfulness practice in a group of experienced meditators, compared to a group of untrained control subjects who engaged in quiet non-meditative activities. After eight hours of mindfulness practice, the meditators showed a range of genetic and molecular differences, including altered levels of gene-regulating machinery and reduced levels of pro-inflammatory genes, which in turn correlated with faster physical recovery from a stressful situation ... The observed effects were seen only in the meditators following mindfulness practice ... an outcome providing proof of principle that mindfulness practice can lead to epigenetic alterations of the genome."[478]

Dissociative personality disorder, also known as multiple personality disorder is obviously not a normal condition, however, in the context of the power of the mind, it illustrates very strongly how much the mind can override physiology. In some people with this disorder, one personality can have blue eyes, and another, brown eyes, and this shift from one color to the other can occur within seconds.

In a 2015 case study[479], the authors describe a female patient named B.T. who exhibits 10 unique personalities. B.T. had an accident at the age of 20 which left her blind. "The expert concluded cortical blindness from craniocerebral trauma".

13 years after the accident, B.T. was referred by a psychiatric clinic to a psychotherapist. While undergoing therapy, one of the 10 personalities – an adolescent male, started regaining his vision. With subsequent therapy sessions, more and more of B.T.'s personalities regained their vision, but still others remained blind, and the switch between sight and blindness states alternated within seconds.

The power of belief, whether religious or otherwise, is merely the power of the subconscious mind acting to carry out what it knows to be true. If outwardly you tell yourself one thing, but your subconscious program is saying the opposite, your efforts are doomed to fail. The subconscious mind is programmed through repetition and emotion. For example – if you are a child whose parents repeatedly tell you how smart you are, it will create a positive emotion, and the repetition will manifest into a subconscious program. One day, one of your classmates calls you stupid. It might create a negative emotion, but surely you will know that not to be the case, because your subconscious program knows what it has been programmed to know. Fast forward a few days and two more classmates call you stupid. Now doubt starts to burrow into the subconscious mind, and the old program is overridden with a new one that says "I am stupid".

There is no difference between this scenario and things that you bring yourself to believe, which might not be true, but nevertheless, your subconscious mind believes are facts, and therefore changes your biology to accommodate those "facts".

Knowing how powerful the mind is at controlling physiological conditions and genetic expressions, it is very important to surround yourself with people who will support you with your treatment choices. Negativity, breeding doubt, creating negative emotions within you, will only lead to failure of your treatment.

Likewise, you should do everything in your power to reduce stress in your life. Stress causes cortisol levels to rise. Cortisol is very acidifying to the body and will only feed cancer growth and proliferation. If you have a passion, make time for it. If you don't, find one. Walk in nature, paint, sculpt, listen to music that relaxes you. Don't watch the news. Reduce or eliminate activities that stress you out.

Just as it is important to detox your body of toxins, it is also important to detox your mind. It is very important to purge negative thoughts and negative emotions. If you harbor negativity towards someone else for something that was done to you in the past, forgive this person. Remember, you are not forgiving this person for their sake – you are doing so for your own sake. Let things go. Let things out. Cry if you need to. Be appreciative of what you have. Bring joy into your life. Quiet your mind by practicing meditation. Recite daily affirmations.

3.11   FASTING

Fasting has been a part of cultural and religious practices for thousands of years. It has been known throughout the world for millennia that fasting resets the immune system and greatly improves health. Like with many other ancient medical practices, modern science is now catching up and validating these benefits through scientific research.

A 2014 study[480] in the journal "Cell Stem Cell" demonstrated that prolonged fasting (24 to 120 hours) protects against immune system damage caused by chemotherapy. In addition, prolonged fasting also induced immune system regeneration, shifting stem cells from a dormant state to a state of self-renewal.

In a phase I clinical trial it was demonstrated that 72 hours of prolonged fasting in patients who were receiving 3 different platinum-based chemotherapy medications was associated with normal lymphocyte counts and maintenance of a normal lineage balance in white blood cells, which demonstrates the power of fasting to boost the immune system, even in the face of potent immunosuppressive medications.

According to the authors, "When considering changes in gene expression and metabolism, as well as the levels of various hormones, PF [prolonged fasting] promotes coordinated effects that would be difficult to achieve with any pharmacological or other dietary intervention."[480]

Intermittent fasting of two to four days over a period of 6 months has been shown to kill older and damaged immune cells and generate new ones.

Prof. Valter Longo – one of the study's authors, remarked that "When you starve, the system tries to save energy, and one of the things it can do to save energy is to recycle a lot of the immune cells that are not needed, especially those that may be damaged … What we started noticing in both our human work and animal work is that the white blood cell count goes down with prolonged fasting. Then when you re-feed, the blood cells come back."[481]

Note: Fasting throughout the daytime and engorging at nigh is not only counterproductive, but also harmful to the digestive system, and by extension, to the immune system. When coming out of a fast, one should eat light foods.

Chapter 4

CONCLUSIONS
AND RECOMMENDATIONS

The state of our food, our environment, our minds, and by extension our health has been on a downward spiral for quite a long time. We've made many scientific discoveries, and we've achieved much scientific progress, but we've also gone down many bad paths as a result of errors in judgement, deep-rooted scientific dogmas, greed and corruption. The nutritional recommendations made by most scientific organizations and governments are based more on subsidies of staple crops, lowering of production costs, and increasing profits rather than on true scientific discovery. Nearly all of the pharmaceutical medications that we are being prescribed, including pharmaceutical-grade vitamins, which most times are synthetic or produced with genetically engineered bacteria, and are isolates (not complex with other vitamins and minerals which are essential for absorption and assimilation), are toxic. This is actually a key feature of the business plan of pharmaceutical companies – to create life-long customers. The FDA are aware of this, and are complicit.

We have been told that many of the toxic chemicals which are used on our crops, in our water, in food preparation, on our lawns, and everywhere in between have been tested for health safety and are perfectly innocuous, however, what is discovered in a lab and what is communicated to the public are two very different things, and even more frightening, most of those chemicals have never been tested at all. Furthermore, many chemicals that we were told are perfectly safe, and which were used extensively on our food supply and in consumer products are now banned due to their extreme toxicity. Many more have been shown to be extremely toxic, but corporate interests are keeping those chemicals on the market and in our food supply.

Our nations' soils are being depleted and destroyed with monocultures and toxic chemicals, depleting the nutritional value of our foods and poisoning our bodies with noxious chemicals. The very nature of our food crops is being altered with genetic engineering, leading to all sorts of toxic, allergenic, and anti-nutritional effects which are difficult and even impossible to detect. The toxic soup of chemicals that are used in conjunction with those engineered crops are doing a number on our health, which is being hidden from the public through misinformation campaigns by the industry and our governments in favor of profits.

Still, there are many good scientists who are truly committed to integrity in science and using it to benefit the world rather than to enrich multinational corporations. The scientific literature is littered with studies of natural plants and substances which show beneficial effects for nearly every ailment, which in almost every case outperform pharmaceutical drugs, and nearly always are devoid of negative side-effects. Unfortunately, most of that science does not make headline news, due to the overwhelming power of multinational corporations, whose advertising dollars keep those news outlets in business.

In today's age of information and access, it is easier than ever to do your own research and not rely on what you are being told. Don't assume that because your doctor went through 12 years of medical school and residency that he or she has not been indoctrinated into a system that is driven purely by profits, and does not have your best interest in mind, knowingly or unknowingly. I cannot tell you how many times

I was given incorrect information by a doctor, that had I not done my own research could have seriously compromised my health.

Do your research. Look for consistency in findings when positive results are reported. Look for conflicts of interest when negative results are reported. For example, a recent study was published by the American Heart Association demonizing coconut oil[482]. The fact is, the American Heart Association receives millions of dollars in grant money from corn, soy, and canola growers' associations, as well as from junk food companies and pharmaceutical companies, and coconuts are not a domestic crop. Not to mention all of the studies that show the extensive health benefits of coconut oil. What do they recommend instead? canola oil, corn oil, soybean oil, peanut oil, safflower oil, sunflower oil, and walnuts. Canola, corn, and soybeans are almost entirely GMO, and all of the oils they recommend are highly processed in ways that render them toxic.

Everyone is different and each person responds to treatment differently. If you look at it from an engineering perspective, if you have a device which is comprised of two parts, the possible failure modes are very limited. However, if you have a machine that is comprised of thousands of parts of different functions, made of different materials, and having different mechanical, thermal, and resonant properties, the number of possible interactions and potential modes of failure increase exponentially. The human body is incredibly complex, comprised of trillion of cells, forming various organs and tissues of varying functions, and requiring nutrients at different quantities at different times. Microbes in the human body outnumber cells 10 to 1, and those microbes play essential roles in digestion, synthesis and other functions. Those microbes are a part of us and without them we could not sustain life, and therefore, their health needs to be considered as well. Diet, physical activity, injury, environmental exposures, psychological states and many other internal and external factors modulate the function or dysfunction of those cells, organs, tissues, and microorganisms.

Those influencers modulate the release of different hormones, which affect the function of all the systems within the body, changing the way we assimilate nutrients, changing the energy distribution of the body; where the blood is sent to and which systems are prioritized before others. All of these parameters change the way that medicine, whether synthetic or natural, work within the body and how effective they are at doing their job (although synthetic medications add many more layers of dysfunction, since the body recognizes them as foreign and toxic in most cases). For this reason, one course of treatment which might work for one or many individuals might not work for you. This is why it is crucial that first, you create a plan and identify the remedies or protocols that have been shown to be effective for the type of cancer (or another ailment) that you have. Remember that the remedies and protocols mentioned in this book are but a few examples and there are many more, so do your research. Then, consult a naturopathic doctor or herbalist to help you narrow down the combination of treatments to use. Remember that disease does not just happen - your natural defenses have to be weak, and your environment (including food) has to be deficient and toxic in order for you to become ill, even from viruses and bacteria. So it is crucial that you not just treat the disease, but treat the whole body. That means looking at your diet and making changes that will give your body the best opportunity to heal. Increase good nutrition (don't look to your medical doctor for advice in this regard because most of them are clueless). Buy organic as much as possible, and learn which fruits and vegetables are at a higher likelihood of being sprayed with chemicals, and avoid them entirely if not organic. It is impossible for me to write about every chemical that is used in the food supply, so do some research on your own. Reduce or eliminate bad influencers (dietary, environmental, psychological, etc.), which will give your body the opportunity to heal itself.

Biology, whether of humans or plants, etc. is unbelievably complex and beautifully orchestrated. Do some research on cell biology and you will be awe-struck at the beauty and near-perfection of how it all functions. I say near-perfection because we can still fake it out and make it not work as intended, unfortunately. But it is nevertheless amazing in the way that nearly every possibility is planned for and cells know exactly what to do and how to do it.

It is important that once you select a course of treatment that you stick to it and not jump around. You do however need to monitor your progress. If you discover that your treatment is not working, you might need to change gears and try something else. Although I have been pretty harsh on the orthodox medical community, they do serve their purpose. Diagnostic tools, like bloodwork, x-ray, CT scan, MRI, ultrasonography, etc. are important, and you should use them as needed to set a course and monitor the progress of your treatment. Don't let your doctor however pressure you into a treatment that you do not want or need. Remember that every organ in your body has a function, and removing any organ will have a negative cascade effect on your health. Obviously, if an organ is seriously damaged and poses an immediate threat to your life, operation might be necessary, but most organs which are removed in this country are removed unnecessarily.

If there is just one thing that you remember from reading this book it should be this – the medical industry operates on fear; especially oncologists. They will try to force you into submitting to their course of treatment immediately and without thinking. They will make it sound like if you do not act immediately you will die. Ironically, studies show that those who do nothing to treat their cancer live a lot longer, and with better quality of life than those who undergo chemo and/or radiation. Surgeries are not so innocent either, for they often lead to metastasis, making treatment a lot more difficult. If there is ever a time to stop and think about your options it's when you are confronted with cancer. Other than the rare case where a tumor is pressing on an artery, or another vital organ and poses immediate danger to life, at which case emergency surgery to debulk or remove the tumor might be the best course of action, there is no cancer that grows so rapidly that a few days of rational thinking would change the prognosis.

REFERENCES

Because websites are updated regularly, the links that are provided may or may not work in the future. For that reason, if a link is no longer valid, a web search of the title of the referenced document should lead you to its new location.

1.   Gilles Eric Séralini, Toxicity of GMOs and Pesticides: Séralini's Team Wins Defamation and Forgery Court Cases; Global Research, 2015.
     http://www.globalresearch.ca/toxicity-of-gmos-and-pesticides-seralinis-team-wins-defamation-and-forgery-court-cases/5492480

2.   Gary Ruskin, Why You Can't Trust Henry Miller; U.S. Right to Know, 2015.
     http://usrtk.org/hall-of-shame/why-you-cant-trust-henry-miller-on-gmos/

3.   Andrew Rowell, The sinister sacking of the world's leading GM expert and the trail that leads to Tony Blair and the White House; GMWatch.
     http://www.gmwatch.org/latest-listing/42-2003/4305

4.   L. Flynn, M.S. Gillard, Pro-GM food scientist 'threatened editor'; the Guardian, 31 Oct. 1999.
     https://www.theguardian.com/science/1999/nov/01/gm.food

5.   Dr. Oz Breaks His Silence; The Dr. Oz Show, 4/23/2015.
     http://www.doctoroz.com/episode/dr-oz-fights-back-his-exclusive-reaction-his-critics

6.   Elahe Izadi, Dr. Oz responds after prominent physicians call for his firing from Columbia University; The Washington Post, 4/18/2015.
     https://www.washingtonpost.com/news/to-your-health/wp/2015/04/16/a-bunch-of-doctors-ask-columbia-university-to-cut-its-ties-with-dr-oz/

7.   Steven M. Druker, The Royal Society's assault on the science of GM foods must cease; The Ecologist, 6/25/2015.
     http://www.theecologist.org/blogs_and_comments/commentators/2921277/the_royal_societys_assault_on_the_science_of_gm_foods_must_cease.html

8.   Y. Tantamango-Bartley et al., Vegetarian Diets and the Incidence of Cancer in a Low-risk Population; Cancer Epidemiology, Biomarkers & Prevention; 11/20/2012. doi:10.1158/1055-9965.EPI-12-1060.
     http://cebp.aacrjournals.org/content/22/2/286.long

9.   T.J. Key et al., Cancer incidence in British vegetarians; British Journal of Cancer, 2009. doi:10.1038/sj.bjc.6605098.
     http://www.nature.com/bjc/journal/v101/n1/full/6605098a.html

10. Food, Nutrition, and Physical Activity, and the Prevention of Cancer: a Global Perspective. World Cancer Research Fund, American Institute for Cancer Research. http://www.wcrf.org/sites/default/files/english.pdf

11. Department of Commerce Bureau of the Census, Mortality from Cancer and Other Malignant Tumors in the Registration Area of the United States, 1914.
     https://www.cdc.gov/nchs/data/vsushistorical/mortcancer_1914.pdf

12. The New England Medical Gazette, Vol. LI, Jan. 1916, p.112;
     https://archive.org/stream/newenglandmedica51bost#page/112/mode/2up/search/52%2C420

13. American Cancer Society. Cancer Facts and Figures 2014.
http://www.cancer.org/acs/groups/content/@research/documents/webconte
nt/acspc-042151.pdf

14. AACR Cancer Progress Report 2015.
http://cancerprogressreport.org/2015/Documents/AACR_CPR2015.pdf

15. U.S. Patents fraudulently filed for the U.S. Department of Health and
Human Services for cures for cancer developed by and stolen from Dr.
Stanislaw Burzynski; U.S. patent numbers US6037376 A, US5635532 A,
US5605930 A, US5852056 A, US5654333 A, US5661179 A, US5635533 A,
US5710178 A, US5843994 A, US5877213 A

16. Vitamin B17 Controversy: Poison or Cancer Treatment?; Dr. Axe.
https://draxe.com/vitamin-b17/

17. Acrylamide in Food and Cancer Risk; National Cancer Institute.
http://www.cancer.gov/about-cancer/causes-
prevention/risk/diet/acrylamide-fact-sheet#q2

18. Hazard Summary or Propylene oxide; EPA.
https://www3.epa.gov/ttn/atw/hlthef/prop-oxi.html

19. A look back at 2009: one step forward, two steps back. Prescriere
International, Apr. 2010. PMID: 20568499.
http://www.ncbi.nlm.nih.gov/pubmed/20568499

20. National Vital Statistics Reports, Volume 63, Number 5; September 24, 2014;
International Comparisons of Infant Mortality and Related Factors: United
States and Europe, 2010.
http://www.cdc.gov/nchs/data/nvsr/nvsr63/nvsr63_05.pdf

21. Myra L. Karstadt. Testing Needed for Acesulfame Potassium, an Artificial
Sweetener; Environ Health Perspectives, Sep. 2006. PMCID: PMC1570055.
http://www.ncbi.nlm.nih.gov/pmc/articles/PMC1570055/

22. S.S. Schiffman, K.I. Rother. Sucralose, A Synthetic Organochlorine
Sweetener: Overview of Biological Issues; Journal of Toxicology and
Environmental Health. Part B, Critical Reviews; Sep. 2013. doi:
10.1080/10937404.2013.842523.
http://www.ncbi.nlm.nih.gov/pmc/articles/PMC3856475/

23. M. Soffritti et al. Life-span exposure to low doses of aspartame beginning
during prenatal life increases cancer effects in rats; Environmental Health
Perspectives, Sep. 2007. doi: 10.1289/ehp.10271.
http://www.ncbi.nlm.nih.gov/pubmed/?term=17805418

24. F. Belpoggi et al. Results of long-term carcinogenicity bioassay on Sprague-
Dawley rats exposed to aspartame administered in feed; Annals of the New
York Academy of Sciences, Sep. 2006. doi: 10.1196/annals.1371.080.
http://www.ncbi.nlm.nih.gov/pubmed/?term=17119233

25. M. Soffritti et al. Life-span exposure to low doses of aspartame beginning
during prenatal life increases cancer effects in rats; Environmental Health
Perspectives, Sep. 2007. doi: 10.1289/ehp.10271.
http://www.ncbi.nlm.nih.gov/pubmed/?term=17805418

26. F. Belpoggi et al. Results of long-term carcinogenicity bioassay on Sprague-
Dawley rats exposed to aspartame administered in feed; Annals of the New
York Academy of Sciences, Sep. 2006. doi: 10.1196/annals.1371.080.
http://www.ncbi.nlm.nih.gov/pubmed/?term=17119233

27. M. Soffritti et al. Aspartame administered in feed, beginning prenatally through life span, induces cancers of the liver and lung in male Swiss mice; American Journal of Industrial Medicine, Dec. 2010. doi: 10.1002/ajim.20896. http://www.ncbi.nlm.nih.gov/pubmed/?term=20886530

28. M. Soffritti et al. The carcinogenic effects of aspartame: The urgent need for regulatory re-evaluation; American Journal of Industrial Medicine, Apr. 2014. doi: 10.1002/ajim.22296. http://www.ncbi.nlm.nih.gov/pubmed/?term=24436139

29. E.S. Schernhammer et al. Consumption of artificial sweetener- and sugar-containing soda and risk of lymphoma and leukemia in men and women; The American Journal of Clinical Nutrition, Dec. 2012. doi: 10.3945/ajcn.111.030833. http://www.ncbi.nlm.nih.gov/pubmed/?term=23097267

30. Safety of artificial sweetener called into question by MP; The Guardian, 12/15/2005. http://www.theguardian.com/politics/2005/dec/15/foodanddrink.immigrationpolicy

31. Melanie Warner. The Lowdown on Sweet?; The New York Times, 2/12/2006. http://www.nytimes.com/2006/02/12/business/yourmoney/the-lowdown-on-sweet.html

32. Aspartame. SourceWatch. http://www.sourcewatch.org/index.php/Aspartame#cite_note-89

33. A. Noorafshan, M. Erfanizadeh, S. Karbalay-Doust. Sodium benzoate, a food preservative, induces anxiety and motor impairment in rats; Neurosciences (Riyadh, Saudi Arabia), Jan. 2014. PMID: 24419445. http://www.ncbi.nlm.nih.gov/pubmed/?term=24419445

34. N. Zengin et al. The evaluation of the genotoxicity of two food preservatives: sodium benzoate and potassium benzoate; Food and Chemical Toxicology, Apr. 2011. doi: 10.1016/j.fct.2010.11.040. http://www.ncbi.nlm.nih.gov/pubmed/?term=21130826

35. D. McCann et al. Food additives and hyperactive behaviour in 3-year-old and 8/9-year-old children in the community: a randomised, double-blinded, placebo-controlled trial; Lancet, 11/3/2007. doi: 10.1016/S0140-6736(07)61306-3. http://www.ncbi.nlm.nih.gov/pubmed/?term=17825405

36. B. Bateman et al. The effects of a double blind, placebo controlled, artificial food colourings and benzoate preservative challenge on hyperactivity in a general population sample of preschool children; Archives of Disease in Childhood, Jun. 2004. PMCID: PMC1719942. http://www.ncbi.nlm.nih.gov/pubmed/?term=15155391

37. Wikipedia, Tuskegee syphilis experiment. https://en.wikipedia.org/wiki/Tuskegee_syphilis_experiment

38. CBS News, Secret Cold War tests in St. Louis cause worry. http://www.cbsnews.com/news/secret-cold-war-tests-in-st-louis-cause-worry/

39. Huffington Post, Secret Cold War Tests In St. Louis Raise Concerns. http://www.huffingtonpost.com/2012/10/03/secret-cold-war-tests_n_1937613.html

40. W. Bogdanich, E. Koli - The New York Times. 2 Paths of Bayer Drug in 80's: Riskier One Steered Oversea; 5/22/2003.
shttp://www.nytimes.com/2003/05/22/business/2-paths-of-bayer-drug-in-80-s-riskier-one-steered-overseas.html?pagewanted=print

41. B. Meier - The New York Times. Blood, Money and AIDS: Hemophiliacs Are Split;Liability Cases Bogged Down in Disputes; 6/11/1996.
http://www.nytimes.com/1996/06/11/business/blood-money-aids-hemophiliacs-are-split-liability-cases-bogged-down-disputes.html

42. Wikiepedia - Contaminated haemophilia blood products.
https://en.wikipedia.org/wiki/Contaminated_haemophilia_blood_products

43. Gilbert C. White, II, M.D. Hemophilia: An Amazing 35-Year Journey from the Depths of HIV to the Threshold of Cure; American Clinical and Climatological Association, 2010. PMC2917149.
https://www.ncbi.nlm.nih.gov/pmc/articles/PMC2917149/

44. Nathaniel Rich - The New York Times. The Lawyer Who Became DuPont's Worst Nightmare; 1/6/2016.
https://www.nytimes.com/2016/01/10/magazine/the-lawyer-who-became-duponts-worst-nightmare.html

45. T. Colin Campbell, PhD. Animal vs. Plant Protein; Center for Nutrition Studies, 10/29/2013.   http://nutritionstudies.org/animal-vs-plant-protein/

46. James, John T. PhD. A New, Evidence-based Estimate of Patient Harms Associated with Hospital Care; Journal of Patient Safety: September 2013 - Volume 9 - Issue 3 - p 122–128. doi: 10.1097/PTS.0b013e3182948a69.
http://journals.lww.com/journalpatientsafety/Fulltext/2013/09000/A_New,_Evidence_based_Estimate_of_Patient_Harms.2.aspx

47. J.K. Fauser et al. Induction of apoptosis by the medium-chain length fatty acid lauric acid in colon cancer cells due to induction of oxidative stress; Chemotherapy, 2013. doi: 10.1159/000356067.
https://www.ncbi.nlm.nih.gov/pubmed/?term=24356281

48. O. LeGendre, P.A.S. Breslin, D.A. Foster. (-)-Oleocanthal rapidly and selectively induces cancer cell death via lysosomal membrane permeabilization; Molecular & Cellular Oncology, Oct-Dec 2015. doi: 10.1080/23723556.2015.1006077.
https://www.ncbi.nlm.nih.gov/pmc/articles/PMC4568762/

49. P. Pérez-Martínez et al. Mediterranean diet rich in olive oil and obesity, metabolic syndrome and diabetes mellitus; Current Pharmaceutical Design, 2011. PMID: 21443484.
https://www.ncbi.nlm.nih.gov/pubmed/?term=21443484

50. C. Virruso et al. Nutraceutical properties of extra-virgin olive oil: a natural remedy for age-related disease?; Rejuvination Research, Apr. 2014. doi: 10.1089/rej.2013.1532.
https://www.ncbi.nlm.nih.gov/pubmed/?term=24219356

51. Youn K. Shim et al. Parental Exposure to Pesticides and Childhood Brain Cancer: U.S. Atlantic Coast Childhood Brain Cancer Study. PMCID: PMC2702394. http://www.ncbi.nlm.nih.gov/pmc/articles/PMC2702394/

52. Leah S., Maria E.L. Non-Hodgkin Lymphoma and Occupational Exposure to Agricultural Pesticide Chemical Groups and Active Ingredients: A Systematic Review and Meta-Analysis. doi:10.3390/ijerph110404449.
http://www.mdpi.com/1660-4601/11/4/4449

53. Nancy L.S., Andre L., Jon A., Bradley W. Genetically engineered crops, glyphosate and the deterioration of health in the United States of America. Journal of Organic Systems, 9(2), 2014.
https://people.csail.mit.edu/seneff/Swanson_et_al_2014.pdf

54. Ian Forrest Robey. Examining the relationship between diet-induced acidosis and cancer; Nutrition & Metabolism, 2012. doi: 10.1186/1743-7075-9-72.
https://nutritionandmetabolism.biomedcentral.com/articles/10.1186/1743-7075-9-72

55. G.K. Schwalfenberg, The Alkaline Diet: Is There Evidence That an Alkaline pH Diet Benefits Health?; Journal of Environmental and Public Health, 2012.
http://www.ncbi.nlm.nih.gov/pmc/articles/PMC3195546/

56. D. Piepenburg, Acid – Alkaline Balance and Cancer: The Truth Behind the Myth; Minnesota Oncology, 4/1/2014. http://mnoncology.com/about-us/practice-news/acid-alkaline-balance-and-cancer-the-truth-behind-the-myth/

57. Woodrow C. Monte, Ph.D., R.D. Aspartame: Methanol and the Public Health; Journal of Applied Nutrition, Volume 36, Number 1, 1984.
http://www.mpwhi.com/aspartame_methanol_and_public_health.pdf

58. Aspartame: By Far the Most Dangerous Substance Added to Most Foods Today; mercola.com, 11/6/2011.
http://articles.mercola.com/sites/articles/archive/2011/11/06/aspartame-most-dangerous-substance-added-to-food.aspx

59. Netherwood T, Martin-Orue SM, O'Donnell AG, et al. Assessing the survival of transgenic plant DNA in the human gastrointestinal tract. Nat Biotechnol. 2004;22:204–209. doi:10.1038/nbt934.
http://www.nature.com/nbt/journal/v22/n2/full/nbt934.html

60. Mike Zelina et al. The Health Effects of Genetically Engineered Crops On San Luis Obispo County; A Citizen Response to the SLO Health Commission GMO Task Force Report.
http://www.slocounty.ca.gov/Assets/PH/HealthCommission/GMOTaskForce/Citizen+Response+on+the+Health+Effects+of+GE+Crops.pdf

61. The New York Times, The Rise of Antibiotic Resistance. May 10, 2014.
http://mobile.nytimes.com/2014/05/11/opinion/sunday/the-rise-of-antibiotic-resistance.html?referer=&_r=1

62. Huffington Post, Major Poultry Farms Routinely Feed Antibiotics To Chickens. Sep. 15, 2014.
http://www.huffingtonpost.com/2014/09/15/poultry-farms-antibiotics-chickens_n_5822438.html?utm_hp_ref=green

63. Steven M. Druker, Altered Genes, Twisted Truth: How the Venture to Genetically Engineer Our Food Has Subverted Science, Corrupted Government, and Systematically Deceived the Public (Clear River Press)

64. Caughey B, Baron GS. Prions and their partners in crime. Nature. 2006;443:803-10. doi:10.1038/nature05294.
http://www.nature.com/nature/journal/v443/n7113/full/nature05294.html

65. S.Z. Agapito-Tenfen, M.P. Guerra, O-G Wikmark, R.O. Nodari. Comparative proteomic analysis of genetically modified maize grown under different agroecosystems conditions in Brazil. Proteome Sci. 2013;11(1):46. doi:10.1186/1477-5956-11-46. http://www.proteomesci.com/content/11/1/46

66. Padgette SR, Taylor NB, Nida DL, et al. The composition of glyphosate-tolerant soybean seeds is equivalent to that of conventional soybeans. J Nutr. 1996;126:702-16, PubMed ID: 8598556. https://www.ncbi.nlm.nih.gov/pubmed/?term=8598556

67. Freese W, Schubert D. Safety testing and regulation of genetically engineered foods. Biotechnology and Genetic Engineering Reviews. Vol. 21, November 2004. http://www.centerforfoodsafety.org/files/freese_safetytestingandregulation ofgeneticallyebgineeredfoods_nov212004_62269.pdf

68. Kahl L. Memorandum to Dr James Maryanski, FDA biotechnology coordinator, about the Federal Register document, "Statement of policy: Foods from genetically modified plants." US Food & Drug Administration; 1992. Available at: http://www.biointegrity.org/FDAdocs/01/01.pdf

69. Guest GB. Memorandum to Dr James Maryanski, biotechnology coordinator: Regulation of transgenic plants – FDA Draft Federal Register Notice on Food Biotechnology. US Department of Health & Human Services; 1992. Available at: http://www.biointegrity.org/FDAdocs/08/08.pdf

70. Matthews EJ. Memorandum to toxicology section of the Biotechnology Working Group: "Safety of whole food plants transformed by technology methods." US Food & Drug Administration; 1991. Available at: http://www.biointegrity.org/FDAdocs/02/02.pdf

71. Shibko SL. Memorandum to James H. Maryanski, biotechnology coordinator, CFSAN: Revision of toxicology section of the "Statement of policy: Foods derived from genetically modified plants." US Food & Drug Administration; 1992. Available at: http://www.biointegrity.org/FDAdocs/03/03.pdf

72. Pribyl LJ. Comments on the March 18, 1992 version of the Biotechnology Document. US Food & Drug Administration; 1992. Available at: http://www.biointegrity.org/FDAdocs/12/ljpp.pdf

73. Pribyl LJ. Comments on Biotechnology Draft Document, 2/27/92. US Food & Drug Administration; 1992. Available at: http://www.biointegrity.org/FDAdocs/04/04.pdf

74. 2014 USDA report titled "Genetically Engineered Crops in the United States". http://www.ers.usda.gov/media/1282246/err162.pdf

75. Benbrook C. Impacts of genetically engineered crops on pesticide use in the US – The first sixteen years. Environ Sci Eur. 2012;24. doi:10.1186/2190-4715-24-24. http://www.enveurope.com/content/24/1/24

76. Mortensen DA, Egan JF, Maxwell BD, Ryan MR, Smith RG. Navigating a critical juncture for sustainable weed management. BioScience. 2012;62(1):75-84. http://bioscience.oxfordjournals.org/content/62/1/75.full.pdf

77. Benbrook CM. Rust, resistance, run down soils, and rising costs – Problems facing soybean producers in Argentina. Technical Paper No 8. AgBioTech InfoNet; 2005. https://www.organic-center.org/reportfiles/rust-resistence-run-down-soi.pdf

78. Pengue W. El glifosato y la dominación del ambiente. Biodiversidad. 2003;37. http://www.grain.org/biodiversidad/?id=208

79. MECON (Ministerio de Economia Argentina). Mercado argentino de fitosanitarios – Año 2001. http://bit.ly/1eqMudL

80. CASAFE. Mercado Argentino de productos fitosanitarios; 2012. http://www.casafe.org/pdf/estadisticas/Informe%20Mercado%20Fitosanitario%202012.pdf

81. regulations.gov, Pesticide Tolerances: Glyphosate. http://www.regulations.gov/#!documentDetail;D=EPA-HQ-OPP-2012-0132-0009

82. Gurian-Sherman D. Failure to yield: Evaluating the performance of genetically engineered crops. Cambridge, MA: Union of Concerned Scientists; 2009.
http://www.ucsusa.org/assets/documents/food_and_agriculture/failure-to-yield.pdf

83. The Organic & Non-GMO Report, Farmers' seed options drastically reduced in GMO-producing countries. http://www.non-gmoreport.com/articles/march2013/farmers-seed-options-GMO-producing-countries.php

84. DailyMail.com, The GM genocide: Thousands of Indian farmers are committing suicide after using genetically modified crops. www.dailymail.co.uk/news/article-1082559/The-GM-genocide-Thousands-Indian-farmers-committing-suicide-using-genetically-modified-crops.html

85. Mercola.com, The "Massive Con" Causing a Suicide Every 30 Minutes. http://articles.mercola.com/sites/articles/archive/2012/04/03/gmo-crops-affect-farmers.aspx

86. W.E. Huffman at al., Consumer Willingness to Pay for Genetically Modified Food Labels in a Market with Diverse Information: Evidence from Experimental Auctions. http://www.waeaonline.org/jareonline/archives/28.3%20-%20December%202003/JARE,Dec2003,pp481,Huffman.pdf

87. J.R. Latham, A.K. Wilson, R.A. Steinbrecher, The Mutational Consequences of Plant Transformation.
doi: 10.1155/JBB/2006/25376.
http://www.ncbi.nlm.nih.gov/pmc/articles/PMC1559911/

88. M. Bardini, M. Labra, M. Winfield, F. Sala, Antibiotic-induced DNA methylation changes in calluses of Arabidopsis thaliana. Plant Cell, Tissue and Organ Culture February 2003, Volume 72, Issue 2, pp 157-162. http://link.springer.com/article/10.1023/A:1022208302819

89. Hidden Dangers in Kids' Meals: Genetically Engineered Foods;
Part 1: https://www.youtube.com/watch?v=oqc9-6dGWOw
Part 2: https://www.youtube.com/watch?v=B5ydsjKyBZA
Part 3: https://www.youtube.com/watch?v=SH6rStYRm_M

90. Jane Goodall, Harvest for Hope: A Guide to Mindful Eating

91. Collectors Weekly; What Were We Thinking? The Top 10 Most Dangerous Ads. http://www.collectorsweekly.com/articles/the-top-10-most-dangerous-ads/

92. United States Environmental Protection Agency; DDT Ban Takes Effect, 1972. http://www.epa.gov/aboutepa/ddt-ban-takes-effect

93. Pesticide Action Network - North America; The DDT Story. http://www.panna.org/resources/ddt-story

94. The Nuremberg Code. http://www.nj.gov/health/irb/documents/nuremburg_code.pdf

95. A. Aris, S. Leblanc, Maternal and fetal exposure to pesticides associated to genetically modified foods in Eastern Townships of Quebec, Canada. Elsevier, Reproductive Toxicology. PubMed ID: 21338670 https://www.uclm.es/Actividades/repositorio/pdf/doc_3721_4666.pdf

96. Mazza R, Soave M, Morlacchini M, Piva G, Marocco A. Assessing the transfer of genetically modified DNA from feed to animal tissues. Transgenic Res. 2005;14:775–84. doi:10.1007/s11248-005-0009-5. PubMed ID: 16245168: http://www.ncbi.nlm.nih.gov/pubmed/16245168

97. Sharma R, Damgaard D, Alexander TW, et al. Detection of transgenic and endogenous plant DNA in digesta and tissues of sheep and pigs fed Roundup Ready canola meal. J Agric Food Chem. 2006;54:1699–1709. doi:10.1021/jf052459o. PubMed ID: 16506822: http://www.ncbi.nlm.nih.gov/pubmed/16506822

98. Chainark P, Satoh S, Hirono I, Aoki T, Endo M. Availability of genetically modified feed ingredient: investigations of ingested foreign DNA in rainbow trout Oncorhynchus mykiss. Fish Sci. 2008;74:380–390. http://onlinelibrary.wiley.com/doi/10.1111/j.1444-2906.2008.01535.x/abstract

99. Ran T, Mei L, Lei W, Aihua L, Ru H, Jie S. Detection of transgenic DNA in tilapias (Oreochromis niloticus, GIFT strain) fed genetically modified soybeans (Roundup Ready). Aquac Res. 2009;40:1350–1357. http://onlinelibrary.wiley.com/doi/10.1111/j.1365-2109.2009.02187.x/abstract

100. Lin Zhang at al. Exogenous plant MIR168a specifically targets mammalian LDLRAP1: evidence of cross-kingdom regulation by microRNA. doi:10.1038/cr.2011.158. http://www.nature.com/cr/journal/v22/n1/abs/cr2011158a.html

101. Mercola.com; Why Did Officials Approve this Bt-toxin Corn Chip that Creates a 'Pesticide Factory' in Your Gut? 10/8/2010. http://articles.mercola.com/sites/articles/archive/2010/10/08/a-pesticide-factory-in-your-stomach-think-corn-chips.aspx

102. Székács A, Darvas B. Comparative aspects of Cry toxin usage in insect control. In: Ishaaya I, Palli SR, Horowitz AR, eds. Advanced Technologies for Managing Insect Pests. Dordrecht, Netherlands: Springer; 2012:195–230. https://link.springer.com/chapter/10.1007/978-94-007-4497-4_10

103. Séralini GE, Mesnage R, Clair E, Gress S, de Vendômois JS, Cellier D. Genetically modified crops safety assessments: Present limits and possible improvements. Environ Sci Eur. 2011;23. doi:10.1186/2190-4715-23-10. http://www.enveurope.com/content/23/1/10

104. Li H, Buschman LL, Huang F, Zhu KY, Bonning B, Oppert BA. Resistance to Bacillus thuringiensis endotoxins in the European corn borer. Biopesticide International. 2007;3:96–107.
http://www.connectjournals.com/toc2.php?abstract=104102H_096-107_abs.htm&&bookmark=CJ-023217&&issue_id=02&&yaer=

105. Carman JA, Vlieger HR, Ver Steeg LJ, et al. A long-term toxicology study on pigs fed a combined genetically modified (GM) soy and GM maize diet. J Org Syst. 2013;8:38–54. http://www.organic-systems.org/journal/81/8106.pdf

106. Glyphosate: Unsafe on Any Plate, Food Testing Results and Scientific Reasons for Concern; Report by Food Democracy Now! and The Detox Project.
https://s3.amazonaws.com/media.fooddemocracynow.org/images/FDN_Glyphosate_FoodTesting_Report_p2016.pdf

107. Heritage J. The fate of transgenes in the human gut. Nat Biotechnol. 2004;22:170-2. doi:10.1038/nbt0204-170.
http://www.nature.com/nbt/journal/v22/n2/full/nbt0204-170.html
http://www.somosbacteriasyvirus.com/humangut.pdf

108. Poulsen M, Kroghsbo S, Schrøder M, et al. A 90-day safety study in Wistar rats fed genetically modified rice expressing snowdrop lectin Galanthus nivalis (GNA). Food Chem Toxicol. 2007;45:350-63. doi:10.1016/j.fct.2006.09.002.
http://www.ncbi.nlm.nih.gov/pubmed/17052828

109. Schrøder M, Poulsen M, Wilcks A, et al. A 90-day safety study of genetically modified rice expressing Cry1Ab protein (Bacillus thuringiensis toxin) in Wistar rats. Food Chem Toxicol. 2007;45:339-49. doi:10.1016/j.fct.2006.09.001.
http://www.ncbi.nlm.nih.gov/pubmed/17050059

110. Sahar El Aidy, Timothy G. Dinan, John F. Cryan. Immune modulation of the brain-gut-microbe axis.
http://journal.frontiersin.org/article/10.3389/fmicb.2014.00146/full

111. Elaine Y. Hsiao, Sara W. McBride, Sophia Hsien, Gil Sharon, Embriette R. Hyde, Tyler McCue, Julian A. Codelli, Janet Chow, Sarah E. Reisman, Joseph F. Petrosino, Paul H. Patterson, Sarkis K. Mazmanian. The microbiota modulates gut physiology and behavioral abnormalities associated with autism. doi: 10.1016/j.cell.2013.11.024.
http://www.ncbi.nlm.nih.gov/pmc/articles/PMC3897394/

112. Desbonnet L, Garrett L, Clarke G, Kiely B, Cryan JF, Dinan TG. Effects of the probiotic Bifidobacterium infantis in the maternal separation model of depression. doi: 10.1016/j. PebMed ID: 20696216.
http://www.ncbi.nlm.nih.gov/pubmed/20696216

113. J.A. Bravo et al. Ingestion of Lactobacillus strain regulates emotional behavior and central GABA receptor expression in a mouse via the vagus nerve; PNAS, 8/29/2011. doi: 10.1073/pnas.1102999108.
http://www.pnas.org/content/108/38/16050

114. Kristin Schmidt, Philip J. Cowen, Catherine J. Harmer, George Tzortzis, Steven Errington, Philip W. J. Burnet. Prebiotic intake reduces the waking cortisol response and alters emotional bias in healthy volunteers. doi: 10.1007/s00213-014-3810-0. PMCID: PMC4410136.
http://www.ncbi.nlm.nih.gov/pmc/articles/PMC4410136/

115. Kirsten Tillisch, Jennifer Labus, Lisa Kilpatrick, Zhiguo Jiang, Jean Stains, Bahar Ebrat, Denis Guyonnet, Sophie Legrain–Raspaud, Beatrice Trotin, Bruce Naliboff, Emeran A. Mayer. Consumption of Fermented Milk Product With Probiotic Modulates Brain Activity. doi: 10.1053/j.gastro.2013.02.043. PMCID: PMC3839572.
http://www.ncbi.nlm.nih.gov/pmc/articles/PMC3839572/

116. Mark Lyte. Microbial Endocrinology in the Microbiome-Gut-Brain Axis: How Bacterial Production and Utilization of Neurochemicals Influence Behavior. DOI: 10.1371/journal.ppat.1003726.
http://journals.plos.org/plospathogens/article?id=10.1371/journal.ppat.10037 26

117. R. M. Stilling, T. G. Dinan, J. F. Cryan. Microbial genes, brain & behaviour – epigenetic regulation of the gut–brain axis. DOI: 10.1111/gbb.12109.
http://onlinelibrary.wiley.com/doi/10.1111/gbb.12109/abstract;jsessionid=F9 A259194D111B1544816067055A05B7.f04t02

118. A.A. Shehata et al. The effect of glyphosate on potential pathogens and beneficial members of poultry microbiota in vitro; Current Microbiology, Apr. 2013. doi: 10.1007/s00284-012-0277-2.
https://www.ncbi.nlm.nih.gov/pubmed/23224412

119. Richard Strohman, Toward a new paradigm for life Beyond genetic determinism. http://www.psrast.org/strohmnewgen.htm

120. ALLIANCE FOR BIO-INTEGRITY, et al. Plaintiffs v. DONNA SHALALA, et al. Defendants. http://www.mindfully.org/GE/Richard-Lacey-FDA-Suit-28may99.htm

121. IU Bloomington News, Study of complete RNA collection of fruit fly uncovers unprecedented complexity, March 17, 2014.
http://news.indiana.edu/releases/iu/2014/03/drosophila-transcriptome-diversity-uncovered.shtml

122. K.Z. Guyton at al. Carcinogenicity of tetrachlorvinphos, parathion, malathion, diazinon, and glyphosate, The Lancet Oncology, 2015.
http://dx.doi.org/10.1016/S1470-2045(15)70134-8

123. Moms Across America, Glyphosate Testing Report: Findings in American Mothers' Breast Milk, Urine and Water.
http://www.momsacrossamerica.com/glyphosate_testing_results

124. M Krüger at al. Detection of Glyphosate Residues in Animals and Humans; Environmental & Analytical Toxicology, 2014.
http://dx.doi.org/10.4172/2161-0525.1000210

125. Medical Laboratory Bremen, Determination of Glyphosate residues in human urine samples from 18 European countries, 2013.
http://www.foeeurope.org/sites/default/files/glyphosate_studyresults_june1 2.pdf

126. IARC Monographs Volume 112: evaluation of five organophosphate insecticides and herbicides; 2015. http://www.iarc.fr/en/media-centre/iarcnews/pdf/MonographVolume112.pdf

127. Samsel A, Seneff S. Glyphosate's suppression of cytochrome P450 enzymes and amino acid biosynthesis by the gut microbiome: Pathways to modern diseases. Entropy. 2013;15:1416-1463. http://www.mdpi.com/1099-4300/15/4/1416

128. Gilles-Eric Séralini, et al. RETRACTED: Long term toxicity of a Roundup herbicide and a Roundup-tolerant genetically modified maize. doi:10.1016/j.fct.2012.08.005.
http://www.sciencedirect.com/science/article/pii/S0278691512005637

129. Soso AB, Barcellos LJG, Ranzani-Paiva MJ, et al. Chronic exposure to sublethal concentration of a glyphosate-based herbicide alters hormone profiles and affects reproduction of female Jundiá (Rhamdia quelen). Environ Toxicol Pharmacol. 2007;23:308–313.
http://www.sciencedirect.com/science/article/pii/S1382668906001578

130. Walsh LP, McCormick C, Martin C, Stocco DM. Roundup inhibits steroidogenesis by disrupting steroidogenic acute regulatory (StAR) protein expression. Env Health Perspect. 2000;108:769-76.
http://www.ncbi.nlm.nih.gov/pmc/articles/PMC1638308/

131. Romano RM, Romano MA, Bernardi MM, Furtado PV, Oliveira CA. Prepubertal exposure to commercial formulation of the herbicide Glyphosate alters testosterone levels and testicular morphology. Arch Toxicol. 2010;84:309-317. http://link.springer.com/article/10.1007/s00204-009-0494-z

132. Gasnier C, Dumont C, Benachour N, Clair E, Chagnon MC, Séralini GE. Glyphosate-based herbicides are toxic and endocrine disruptors in human cell lines. Toxicology. 2009;262:184-91. doi:10.1016/j.tox.2009.06.006.
http://www.sciencedirect.com/science/article/pii/S0300483X09003047

133. Hokanson R, Fudge R, Chowdhary R, Busbee D. Alteration of estrogen-regulated gene expression in human cells induced by the agricultural and horticultural herbicide glyphosate. Hum Exp Toxicol. 2007;26:747-52. doi:10.1177/0960327107083453.
http://het.sagepub.com/content/26/9/747.short

134. Thongprakaisang S, Thiantanawat A, Rangkadilok N, Suriyo T, Satayavivad J. Glyphosate induces human breast cancer cells growth via estrogen receptors. Food Chem Toxicol. 2013. doi:10.1016/j.fct.2013.05.057.
http://www.sciencedirect.com/science/article/pii/S0278691513003633

135. Robin Mesnage et al. Transcriptome profile analysis reflects rat liver and kidney damage following chronic ultra-low dose Roundup exposure. doi:10.1186/s12940-015-0056-1.
http://www.ehjournal.net/content/pdf/s12940-015-0056-1.pdf

136. Prescott VE, Campbell PM, Moore A, et al. Transgenic expression of bean alpha-amylase inhibitor in peas results in altered structure and immunogenicity. J Agric Food Chem. 2005;53:9023–30. doi:10.1021/jf050594v.
http://pubs.acs.org/doi/abs/10.1021/jf050594v

137. James C. Global status of commercialized biotech/GM crops: 2012. ISAAA; 2012.
http://www.isaaa.org/resources/publications/briefs/44/download/isaaa-brief-44-2012.pdf

138. USDA Economic Research Service. Recent trends in GE adoption. 2013. Available at: http://www.ers.usda.gov/data-products/adoption-of-genetically-engineered-crops-in-the-us/recent-trends-in-ge-adoption.aspx#.UzgPocfc26w

139. L. Hardell, M. Eriksson, M. Nordstrom. Exposure to pesticides as risk factor for non-Hodgkin's lymphoma and hairy cell leukemia: pooled analysis of two Swedish case-control studies; Leukemia & Lymphoma, May 2002. PMID: 12148884. https://www.ncbi.nlm.nih.gov/pubmed/?term=12148884

140. S. Thongprakaisang et al. Glyphosate induces human breast cancer cells growth via estrogen receptors; Food and Chemical Toxicology, Sep. 2013. doi: 10.1016/j.fct.2013.05.057. https://www.ncbi.nlm.nih.gov/pubmed/?term=23756170

141. John D. Beard at al. Pesticide Exposure and Depression among Male Private Pesticide Applicators in the Agricultural Health Study. doi: 10.1289/ehp.1307450.http://ehp.niehs.nih.gov/wp-content/uploads/122/9/ehp.1307450.pdf

142. NPR Shots, Scientists Give Genetically Modified Organisms A Safety Switch, 1/21/2015. http://www.npr.org/sections/health-shots/2015/01/21/378820888/scientists-give-genetically-modified-organisms-a-safety-switch

143. Tokar B. Deficiencies in federal regulatory oversight of genetically engineered crops. Institute for Social Ecology Biotechnology Project; 2006. http://environmentalcommons.org/RegulatoryDeficiencies.html

144. Jeffrey A Allen et al. Post-epidemic eosinophilia myalgia syndrome associated with L-Tryptophan. doi: 10.1002/art.30514. http://www.ncbi.nlm.nih.gov/pmc/articles/PMC3848710/

145. American Academy of Environmental Medicine, Genetically Modified Foods (Position Paper). https://www.aaemonline.org/gmo.php

146. IFOAM Organics International; Monsanto on Trial for Crimes Against Human Health and the Environment in the International People's Court. http://www.ifoam.bio/en/news/2016/01/22/monsanto-trial-crimes-against-human-health-and-environment-international-peoples

147. Robert E. Brackett, Ph.D., Director of Center for Food Safety and Applied Nutrition – Bioengineered Foods; FDA hearing before the Senate Committee on Agriculture, Nutrition and Forestry, June 14, 2005. http://www.fda.gov/NewsEvents/Testimony/ucm112927.htm

148. S. L. Greene, S. R. Kesoju, R. C. Martin, M. Kramer Occurrence of Transgenic Feral Alfalfa (Medicago sativa subsp. sativa L.) in Alfalfa Seed Production Areas in the United States. doi: 10.1371/journal.pone.0143296. http://journals.plos.org/plosone/article?id=10.1371/journal.pone.0143296

149. GMWatch, Judge declares GM crop illegal, 2007. http://www.gmwatch.org/news/archive/2007/7001-judge-declares-gm-crop-illegal-752007

150. Everything.Explained.Today, Genetically modified tree explained. http://everything.explained.today/Genetically_modified_tree/

151. M. Perkowski, Capital Press, USDA cannot restrict GMO pine; Jan. 28, 2015. http://www.capitalpress.com/Timber/20150128/usda-cannot-restrict-gmo-pine

152. Benbrook C. Impacts of genetically engineered crops on pesticide use in the US – The first sixteen years. Environ Sci Eur. 2012;24. http://www.enveurope.com/content/pdf/2190-4715-24-24.pdf

153. Binimelis R, Pengue W, Monterroso I. Transgenic treadmill: Responses to the emergence and spread of glyphosate-resistant johnsongrass in Argentina. Geoforum. 2009;40:623–633. http://www.sciencedirect.com/science/article/pii/S0016718509000360

154. The Organic & Non-GMO Report, Scientist warns of dire consequences with widespread use of glyphosate. http://www.non-gmoreport.com/articles/may10/consequenceso_widespread_glyphosate_use.php

155. Selim Eker et al. Foliar-Applied Glyphosate Substantially Reduced Uptake and Transport of Iron and Manganese in Sunflower (Helianthus annuus L.) Plants. doi: 10.1021/jf0625196. http://pubs.acs.org/doi/abs/10.1021/jf0625196

156. Bill Freese, Food Safety Review, a publication of the Center for Food Safety; Going Backwards: Dow ' s 2,4-D-Resistant Crops and a More Toxic Future. http://www.centerforfoodsafety.org/files/fsr_24-d.pdf

157. R. Polonetsky, G. Null, Seeds of Death Documentary, 50:18. https://www.youtube.com/watch?v=aFVF3MJNOHg

158. Majewski M.S. et al., US Geological Survey. Pesticides in Mississippi air and rain: a comparison between 1995 and 2007. Enviromental Toxicology and Chemistry, June 2014. PMID: 24549493. http://www.ncbi.nlm.nih.gov/pubmed/24549493

159. Percy Schmeiser David versus Monsanto, Denkmal Film. https://www.youtube.com/watch?v=IvkNda-_jdc

160. Groves M. Plant researchers offer bumper crop of humanity. LA Times; December 1997. http://articles.latimes.com/1997/dec/26/news/mn-2352

161. Gathura G. GM technology fails local potatoes. The Daily Nation (Kenya); January 2004. http://bit.ly/KPQPxL

162. New Scientist. Monsanto failure. 2004;181(2433). http://bit.ly/MHPG9W

163. Donald Danforth Plant Science Center. Danforth Center cassava viral resistance review update; 2006. http://bit.ly/1ry2DUC

164. Aaron deGrassi. Genetically modified crops and sustainable poverty alleviation in Sub-Saharan Africa: An assessment of current evidence. Third World Network – Africa; 2003. http://www.mindfully.org/GE/2003/Sustainable-Poverty-deGrassiJun03.htm

165. International Institute of Tropical Agriculture (IITA). Farmers get better yields from new drought-tolerant cassava; November 2008. http://www.cgiar.org/web-archives/www-cgiar-org-newsroom-releases-news-asp-idnews-797/

166. Paul H, Steinbrecher R. Hungry Corporations: Transnational biotech companies colonise the food chain. In: London, UK: Zed Books; 2003:3

167. Sustainable Pulse, GM Crops Now Banned in 38 Countries Worldwide – Sustainable Pulse Research; Oct. 22, 2015. http://sustainablepulse.com/2015/10/22/gm-crops-now-banned-in-36-countries-worldwide-sustainable-pulse-research/#.Vui34eY5v7w

168. Monbiot G. Organic farming will feed the world. The Guardian (UK); August 2000. http://www.monbiot.com/2000/08/24/organic-farming-will-feed-the-world/

169. Pollan M. Playing God in the garden. New York Times Magazine.; October 25, 1998. http://www.nytimes.com/1998/10/25/magazine/playing-god-in-the-garden.html

170. US Food and Drug Administration (FDA). Statement of policy: Foods derived from new plant varieties. FDA Fed Regist. 1992;57(104):22984. http://www.fda.gov/Food/GuidanceRegulation/GuidanceDocumentsRegulatoryInformation/Biotechnology/ucm096095.htm

171. European Food Safety Authority (EFSA). Frequently asked questions on EFSA GMO risk assessment. 2006. http://www.cibpt.org/docs/faq-efsa-gmo-risk-assessment.pdf

172. Biotechnology Consultation Agency Response Letter BNF No. 000034, September 25, 1996 https://www.fda.gov/Food/IngredientsPackagingLabeling/GEPlants/Submissions/ucm161107.htm

173. Mindfully.org, Lawsuit Challenges FDA Policy on Genetically Engineered Foods. http://www.mindfully.org/GE/Lawsuit-FDA-Policy-Foods.htm

174. National Research Council; Safety of Genetically Engineered Foods: Approaches toAssessing Unintended Health Effects. doi:10.17226/10977. http://www.nap.edu/read/10977/chapter/1

175. Henry-York Steiner et al., Editor's Choice: Evaluating the Potential for Adverse Interactions within Genetically Engineered Breeding Stacks, Plant Physiology April 2013. PMCID: PMC3613440. http://www.ncbi.nlm.nih.gov/pmc/articles/PMC3613440/

176. Stephen Wilson, We're not ready for genetic engineering. http://lockstep.com.au/blog/2011/01/15/not-ready-for-gm

177. Royal Commission on Genetic Modification; July 2001 Report. https://www.mfe.govt.nz/sites/default/files/Royal Commission on GM in NZ.pdf

178. Steven M. Druker; How the report of the Royal Commission on Genetic Modification Presents a False and Unjustifiable Favorable Picture of Bioengineered Foods. http://www.gefree.org.nz/gm-royal-commission-false-picture-bioengineered-foods

179. Steven M. Druker, JD, Executive Director Alliance for Bio - Integrity; An Open Letter - And a Challenge to the Royal Society. http://beyond-gm.org/wp-content/uploads/2015/03/DRUKER_OPEN-LETTER-TO-THE-ROYAL-SOCIETY_Final.pdf

180. Federal Food, Drug, and Cosmetic Act (FD&C Act). http://www.fda.gov/regulatoryinformation/legislation/federalfooddrugandcosmeticactfdcact/

181. Commissioner - Food and Drug Administration, Re: Substances Generally Recognized as Safe (GRAS); Docket No.: FDA-1997-N-0020. https://cspinet.org/new/pdf/GRAS%20Comment%20FINAL.pdf

182. A. Nicolia, A. Manzo, F. Veronesi, D. Rosellini. An overview of the last 10 years of genetically engineered crop safety research; Critical Reviews in Biotechnology, 9/16/2013. doi: 10.3109/07388551.2013.823595. http://www.tandfonline.com/doi/full/10.3109/07388551.2013.823595

183. A. Pusztai, S. Bardocz, S.W.B. Ewen, Genetically Modified Foods: Potential Human Health Effects. https://www.leopold.iastate.edu/sites/default/files/events/Chapter16.pdf

184. Royal Society, Genetically modified plants for food use and human health – an update. February 2002. https://royalsociety.org/~/media/Royal_Society_Content/policy/publications/2002/9960.pdf

185. Royal Society, Review of data on possible toxicity of GM potatoes, June 1999, 3. https://agbiotech.ces.ncsu.edu/wp-content/uploads/2015/08/Review-of-data-on-possible-toxicity-of-GM-potatoes.pdf?fwd=no

186. Gilles-Eric Séralini, et al. Republished study: long-term toxicity of a Roundup herbicide and a Roundup-tolerant genetically modified maize, Environmental Sciences Europe, 2014. doi:10.1186/s12302-014-0014-5. http://www.enveurope.com/content/26/1/14

187. Robinson C, Latham J. The Goodman affair: Monsanto targets the heart of science. Independent Science News. 2013. Available at: http://www.independentsciencenews.org/science-media/the-goodman-affair-monsanto-targets-the-heart-of-science/

188. Elsevier announces article retraction from Journal Food and Chemical Toxicology: https://www.elsevier.com/about/press-releases/research-and-journals/sthash.VfY74Y24.dpuf

189. Committee on Publication Ethics (COPE). Retraction guidelines, 2009. http://publicationethics.org/files/retraction%20guidelines.pdf

190. Committee on Publication Ethics (COPE). Members: Food and Chemical Toxicology. http://publicationethics.org/members/food-and-chemical-toxicology

191. David Schubert, Science study controversy impacts world health: The San Diego Union-Tribune, 2014. http://www.sandiegouniontribune.com/news/2014/jan/08/science-food-health/

192. Food and Chemical Toxicology Editor-in-Chief, A. Wallace Hayes, Publishes Response to Letters to the Editors; Elsevier, 2013. http://www.elsevier.com/about/press-releases/research-and-journals/food-and-chemical-toxicology-editor-in-chief,-a.-wallace-hayes,-publishes-response-to-letters-to-the-editors#sthash.tTW2LCGq.dpuf

193. Dr. S.W.B. Ewen, A. Pusztai, PhD, Effect of diets containing genetically modified potatoes expressing Galanthus nivalis lectin on rat small intestine; The Lancet, 1999. http://dx.doi.org/10.1016/S0140-6736(98)05860-7

194. Jeffrey M. Smith: Monsanto, GMO Seeds of Destruction, 19:40. https://www.youtube.com/watch?v=LSDEkoPwMfk

195. Interview with Dr. Arpad Pusztai: The Scientist Whose Research Has All But Brought GE Foods to a Halt in Britain; Organic Consumers Association. https://www.organicconsumers.org/old_articles/ge/pusztaihalt.php

196. Editorial: Health risks of genetically modified foods; The Lancet Vol. 353, No. 9167, p1811, 29 May 1999. http://www.thelancet.com/journals/lancet/article/PIIS0140-6736%2899%2900093-8/fulltext

197. How to Know if Your Weed Killer Could Cause Cancer; The Dr. Oz Show, 4/7/2015. http://www.doctoroz.com/episode/how-outsmart-identity-thieves-after-your-money-and-medical-data?video_id=4158724753001

198. Dr. Oz Explains Genetically Modified Apples; The Dr. Oz Show, 3/10/2015. http://www.doctoroz.com/episode/non-browning-gmo-apple-it-safe

199. WikiLeaks; France and the WTO AG Biotech Case, 07PARIS4723_a.
https://www.wikileaks.org/plusd/cables/07PARIS4723_a.html

200. Global GMO Scandal - American Nutrition Association, Nutrition Digest,
Vol. 38, No. 2. http://americannutritionassociation.org/newsletter/gmo-
foods-world-wide-scandal

201. Kurt Eichenwald, Biotechnology Food: From the Lab to a Debacle; The New
York Times, 1/25/2001.
http://www.nytimes.com/2001/01/25/business/25FOOD.html?pagewanted=a
ll

202. StarLink corn recall; Wikipedia.
https://en.wikipedia.org/wiki/StarLink_corn_recall

203. Ronnie Cummins, Monsanto's Permit to Poison Us; The Hufington Post,
5/25/2011. http://www.huffingtonpost.com/ronnie-cummins/monsantos-
permit-to-poiso_b_649568.html

204. Biotechnology Consultation Agency Response Letter BNF No. 000080; U.S.
Food and Drug Administration.
http://www.fda.gov/Food/FoodScienceResearch/GEPlants/Submissions/ucm
155752.htm

205. Biotechnology Consultation Agency Response Letter BNF No. 000116; U.S.
Food and Drug Administration.
http://www.fda.gov/Food/FoodScienceResearch/GEPlants/Submissions/ucm
240079.htm

206. Biotechnology Consultation Agency Response Letter BNF No. 000117; U.S.
Food and Drug Administration.
http://www.fda.gov/Food/FoodScienceResearch/GEPlants/Submissions/ucm
314243.htm

207. Biotechnology Consultation Agency Response Letter BNF No. 000121; U.S.
Food and Drug Administration.
http://www.fda.gov/Food/FoodScienceResearch/GEPlants/Submissions/ucm
242539.htm

208. Biotechnology Consultation Agency Response Letter BNF No. 000125; U.S.
Food and Drug Administration.
http://www.fda.gov/Food/FoodScienceResearch/GEPlants/Submissions/ucm
282993.htm

209. Biotechnology Consultation Agency Response Letter BNF No. 000126; U.S.
Food and Drug Administration.
http://www.fda.gov/Food/FoodScienceResearch/GEPlants/Submissions/ucm
304083.htm

210. Biotechnology Consultation Agency Response Letter BNF No. 000135; U.S.
Food and Drug Administration.
http://www.fda.gov/Food/FoodScienceResearch/GEPlants/Submissions/ucm
352956.htm

211. Biotechnology Consultation Agency Response Letter BNF 000144; U.S. Food
and Drug Administration.
http://www.fda.gov/Food/FoodScienceResearch/GEPlants/Submissions/UC
M451465

212. Biotechnology Consultation Agency Response Letter BNF 000148; U.S. Food and Drug Administration.
http://www.fda.gov/Food/FoodScienceResearch/GEPlants/Submissions/ucm493311.htm

213. Eisenhower's Farewell Address to the Nation; January 17, 1961
http://mcadams.posc.mu.edu/ike.htm

214. Ken Yamada, Wall Street Journal, Genetic Vegomatics Splice and Dice With Weird Results; April 18, 1992. http://www.mindfully.org/GE/Vegomatics-Splice-Dice18apr92.htm

215. Smallholders, food security, and the environment; UNEP & IFAD, 2013.
https://www.ifad.org/documents/10180/666cac24-14b6-43c2-876d-9c2d1f01d5dd

216. Reaping the benefits, Science and the sustainable intensification of global agriculture, October 2009; The Royal Society.
https://royalsociety.org/~/media/Royal_Society_Content/policy/publications/2009/4294967719.pdf

217. Steven Franzel. Financial analysis of agroforestry practices. In Valuing agroforestry systems, ed. J.R.R. Alavalapati and D. Mercer, 9-37; 2004.
http://link.springer.com/chapter/10.1007/1-4020-2413-4_2

218. S. Franzel,D. Phiri, F. Kwesiga. Trees on the farm: assessing the adoption potential of agroforestry practices in Africa; 2002. doi: 10.1079/9780851995618.0037.
http://www.cabi.org/cabebooks/ebook/20023147398

219. O.C. Ajayi et al. Labour inputs and financial profitability of conventional and agroforestry-based soil fertility management practices in Zambia; AgEcon, 9/30/2009. http://purl.umn.edu/55046

220. Push–pull agricultural pest management. Wikipedia.
https://en.wikipedia.org/wiki/Push%E2%80%93pull_agricultural_pest_management

221. The Farming System Trial, Celebrating 30 Years; Rodale Institute, 2011.
http://rodaleinstitute.org/assets/FSTbooklet.pdf

222. George Monbiot. Organic Farming Will Feed the World. 8/24/2000.
http://www.monbiot.com/2000/08/24/organic-farming-will-feed-the-world/

223. Global Research - Center for Research on Globalization; American Farmers Abandoning Genetically Modified Seeds: "Non-GMO Crops are more Productive and Profitable". http://www.globalresearch.ca/american-farmers-abandoning-genetically-modified-seeds-non-gmo-crops-are-more-productive-and-profitable/5366365

224. Center for Food Safety; International Labeling Laws.
http://www.centerforfoodsafety.org/issues/976/ge-food-labeling/international-labeling-laws

225. P. Quillin, PHD, RD, CNS, Cancer's Sweet Tooth.
http://www.mercola.com/article/sugar/sugar_cancer.htm

226. The Futility of Conventional Cancer Treatments; Dr. Axe.
http://draxe.com/the-futility-of-conventional-cancer-treatments/

227. American Cancer Society; Cancer Treatment & Survivorship Facts & Figures, 2012-2013.
http://www.cancer.org/acs/groups/content/@epidemiologysurveilance/documents/document/acspc-033876.pdf

228. Wikipedia; History of cancer chemotherapy.
https://en.wikipedia.org/wiki/History_of_cancer_chemotherapy

229. Wikipedia; Chemotherapy. https://en.wikipedia.org/wiki/Chemotherapy

230. G. Morgan, R. Ward , M. Barton, The Contribution of Cytotoxic Chemotherapy to 5-year Survival in Adult Malignancies; Clinical Oncology, 2004. doi:10.1016/j.clon.2004.06.007.
https://www.burtongoldberg.com/home/burtongoldberg/contribution-of-chemotherapy-to-five-year-survival-rate-morgan.pdf

231. American Society of Clinical Oncology. Meta-analysis of randomized trials testing the biochemical modulation of fluorouracil by methotrexate in metastatic colorectal cancer. Advanced Colorectal Cancer Meta-Analysis Project; Journal of Clinical Oncology, 1994. PMID: 8164048.
http://jco.ascopubs.org/content/12/5/960.abstract

232. Dying Well – The Final Stage of Survivorship; National Coalition for Cancer Survivorship. http://www.canceradvocacy.org/resources/cancer-survival-toolbox/special-topics/dying-well/?gclid=Cj0KCQjwiqTNBRDVARIsAGsd9MpQfWZIloIdCKpQI6qVuvoSUM24XqilZ_PJWyZoPtzvUP73-4niX7kaAh5GEALw_wcB

233. Global Pharmaceutical Industry - Statistics & Facts; Statista.
http://www.statista.com/topics/1764/global-pharmaceutical-industry/

234. M. Al-Hajj et al., Prospective identification of tumorigenic breast cancer cells. doi: 10.1073/pnas.0530291100.
http://www.pnas.org/content/100/7/3983.long

235. Charafe-Jauffret E. et al., Cancer Stem Cells in Breast: Current Opinion and Future Challenges; Pathobiology, 2008. doi:10.1159/000123845.
http://www.karger.com/Article/FullText/123845

236. D. Bhuvanesh, J. Chang, Treatment Resistance in Stem Cells and Breast Cancer; Journal of Mammary Gland Biology and Neoplasia, 2009. doi:10.1007/s10911-009-9117-9.

237. Wikipedia; Phytoestrogens. https://en.wikipedia.org/wiki/Phytoestrogens

238. Report - Glyphosate: Unsafe on Any Plate, Food Testing Results and Scientific Reasons for Concern; Food Democracy Now! and The Detox Project. https://usrtk.org/wp-content/uploads/2016/11/FDN_Glyphosate_FoodTesting_Report_p2016-3.pdf

239. Wikiepedia; Lipid peroxidation.
https://en.wikipedia.org/wiki/Lipid_peroxidation

240. Ayodeji O.F., Ganiyu O, International Journal of Food Science; Thermal Oxidation Induces Lipid Peroxidation and Changes in the Physicochemical Properties and β-Carotene Content of Arachis Oil.
http://www.hindawi.com/journals/ijfs/2015/806524/

241. Mongabay; Amazon tribe creates 500-page traditional medicine encyclopedia. http://news.mongabay.com/2015/06/amazon-tribe-creates-500-page-traditional-medicine-encyclopedia/

242. Andrew Curry. Archaeology: The milk revolution; Nature, 7/31/2013.
http://www.nature.com/news/archaeology-the-milk-revolution-1.13471

243. The Nobel Prize in Physiology or Medicine 1931; Otto Heinrich Warburg.
http://www.nobelprize.org/nobel_prizes/medicine/laureates/1931/

244. Otto Warburg, The Metabolism of Carcinoma Cells; 1925.
http://wp.nyu.edu/biochemistry2016_2/wp-
content/uploads/sites/3323/2016/01/J-Cancer-Res-1925-Warburg-148-63.pdf

245. S.A. Cunningham, J.D. Ruben, K.M. Venkat Narayan. Health of foreign-
born people in the United States: A review; Health & Place, Vol. 14, Issue 4,
Dec. 2008, P.623-635. doi: 10.1016/j.healthplace.2007.12.002.
http://www.sciencedirect.com/science/article/pii/S135382920700113X

246. Sevcan Mamur et al., Does potassium sorbate induce genotoxic or
mutagenic effects in lymphocytes?; Elsevier Toxicology in Vitro.
doi:10.1016/j.tiv.2009.12.021.
http://www.sciencedirect.com/science/article/pii/S0887233309003853

247. K. Kitano et al., Mutagenicity and DNA-damaging activity caused by
decomposed products of potassium sorbate reacting with ascorbic acid in
the presence of Fe salt; Elsevier Food and Chemical Toxicology.
doi:10.1016/S0278-6915(02)00119-9.
http://www.sciencedirect.com/science/article/pii/S0278691502001199

248. N. Zengin et al., The evaluation of the genotoxicity of two food
preservatives: Sodium benzoate and potassium benzoate; Elsevier Food and
Chemical Toxicology. doi:10.1016/j.fct.2010.11.040.
http://www.sciencedirect.com/science/article/pii/S0278691510006988

249. P.J. Hughes et al., Estrogenic Alkylphenols Induce Cell Death by Inhibiting
Testis Endoplasmic Reticulum Ca2+ Pumps; Biochem. & Biophys. Res.
Comm., 11/2/2000. doi:10.1006/bbrc.2000.3710
http://www.sciencedirect.com/science/article/pii/S0006291X00937100

250. Two Preservatives to Avoid?; Berkley Wellness, 2/1/2011.
http://www.berkeleywellness.com/healthy-eating/food-safety/article/two-
preservatives-avoid

251. D. Thompson, P. Moldéus, Cytotoxicity of butylated hydroxyanisole and
butylated hydroxytoluene in isolated rat hepatocytes; Biochemical
Pharmacology, 6/1/1988. doi:10.1016/0006-2952(88)90582-5.
http://www.sciencedirect.com/science/article/pii/0006295288905825

252. Safer AM, al-Nughamish AJ, Hepatotoxicity induced by the anti-oxidant
food additive, butylated hydroxytoluene (BHT), in rats: an electron
microscopical study; Histol Histopathol., 4/14/1999. PMID: 10212800.
http://www.ncbi.nlm.nih.gov/pubmed/10212800

253. S. Kobylewskia & M.F. Jacobsonb, Toxicology of food dyes; International
Journal of Occupational and Environmental Health. doi:
10.1179/1077352512Z.00000000034.
http://www.tandfonline.com/doi/abs/10.1179/1077352512Z.00000000034?jou
rnalCode=yjoh20

254. Vânia Paula Salviano dos Santos et al., Benzene as a Chemical Hazard in
Processed Foods; Int'l J. of Food Science, 2015. doi:10.1155/2015/545640
http://www.hindawi.com/journals/ijfs/2015/545640/

255. E. Lichtblau, S. Shane, Vast F.D.A. Effort Tracked E-Mails of Its Scientists;
The New York Times, 7/14/2012.
http://www.nytimes.com/2012/07/15/us/fda-surveillance-of-scientists-
spread-to-outside-critics.html?pagewanted=all&_r=0

256. Luo KW et al., In vivo and in vitro anti-tumor and anti-metastasis effects of Coriolus versicolor aqueous extract on mouse mammary 4T1 carcinoma; Phytomedicine, 2014. doi:10.1016/j.phymed.2014.04.020. http://www.ncbi.nlm.nih.gov/pubmed/24856767

257. J. Jiang, BreastDefend™ prevents breast-to-lung cancer metastases in an orthotopic animal model of triple-negative human breast cancer; Oncology Reports, 7/26/2012. doi:10.3892/or.2012.1936. https://www.spandidos-publications.com/or/28/4/1139

258. Lj. Harhaji et al., Anti-tumor effect of Coriolus versicolor methanol extract against mouse B16 melanoma cells: In vitro and in vivo study; Food & Chem. Tox., May 2008. doi:10.1016/j.fct.2008.01.027. http://www.ncbi.nlm.nih.gov/pubmed/18313195

259. CY Ho et al., Coriolus versicolor (Yunzhi) extract attenuates growth of human leukemia xenografts and induces apoptosis through the mitochondrial pathway; Oncology Reports, 9/1/2006. doi:10.3892/or.16.3.609. https://www.spandidos-publications.com/or/16/3/609

260. E. Vetchinkina et al. Antitumor Activity of Extracts from Medicinal Basidiomycetes Mushrooms; Int'l J. of Medicinal Mushrooms, 2016. doi: 10.1615/IntJMedMushrooms.v18.i11.10. https://www.ncbi.nlm.nih.gov/pubmed/28008808

261. K. Na et al. Anticarcinogenic effects of water extract of sporoderm-broken spores of Ganoderma lucidum on colorectal cancer in vitro and in vivo; Int'l J. of Oncology, May 2017. doi: 10.3892/ijo.2017.3939. https://www.ncbi.nlm.nih.gov/pubmed/28358412

262. Y. Yang et al. Feeding of the water extract from Ganoderma lingzhi to rats modulates secondary bile acids, intestinal microflora, mucins, and propionate important to colon cancer; Bioscience, Biotechnology, and Biochemistry, 6/29/2017. doi: 10.1080/09168451.2017.1343117. https://www.ncbi.nlm.nih.gov/pubmed/28661219

263. Moringa oleifera; Wikipedia. https://en.wikipedia.org/wiki/Moringa_oleifera

264. A.K. Al-Asmari et al., Moringa oleifera as an Anti-Cancer Agent against Breast and Colorectal Cancer Cell Lines; PLOS One, 8/19/2015. http://dx.doi.org/10.1371/journal.pone.0135814

265. E.A. Elsayed et al., In vitro Evaluation of Cytotoxic Activities of Essential Oil from Moringa oleifera Seeds on HeLa, HepG2, MCF-7, CACO-2 and L929 Cell Lines; Asian Pac J Cancer Prev., 2015. PMID: 26107222. http://www.ncbi.nlm.nih.gov/pubmed/26107222

266. I.L. Jung. Soluble Extract from Moringa oleifera Leaves with a New Anticancer Activity; PLOS One, 4/18/2014. http://dx.doi.org/10.1371/journal.pone.0095492

267. F.C. Maiyo, R. Moodley, M. Singh, Cytotoxicity, Antioxidant and Apoptosis Studies of Quercetin-3-O Glucoside and 4-(β-D-Glucopyranosyl-1$\rightarrow$4-α-L-Rhamnopyranosyloxy)-Benzyl Isothiocyanate from Moringa oleifera; Bentham Science - Anti-Cancer Agents in Medicinal Chemistry, 2016. doi:10.2174/1871520615666151002110424. http://www.eurekaselect.com/135459/article

268. I.L. Jung, J.H. Lee, S.C. Kang, A potential oral anticancer drug candidate, Moringa oleifera leaf extract, induces the apoptosis of human hepatocellular carcinoma cells; Oncology Letters, 2015. doi:10.3892/ol.2015.3482. http://www.ncbi.nlm.nih.gov/pmc/articles/PMC4533244/

269. P.T. Krishnamurthy et al., Identification and characterization of a potent anticancer fraction from the leaf extracts of Moringa oleifera L; Indian Journal of Experimental Biology, 2015. PMID: 25757240. http://www.ncbi.nlm.nih.gov/pubmed/25757240

270. E.O. Akanni et al., Chemopreventive and anti-leukemic effects of ethanol extracts of Moringa oleifera leaves on wistar rats bearing benzene induced leukemia; Bentham Science - Current Pharmaceutical Biotechnology, 2014. PMID: 25051949. http://www.ncbi.nlm.nih.gov/pubmed/25051949

271. D. Brunelli et al., The isothiocyanate produced from glucomoringin inhibits NF-kB and reduces myeloma growth in nude mice in vivo; Biochemical Pharmacology, 4/15/2010. doi: 10.1016/j.bcp.2009.12.008. http://www.ncbi.nlm.nih.gov/pubmed/20006591

272. A. Shaban et al., In Vitro Cytotoxicity of Moringa Oleifera Against Different Human Cancer Cell Lines; Asian Journal of Pharmaceutical and Clinical Research, 2012. http://www.ajpcr.com/Vol5Suppl4/1488.pdf

273. A.F. Abdull Razis et al., Mini-Review: Health Benefits of Moringa Oleifera; Asian Pacific Journal of Cancer Prevention, 2014. doi: 10.7314/APJCP.2014.15.20.8571. https://www.researchgate.net/publication/267932962_Health_Benefits_of_Moringa_oleifera

274. Jed W. Fahey, Sc.D., Moringa oleifera : A Review of the Medical Evidence for Its Nutritional, Therapeutic, and Prophylactic Properties. Part 1; Trees for Life Journal, 12/1/2005. http://www.tfljournal.org/article.php/20051201124931586

275. I. Nath, S. Paul, B. Nath, Moringa Oleifera: Bio-Inspired Approaches to Plant Based Nonomedicine, a Mini-Review; European Journal of Molecular Biology and Biochemistry, 2015. http://mcmed.us/downloads/144205064489%28ejmbb%29.pdf

276. P. Karna et al., Benefits of whole ginger extract in prostate cancer; British Journal of Nutrition, 2012. doi:10.1017/S0007114511003308. http://www.ncbi.nlm.nih.gov/pubmed/21849094

277. E. Langner, S. Greifenberg, J. Gruenwald, Ginger: history and use; Advances in Therapy, 1998. PMID: 10178636. http://www.ncbi.nlm.nih.gov/pubmed/10178636

278. C. Nordqvist, Ginger Kills Ovarian Cancer Cells; Medical News Today, 4/17/2006. http://www.medicalnewstoday.com/articles/41747.php

279. S.H.M Habib et al., Ginger Extract (Zingiber Officinale) has Anti-Cancer and Anti-Inflammatory Effects on Ethionine-Induced Hepatoma Rats; Clinics, 2008. doi:10.1590/S1807-59322008000600017. http://www.ncbi.nlm.nih.gov/pmc/articles/PMC2664283/

280. N. Rastogi et al., Proteasome inhibition mediates p53 reactivation and anti-cancer activity of 6-gingerol in cervical cancer cells; Oncotarget 12/22/2015. doi:10.18632/oncotarget.6383. http://www.ncbi.nlm.nih.gov/pubmed/26621832

281. Y.J. Park, [6]-Gingerol induces cell cycle arrest and cell death of mutant p53-expressing pancreatic cancer cells; Yonsei Med. J. 10/31/2006. PMID: 17066513. http://www.ncbi.nlm.nih.gov/pubmed/17066513

282. E.C. Kim, [6]-Gingerol, a pungent ingredient of ginger, inhibits angiogenesis in vitro and in vivo; Biochemical and Biophysical Research Communications, 9/23/2005. doi: 10.1016/j.bbrc.2005.07.076. http://www.sciencedirect.com/science/article/pii/S0006291X05014543

283. K. Jeena et al., Protection against Whole Body γ-Irradiation Induced Oxidative Stress and Clastogenic Damage in Mice by Ginger Essential Oil; Asian Pacific J. of Cancer Prev., 2016. http://www.ncbi.nlm.nih.gov/pubmed/27039766

284. E. Marzbani, The Invisible Arm of Immunity in Common Cancer Chemoprevention Agents; Cancer Prevention Research, 2013. doi: 10.1158/1940-6207.CAPR-13-0036. http://cancerpreventionresearch.aacrjournals.org/content/6/8/764.long

285. S.T. Chien, Galangin, a novel dietary flavonoid, attenuates metastatic feature via PKC/ERK signaling pathway in TPA-treated liver cancer HepG2 cells; Cancer Cell Int., 2/4/2015. PMID: 25698902. http://www.ncbi.nlm.nih.gov/pubmed/25698902

286. Yu-Jen Jou et al., Quantitative phosphoproteomic analysis reveals γ-bisabolene inducing p53-mediated apoptosis of human oral squamous cell carcinoma via HDAC2 inhibition and ERK1/2 activation; Proteomics, Oct. 2015. doi: 10.1002/pmic.201400568. http://www.ncbi.nlm.nih.gov/pubmed/26194454

287. N.H. Oberlies et al., Structure-activity relationships of diverse Annonaceous acetogenins against multidrug resistant human mammary adenocarcinoma (MCF-7/Adr) cells; Journal of Medicinal Chemistry, 6/20/1997. PMID: 9207950. http://www.ncbi.nlm.nih.gov/pubmed/9207950

288. N.H. Oberlies et al., The Annonaceous acetogenin bullatacin is cytotoxic against multidrug-resistant human mammary adenocarcinoma cells; Cancer Letters, 5/1/1997. PMID: 9097981. http://www.ncbi.nlm.nih.gov/pubmed/9097981

289. M.P. Torres et al., Graviola: a novel promising natural-derived drug that inhibits tumorigenicity and metastasis of pancreatic cancer cells in vitro and in vivo through altering cell metabolism; Cancer Letters, 10/1/2012. doi: 10.1016/j.canlet.2012.03.031. http://www.ncbi.nlm.nih.gov/pubmed/22475682

290. K. Geum-soog et al, Two New Mono-Tetrahydrofuran Ring Acetogenins, Annomuricin E and Muricapentocin, from the Leaves of Annona muricata; Journal of Natural Products, 3/11/1998. doi: 10.1021/np970534m. http://pubs.acs.org/doi/pdf/10.1021/np970534m

291. Y. Dai et al., Selective growth inhibition of human breast cancer cells by graviola fruit extract in vitro and in vivo involving downregulation of EGFR expression; Nutrition and Cancer, 2011. doi: 10.1080/01635581.2011.563027. http://www.ncbi.nlm.nih.gov/pubmed/21767082

292. V.C. George et al., Quantitative assessment of the relative antineoplastic potential of the n-butanolic leaf extract of Annona muricata Linn. in normal and immortalized human cell lines; Asian Pacific J. of Cancer Prevention, 2012. PMID: 22524847. http://www.ncbi.nlm.nih.gov/pubmed/22524847

293. Y.M. Ko et al., Annonacin induces cell cycle-dependent growth arrest and apoptosis in estrogen receptor-α-related pathways in MCF-7 cells; J. of Ethnopharmacology, 10/11/2011. doi: 10.1016/j.jep.2011.07.056. http://www.ncbi.nlm.nih.gov/pubmed/21840388

294. C.A. Pieme et al., Antiproliferative activity and induction of apoptosis by Annona muricata (Annonaceae) extract on human cancer cells; BMC Complementary Alternative Medicine, 2014. doi: 10.1186/1472-6882-14-516. http://www.ncbi.nlm.nih.gov/pubmed/25539720

295. V. Kuete et al., Cytotoxicity of methanol extracts of Annona muricata, Passiflora edulis and nine other Cameroonian medicinal plants towards multi-factorial drug-resistant cancer cell lines; SpringerPlus, 9/27/2016. doi: 10.1186/s40064-016-3361-4. https://www.ncbi.nlm.nih.gov/pmc/articles/PMC5039145/

296. K.I. Ahammadsahib et al., Mode of action of bullatacin: a potent antitumor and pesticidal annonaceous acetogenin; Life Sciences, 1993. PMID: 8371627. http://www.ncbi.nlm.nih.gov/pubmed/8371627

297. S. Sun et al., Three new anti-proliferative Annonaceous acetogenins with mono-tetrahydrofuran ring from graviola fruit (Annona muricata); Bioorganic & Medicinal Chemistry Letters, 6/15/2014. http://www.ncbi.nlm.nih.gov/pubmed/24780120

298. C. Yang et al., Synergistic interactions among flavonoids and acetogenins in Graviola (Annona muricata) leaves confer protection against prostate cancer; Oxford Journals Carcinogenesis, 4/11/2015. doi: 10.1093/carcin/bgv046. http://carcin.oxfordjournals.org/content/36/6/656.long

299. G. Deep et al., Graviola inhibits hypoxia-induced NADPH oxidase activity in prostate cancer cells reducing their proliferation and clonogenicity; Scientific Reports, 3/16/2016. doi: 10.1038/srep23135. http://www.ncbi.nlm.nih.gov/pubmed/26979487

300. S.Z. Moghadamtousi et al., Annona muricata leaves induced apoptosis in A549 cells through mitochondrial-mediated pathway and involvement of NF-κB. doi: 10.1186/1472-6882-14-299. http://www.ncbi.nlm.nih.gov/pubmed/25127718

301. S.Z. Moghadamtousi et al., Annona muricata leaves induce G_1 cell cycle arrest and apoptosis through mitochondria-mediated pathway in human HCT-116 and HT-29 colon cancer cells; J. of Ethnopharmacology, 10/28/2014. doi: 10.1016/j.jep.2014.08.011. http://www.ncbi.nlm.nih.gov/pubmed/25195082

302. N. Liu et al., Functional proteomic analysis revels that the ethanol extract of Annona muricataL.induces liver cancer cell apoptosis through endoplasmic reticulum stress pathway; J Ethnopharmacology, 5/17/2016. doi: 10.1016/j.jep.2016.05.045. http://www.ncbi.nlm.nih.gov/pubmed/27224241

303. V.P. Magadi et al., Evaluation of cytotoxicity of aqueous extract of Graviola leaves on squamous cell carcinoma cell-25 cell lines by 3-(4,5-dimethylthiazol-2-Yl) -2,5-diphenyltetrazolium bromide assay and determination of percentage of cell inhibition at G2M phase of cell cycle by flow cytometry: An in vitro study; Contemporary Clinical Dentistry, Oct-Dec 2015. doi: 10.4103/0976-237X.169863. http://www.ncbi.nlm.nih.gov/pubmed/26681860

304. Mayo Clinic, Nearly 7 in 10 Americans are on prescription drugs; ScienceDaily, 19 June 2013.
www.sciencedaily.com/releases/2013/06/130619132352.htm

305. United States Census Bureau, Annual Estimates of the Resident Population for Selected Age Groups by Sex: 4/1/2010 to 7/1/2014.
http://factfinder.census.gov/faces/tableservices/jsf/pages/productview.xhtml?src=bkmk

306. Health, United States, 2015; U.S. Dept. of Health and Human Services, CDC, Nat'l Center for Health Stats., 2015.
http://www.cdc.gov/nchs/data/hus/hus15.pdf#094

307. Making the Vaccine Decision; CDC.
http://www.cdc.gov/vaccines/parents/vaccine-decision/index.html

308. Which vaccines contain human protein and DNA? National Vaccine Information Center. http://www.vaccine-tlc.org/human

309. M-M-R® II (Measles, Mumps, and Rubella Virus Vaccine Live); Merck.
https://www.merck.com/product/usa/pi_circulars/m/mmr_ii/mmr_ii_pi.pdf

310. Helen Branswell. Getting a flu shot every year? More may not be better; STAT, 11/11/2015. https://www.statnews.com/2015/11/11/flu-shots-reduce-effectiveness/

311. A.R. Mawson et al. Pilot comparative study on the health of vaccinated and unvaccinated 6- to 12-year-old U.S. children; Journal of Translational Science, 4/24/2017. doi: 10.15761/JTS.1000186.
http://www.oatext.com/pdf/JTS-3-186.pdf

312. Number of Children & Adolescents Taking Psychiatric Drugs in the U.S.; CCHR International, 2014. https://www.cchrint.org/psychiatric-drugs/children-on-psychiatric-drugs/

313. POP1 Child population: Number of children (in millions) ages 0–17 in the United States by age, 1950–2015 and projected 2016–2050; childstats.gov.
http://www.childstats.gov/americaschildren/tables/pop1.asp

314. T. Remer, Influence of diet on acid-base balance; Seminars in Dialysis, Jul-Aug 2000. PMID: 10923348.
http://www.ncbi.nlm.nih.gov/pubmed/10923348/

315. L. Frassetto, Diet, evolution and aging--the pathophysiologic effects of the post-agricultural inversion of the potassium-to-sodium and base-to-chloride ratios in the human diet; European Journal of Nutrition, Oct. 2001. PMID: 11842945. http://www.ncbi.nlm.nih.gov/pubmed/11842945

316. K.L. Penniston, S.A. Tanumihardjo. The acute and chronic toxic effects of vitamin A; The American Journal of Clinical Nutrition, Feb. 2006, Vol. 83, No. 2, pp 191-201. PMID: 16469975.
http://ajcn.nutrition.org/content/83/2/191.long

317. William C. Roberts, MD. Twenty questions on atherosclerosis; Baylor University Medical Center Proceedings, Apr. 2000, Vol. 13 No. 2, pp 139-143. PMCID: PMC1312295.
https://www.ncbi.nlm.nih.gov/pmc/articles/PMC1312295/

318. P.A. Offit et al. Addressing Parents' Concerns: Do Multiple Vaccines Overwhelm or Weaken the Infant's Immune System?; Pediatrics, Jan. 2002, Vol. 109 / Issue 1.
http://pediatrics.aappublications.org/content/109/1/124.full

319. Zen Honeycutt. Glyphosate in Vaccines Report; Moms Across America, 9/5/2016.
https://d3n8a8pro7vhmx.cloudfront.net/yesmaam/pages/1707/attachments/original/1473130173/FullGlyphosateinVaccinesReport_(6).pdf?1473130173

320. K. Schütz, R. Carle, A. Schieber. Taraxacum—A review on its phytochemical and pharmacological profile; Journal of Ethnopharmacology, 10/11/2006. doi:10.1016/j.jep.2006.07.021.
http://www.sciencedirect.com/science/article/pii/S0378874106003576

321. J.Y. Yoon et al. Novel TRAIL sensitizer Taraxacum officinale F.H. Wigg enhances TRAIL-induced apoptosis in Huh7 cells; Molecular Carcinogenesis, Apr. 2016. PMID: 25647515.
http://www.ncbi.nlm.nih.gov/pubmed/25647515

322. S.J. Chatterjee et al. The efficacy of dandelion root extract in inducing apoptosis in drug-resistant human melanoma cells; Evid Based Complement Alternat Med., 2011. doi: 10.1155/2011/129045.
http://www.ncbi.nlm.nih.gov/pubmed/21234313

323. K. Hata et al. Differentiation-inducing activity of lupeol, a lupane-type triterpene from Chinese dandelion root (Hokouei-kon), on a mouse melanoma cell line; Biological and Pharmaceutical Bulletin, Aug. 2000. PMID: 10963304. http://www.ncbi.nlm.nih.gov/pubmed/10963304

324. S.C. Sigstedt et al. Evaluation of aqueous extracts of Taraxacum officinale on growth and invasion of breast and prostate cancer cells; International Journal of Oncology, May 2008. PMID: 18425335.
http://www.ncbi.nlm.nih.gov/pubmed/18425335

325. J. Jiang, I. Eliaz, D. Sliva. Suppression of growth and invasive behavior of human prostate cancer cells by ProstaCaid™: mechanism of activity; International Journal of Oncology, June 2011. doi: 10.3892/ijo.2011.996.
http://www.ncbi.nlm.nih.gov/pubmed/21468543

326. P. Ovadje et al. Selective induction of apoptosis through activation of caspase-8 in human leukemia cells (Jurkat) by dandelion root extract; Journal of Ethnopharmacology, 1/7/2011. doi: 10.1016/j.jep.2010.09.005.
http://www.ncbi.nlm.nih.gov/pubmed/20849941

327. M. Takasaki et al. Anti-carcinogenic activity of Taraxacum plant. I; Biological and Pharmaceutical Bulletin, June 1999. PMID: 10408234.
http://www.ncbi.nlm.nih.gov/pubmed/10408234

328. M. Takasaki et al. Anti-carcinogenic activity of Taraxacum plant. II; Biological and Pharmaceutical Bulletin, June 1999. PMID: 10408235.
http://www.ncbi.nlm.nih.gov/pubmed/10408235

329. P. Ovadje, C. Hamm, S. Pandey. Efficient induction of extrinsic cell death by dandelion root extract in human chronic myelomonocytic leukemia (CMML) cells; Plos One, 2012. doi: 10.1371/journal.pone.0030604.
http://www.ncbi.nlm.nih.gov/pubmed/22363452

330. P. Ovadje et al. Selective induction of apoptosis and autophagy through treatment with dandelion root extract in human pancreatic cancer cells; Oct. 2012. doi: 10.1097/MPA.0b013e31824b22a2.
http://www.ncbi.nlm.nih.gov/pubmed/22647733

331. A. Rodriguez-Casado. The Health Potential of Fruits and Vegetables Phytochemicals: Notable Examples; Critical Reviews in Food Science and Nutrition, 5/18/2016. PMID: 25225771.
http://www.ncbi.nlm.nih.gov/pubmed/25225771

332. L. Al-Anati et al. Silibinin protects OTA-mediated TNF-α release from perfused rat livers and isolated rat Kupffer cells; Molecular Nutrition & Food Research, 1/20/2009. doi: 10.1002/mnfr.200800110.
https://www.ncbi.nlm.nih.gov/pubmed/19156713

333. R. Jayaraj et al. Hepatoprotective efficacy of certain flavonoids against microcystin induced toxicity in mice; Environmental Toxicology, Oct. 2007. doi: 10.1002/tox.20283.
http://onlinelibrary.wiley.com/doi/10.1002/tox.20283/abstract

334. P.R. Davis-Searles et al. Milk Thistle and Prostate Cancer: Differential Effects of Pure Flavonolignans from Silybum marianum on Antiproliferative End Points in Human Prostate Carcinoma Cells; Cancer Research, 5/15/2005. doi: 10.1158/0008-5472.CAN-04-4662.
http://cancerres.aacrjournals.org/content/65/10/4448.full

335. J. Bosch-Barrera et al. Response of brain metastasis from lung cancer patients to an oral nutraceutical product containing silibinin; Oncotarget, 3/3/2016. doi: 10.18632/oncotarget.7900.
http://www.ncbi.nlm.nih.gov/pubmed/26959886

336. C. Tilley et al. Silibinin and its 2,3-dehydro-derivative inhibit basal cell carcinoma growth via suppression of mitogenic signaling and transcription factors activation; Molecular Carcinogenesis, Jan 2016. doi: 10.1002/mc.22253. http://www.ncbi.nlm.nih.gov/pubmed/25492239

337. J.K. Mastron, K.S. Siveen, G. Sethi, A. Bishayee. Silymarin and hepatocellular carcinoma: a systematic, comprehensive, and critical review; Anti-Cancer Drugs, June 2015. doi: 10.1097/CAD.0000000000000211.
http://www.ncbi.nlm.nih.gov/pubmed/25603021

338. N. Ben Rahal, F.J. Barba, D. Barth, I. Chevalot. Supercritical CO_2 extraction of oil, fatty acids and flavonolignans from milk thistle seeds: Evaluation of their antioxidant and cytotoxic activities in Caco-2 cells; Food and Chemical Toxicology, Sep. 2015. doi: 10.1016/j.fct.2015.07.006.
http://www.ncbi.nlm.nih.gov/pubmed/26172510

339. H.J. Ting et al. Silibinin prevents prostate cancer cell-mediated differentiation of naïve fibroblasts into cancer-associated fibroblast phenotype by targeting TGF β2; Molecular Carcinogenesis, Sep. 2015. doi: 10.1002/mc.22135. http://www.ncbi.nlm.nih.gov/pubmed/24615813

340. K. Jiang et al. Silibinin, a natural flavonoid, induces autophagy via ROS-dependent mitochondrial dysfunction and loss of ATP involving BNIP3 in human MCF7 breast cancer cells; Oncology Reports, June 2015. doi: 10.3892/or.2015.3915. http://www.ncbi.nlm.nih.gov/pubmed/25891311

341. M.B. Pirouzpanah et al. Silibilin-induces apoptosis in breast cancer cells by modulating p53, p21, Bak and Bcl-XL pathways; Asian Pacific Journal of Cancer Prevention, 2015. PMID: 25773855.
http://www.ncbi.nlm.nih.gov/pubmed/25773855

342. F. Li et al. Autophagy induction by silibinin positively contributes to its anti-metastatic capacity via AMPK/mTOR pathway in renal cell carcinoma; International Journal of Molecular Sciences, 4/15/2015. doi: 10.3390/ijms16048415. http://www.ncbi.nlm.nih.gov/pubmed/25884331

343. L. Fan et al. Silymarin induces cell cycle arrest and apoptosis in ovarian cancer cells; European Journal of Pharmacology, 11/15/2014. doi: 10.1016/j.ejphar.2014.09.019. http://www.ncbi.nlm.nih.gov/pubmed/25242120

344. E.N. Simsek, T. Uysal. In vitro investigation of cytotoxic and apoptotic effects of Cynara L. species in colorectal cancer cells; Asian Pacific Journal of Cancer Prevention, Nov. 2013, Vol. 14, Issue 11, P. 6791-6795. PMID: 24377607 . https://www.ncbi.nlm.nih.gov/pubmed/24377607

345. C. Pulito et al. Cynara scolymus affects malignant pleural mesothelioma by promoting apoptosis and restraining invasion; Oncotarget, 7/20/2015. doi: 10.18632/oncotarget.4017. https://www.ncbi.nlm.nih.gov/pubmed/26136339

346. A.M. Mileo et al. Long Term Exposure to Polyphenols of Artichoke (Cynara scolymus L.) Exerts Induction of Senescence Driven Growth Arrest in the MDA-MB231 Human Breast Cancer Cell Line; Oxidative Medicine and Cellular Longevity, Vol. 2015, Article ID 363827. doi: 10.1155/2015/363827. https://www.hindawi.com/journals/omcl/2015/363827/

347. A.M. Mileo et al. Artichoke polyphenols induce apoptosis and decrease the invasive potential of the human breast cancer cell line MDA-MB231; Journal of Cellular Physiology, Sep. 2012. doi: 10.1002/jcp.24029. https://www.ncbi.nlm.nih.gov/pubmed/22170094

348. C. Pereira et al. New insights into the effects of formulation type and compositional mixtures on the antioxidant and cytotoxic activities of dietary supplements based-on hepatoprotective plants; Food & Function, Sept. 2014. doi: 10.1039/c4fo00387j. https://www.ncbi.nlm.nih.gov/pubmed/25089364

349. N.M. Kogan. Cannabinoids and cancer; Mini Reviews in Medicinal Chemistry, Oct. 2005. PMID: 16250836. http://www.ncbi.nlm.nih.gov/pubmed/16250836

350. Marijuana Saves Father's Son (video clip from documentary "The culture high"); YouTube. https://www.youtube.com/watch?v=6XDcsnxrX0g&feature=youtu.be

351. Medical Marijuana Helps My Son With Rare Disease (video); FOX 11 Los Angeles - YouTube. https://www.youtube.com/watch?v=fOa_2Bc-lfY&feature=youtu.be

352. David Bearman, M.D. Cannabis, Cannabinoids - ADD, Tourette's Syndrome, Migraines (video); YouTube. https://www.youtube.com/watch?v=TTeagW1XONI

353. N.M. Kogan, R. Mechoulam. Cannabinoids in health and disease; Dialogues in Clinical Neuroscience, Dec. 2007. PMCID: PMC3202504. http://www.ncbi.nlm.nih.gov/pmc/articles/PMC3202504/#__ffn_sectitle

354. A. Vaccani et al. Cannabidiol inhibits human glioma cell migration through a cannabinoid receptor-independent mechanism; British Journal of Pharmacology, 2/7/2005. doi: 10.1038/sj.bjp.0706134. http://www.ncbi.nlm.nih.gov/pmc/articles/PMC1576089/

355. E. Cudaback, W. Marrs, T. Moeller, N. Stella. The expression level of CB1 and CB2 receptors determines their efficacy at inducing apoptosis in astrocytomas; Plos One, 1/14/2010. doi: 10.1371/journal.pone.0008702. http://www.ncbi.nlm.nih.gov/pubmed/20090845

356. M.A. Friedman. In vivo effects of cannabinoids on macromolecular biosynthesis in Lewis lung carcinomas; Cancer Biochemistry Biophysics, 1977. PMID: 616322. http://www.ncbi.nlm.nih.gov/pubmed/616322

357. S. Jones, J. Howl. Cannabinoid receptor systems: therapeutic targets for tumour intervention; Expert Opinion on Therapeutic Targets, Dec. 2003. doi: 10.1517/14728222.7.6.749.
http://www.ncbi.nlm.nih.gov/pubmed/14640910

358. M. Schley et al. Predominant CB2 receptor expression in endothelial cells of glioblastoma in humans; Brain Research Bulletin, 6/30/2009. doi: 10.1016/j.brainresbull.2009.01.011.
http://www.ncbi.nlm.nih.gov/pubmed/19480992

359. G. Velasco et al. Hypothesis: cannabinoid therapy for the treatment of gliomas?; Neuropharmacology, Spt. 2004. doi: 10.1016/j.neuropharm.2004.04.016.
http://www.ncbi.nlm.nih.gov/pubmed/15275820

360. M.L. López-Rodríguez et al. Involvement of cannabinoids in cellular proliferation; Mini Reviews in Medicinal Chemistry, Jan 2005. PMID: 15638794. http://www.ncbi.nlm.nih.gov/pubmed/15638794

361. A. Carracedo et al. Cannabinoids induce apoptosis of pancreatic tumor cells via endoplasmic reticulum stress-related genes; Cancer Research, 7/1/2006. doi: 10.1158/0008-5472.CAN-06-0169.
http://www.ncbi.nlm.nih.gov/pubmed/16818650

362. G. Velasco et al. Cannabinoids and gliomas; Molecular Neurobiology, Aug. 2007. doi: 10.1007/s12035-007-0002-5.
http://www.ncbi.nlm.nih.gov/pubmed/17952650

363. M.L. De Jesús et al. Opposite changes in cannabinoid CB1 and CB2 receptor expression in human gliomas; Neurochemistry International, May-Jun 2010. doi: 10.1016/j.neuint.2010.03.007.
http://www.ncbi.nlm.nih.gov/pubmed/20307616

364. A. Carracedo et al. The stress-regulated protein p8 mediates cannabinoid-induced apoptosis of tumor cells; Cancer Cell, Apr. 2006. doi: 10.1016/j.ccr.2006.03.005. http://www.cell.com/cancer-cell/fulltext/S1535-6108(06)00085-7

365. B. Herrera et al. The CB2 cannabinoid receptor signals apoptosis via ceramide-dependent activation of the mitochondrial intrinsic pathway; Experimental Cell Research, 7/1/2006. doi: 10.1016/j.yexcr.2006.03.009. http://www.ncbi.nlm.nih.gov/pubmed/16624285

366. I. Galve-Roperh et al. Anti-tumoral action of cannabinoids: involvement of sustained ceramide accumulation and extracellular signal-regulated kinase activation; Nature Medicine, Mar. 2000. doi: 10.1038/73171.
http://www.ncbi.nlm.nih.gov/pubmed/10700234

367. C. Blázquez et al. Down-regulation of tissue inhibitor of metalloproteinases-1 in gliomas: a new marker of cannabinoid antitumoral activity?; Neuropharmacology, Jan. 2008. doi: 10.1016/j.neuropharm.2007.06.021. http://www.ncbi.nlm.nih.gov/pubmed/17675107

368. P. Massi et al. Antitumor effects of cannabidiol, a nonpsychoactive cannabinoid, on human glioma cell lines; Pharmacology & Experimental Therapeutics, Mar. 2004. doi: 10.1124/jpet.103.061002. http://www.ncbi.nlm.nih.gov/pubmed/14617682

369. M. Bifulco, C. Laezza, P. Gazzerro, F. Pentimalli. Endocannabinoids as emerging suppressors of angiogenesis and tumor invasion (review); Oncology Reports, Apt. 2007. PMID: 17342320. http://www.ncbi.nlm.nih.gov/pubmed/17342320

370. M.M. Caffarel et al. Delta9-tetrahydrocannabinol inhibits cell cycle progression in human breast cancer cells through Cdc2 regulation; Cancer Research, 7/1/2006. doi: 10.1158/0008-5472.CAN-05-4566. http://www.ncbi.nlm.nih.gov/pubmed/16818634

371. F. Grotenhermen. Pharmacokinetics and pharmacodynamics of cannabinoids; Clinical Pharmacokinetics, 2003. doi: 10.2165/00003088-200342040-00003. http://www.ncbi.nlm.nih.gov/pubmed/12648025

372. M. Solinas et al. Cannabidiol inhibits angiogenesis by multiple mechanisms; British Journal of Pharmacology, Nov. 2012. doi: 10.1111/j.1476-5381.2012.02050.x. http://www.ncbi.nlm.nih.gov/pubmed/22624859

373. T. Fisher et al. In vitro and in vivo efficacy of non-psychoactive cannabidiol in neuroblastoma; Current Oncology, Mar. 2016. doi: 10.3747/co.23.2893. http://www.ncbi.nlm.nih.gov/pubmed/27022310

374. M. Nikan, S.M. Nabavi, A. Manayi. Ligands for cannabinoid receptors, promising anticancer agents; Life Sciences, 2/1/2016. doi: 10.1016/j.lfs.2015.12.053. http://www.ncbi.nlm.nih.gov/pubmed/26764235

375. S.D. McAllister, L. Soroceanu, P.Y. Desprez. The Antitumor Activity of Plant-Derived Non-Psychoactive Cannabinoids; J Neuroimmune Pharmacology, Jun. 2015. doi: 10.1007/s11481-015-9608-y. https://www.ncbi.nlm.nih.gov/pmc/articles/PMC4470774/

376. G. Aviello et al. Chemopreventive effect of the non-psychotropic phytocannabinoid cannabidiol on experimental colon cancer; Journal of Molecular Medicine (Berlin, Germany), Aug 2012. doi: 10.1007/s00109-011-0856-x. http://www.ncbi.nlm.nih.gov/pubmed/22231745

377. A. Greenhough, H.A. Patsos, A.C. Williams, C. Paraskeva. The cannabinoid delta(9)-tetrahydrocannabinol inhibits RAS-MAPK and PI3K-AKT survival signalling and induces BAD-mediated apoptosis in colorectal cancer cells; Int'l J. of Cancer, 11/15/2007. doi: 10.1002/ijc.22917. http://www.ncbi.nlm.nih.gov/pubmed/17583570

378. F. Borrelli et al. Colon carcinogenesis is inhibited by the TRPM8 antagonist cannabigerol, a Cannabis-derived non-psychotropic cannabinoid; Carcinogenesis, Dec. 2014. doi: 10.1093/carcin/bgu205. http://www.ncbi.nlm.nih.gov/pubmed/25269802

379. B. Romano et al. Inhibition of colon carcinogenesis by a standardized Cannabis sativa extract with high content of cannabidiol; Phytomedicine, 4/15/2014. doi: 10.1016/j.phymed.2013.11.006. http://www.ncbi.nlm.nih.gov/pubmed/24373545

380. C. Sánchez et al. Inhibition of glioma growth in vivo by selective activation of the CB(2) cannabinoid receptor; Cancer Research, 8/1/2001. PMID: 11479216. http://www.ncbi.nlm.nih.gov/pubmed/11479216

381. S. Torres et al. A combined preclinical therapy of cannabinoids and temozolomide against glioma; Molecular Cancer Therapeutics, Jan. 2011. doi: 10.1158/1535-7163.MCT-10-0688. http://www.ncbi.nlm.nih.gov/pubmed/21220494?dopt=Abstract

382. M. Solinas et al. Cannabidiol, a non-psychoactive cannabinoid compound, inhibits proliferation and invasion in U87-MG and T98G glioma cells through a multitarget effect; Plos One, 10/21/2013. doi: 10.1371/journal.pone.0076918. http://www.ncbi.nlm.nih.gov/pubmed/24204703

383. P. Massi et al. Antitumor effects of cannabidiol, a nonpsychoactive cannabinoid, on human glioma cell lines; J of Pharmacology and Experimental Therapeutics, Mar. 2004. doi: 10.1124/jpet.103.061002. http://www.ncbi.nlm.nih.gov/pubmed/14617682

384. P. Massi et al. 5-Lipoxygenase and anandamide hydrolase (FAAH) mediate the antitumor activity of cannabidiol, a non-psychoactive cannabinoid; Journal of Neurochemistry, Feb. 2008. doi: 10.1111/j.1471-4159.2007.05073.x. http://www.ncbi.nlm.nih.gov/pubmed/18028339

385. A. Vaccani et al. Cannabidiol inhibits human glioma cell migration through a cannabinoid receptor-independent mechanism; British J. of Pharmacology, Apr. 2005. doi: 10.1038/sj.bjp.0706134. http://www.ncbi.nlm.nih.gov/pubmed/15700028

386. M. Solinas et al. Cannabidiol, a Non-Psychoactive Cannabinoid Compound, Inhibits Proliferation and Invasion in U87-MG and T98G Glioma Cells through a Multitarget Effect; Plos One, 10/21/2013. doi: 10.1371/journal.pone.0076918. http://journals.plos.org/plosone/article?id=10.1371/journal.pone.0076918

387. L. Soroceanu et al. Id-1 Is a Key Transcriptional Regulator of Glioblastoma Aggressiveness and a Novel Therapeutic Target; Cancer Research, 3/1/2013. doi: 10.1158/0008-5472.CAN-12-1943. http://cancerres.aacrjournals.org/content/73/5/1559

388. C. Blázquez et al. Inhibition of tumor angiogenesis by cannabinoids; FACEB J., Mar. 2003. doi: 10.1096/fj.02-0795fje. http://www.ncbi.nlm.nih.gov/pubmed/12514108

389. C. Blázquez et al. Cannabinoids inhibit the vascular endothelial growth factor pathway in gliomas; Cancer Research, 8/15/2004. doi: 10.1158/0008-5472.CAN-03-3927. http://cancerres.aacrjournals.org/content/64/16/5617.long

390. J.P. Marcu et al. Cannabidiol enhances the inhibitory effects of delta9-tetrahydrocannabinol on human glioblastoma cell proliferation and survival; Molecular Cancer Therapeutics, Jan. 2010. doi: 10.1158/1535-7163.MCT-09-0407. http://mct.aacrjournals.org/content/9/1/180.long

391. G. Velasco et al. Cannabinoids and gliomas; Molecular Neurobiology, Aug.
2007. doi: 10.1007/s12035-007-0002-5.
http://www.ncbi.nlm.nih.gov/pubmed/17952650

392. C. Sánchez et al. Delta9-tetrahydrocannabinol induces apoptosis in C6
glioma cells; FEBS Letters, 9/25/1998. doi: 10.1016/S0014-5793(98)01085-0.
http://onlinelibrary.wiley.com/doi/10.1016/S0014-5793(98)01085-0/full

393. C. Blázquez et al. Cannabinoids inhibit glioma cell invasion by downregulating matrix metalloproteinase-2 expression; Cancer Research,
3/15/2008. doi: 10.1158/0008-5472.CAN-07-5176.
http://cancerres.aacrjournals.org/content/68/6/1945.long

394. M. Salazar et al. Cannabinoid action induces autophagy-mediated cell
death through stimulation of ER stress in human glioma cells; The Journal
of Clinical Investigation, May 2009. doi: 10.1172/JCI37948.
https://www.ncbi.nlm.nih.gov/pmc/articles/PMC2673842/

395. T. Aguado et al. Cannabinoids induce glioma stem-like cell differentiation
and inhibit gliomagenesis; The Journal of Biological Chemistry, 3/2/2007.
doi: 10.1074/jbc.M608900200. http://www.jbc.org/content/282/9/6854.long

396. T. Gómez del Pulgar et al. De novo-synthesized ceramide is involved in
cannabinoid-induced apoptosis; The Biochemical Journal, 4/1/2002. doi:
10.1042/bj3630183. http://www.biochemj.org/content/363/1/183.long

397. P. Massi et al. The non-psychoactive cannabidiol triggers caspase activation
and oxidative stress in human glioma cells; Cellular & Molecular Life
Sciences, Sep. 2006. doi: 10.1007/s00018-006-6156-x.
http://www.ncbi.nlm.nih.gov/pubmed/16909207

398. D. Parolaro, P. Massi. Cannabinoids as potential new therapy for the
treatment of gliomas; Expert Review of Neurotherapeutics, Jan. 2008. doi:
10.1586/14737175.8.1.37. http://www.ncbi.nlm.nih.gov/pubmed/18088200

399. S.D. McAllister et al. Pathways mediating the effects of cannabidiol on the
reduction of breast cancer cell proliferation, invasion, and metastasis; Breast
Cancer Research & Treatment, Aug. 2011. doi: 10.1007/s10549-010-1177-4.
https://www.ncbi.nlm.nih.gov/pmc/articles/PMC3410650/

400. S.D. McAllister et al. Cannabidiol as a novel inhibitor of Id-1 gene
expression in aggressive breast cancer cells; Molecular Cancer Therapeutics,
Nov. 2007. doi: 10.1158/1535-7163.MCT-07-0371.
http://mct.aacrjournals.org/content/6/11/2921.long

401. M.W. Nasser et al. Crosstalk between chemokine receptor CXCR4 and
cannabinoid receptor CB2 in modulating breast cancer growth and invasion;
PLOS One, 2011. doi: 10.1371/journal.pone.0023901.
https://www.ncbi.nlm.nih.gov/pmc/articles/PMC3168464/

402. M.M. Caffarel et al. Cannabinoids: a new hope for breast cancer therapy?;
Cancer Treatment Reviews, Nov. 2012. doi: 10.1016/j.ctrv.2012.06.005.
http://www.ncbi.nlm.nih.gov/pubmed/22776349

403. M.M. Caffarel et al. JunD is involved in the antiproliferative effect of
Delta9-tetrahydrocannabinol on human breast cancer cells; Oncogene,
8/28/2008. doi: 10.1038/onc.2008.145.
http://www.nature.com/onc/journal/v27/n37/full/onc2008145a.html

404. A. Ligresti et al. Antitumor activity of plant cannabinoids with emphasis on the effect of cannabidiol on human breast carcinoma; J. Pharmacology & Experimental Therapeutics, Sep. 2006. doi: 10.1124/jpet.106.105247. http://jpet.aspetjournals.org/content/318/3/1375.long

405. A. Shrivastava, P.M. Kuzontkoski, J.E. Groopman, A. Prasad. Cannabidiol induces programmed cell death in breast cancer cells by coordinating the cross-talk between apoptosis and autophagy; Molecular Cancer Therapeutics, Jul. 2011. doi: 10.1158/1535-7163.MCT-10-1100. http://mct.aacrjournals.org/content/10/7/1161.long

406. M. Haustein, R. Ramer, M. Linnebacher, K. Manda, B. Hinz. Cannabinoids increase lung cancer cell lysis by lymphokine-activated killer cells via upregulation of ICAM-1; Biochemical Pharmacology, 11/15/2014. doi: 10.1016/j.bcp.2014.07.014. http://www.ncbi.nlm.nih.gov/pubmed/25069049

407. R. Ramer et al. Cannabidiol inhibits lung cancer cell invasion and metastasis via intercellular adhesion molecule-1; FASEB J., Apr. 2012. doi: 10.1096/fj.11-198184.

408. L. De Petrocellis et al. Non-THC cannabinoids inhibit prostate carcinoma growth in vitro and in vivo: pro-apoptotic effects and underlying mechanisms; British Journal of Pharmacology, Jan. 2013. doi: 10.1111/j.1476-5381.2012.02027.x. https://www.ncbi.nlm.nih.gov/pmc/articles/PMC3570006/

409. L. Ruiz, Miguel, I. Díaz-Laviada. Delta9-tetrahydrocannabinol induces apoptosis in human prostate PC-3 cells via a receptor-independent mechanism; FEBS Letters, 11/24/1999. doi: 10.1016/S0014-5793(99)01073-X. http://onlinelibrary.wiley.com/doi/10.1016/S0014-5793(99)01073-X/full

410. R.J. McKallip et al. Targeting CB2 cannabinoid receptors as a novel therapy to treat malignant lymphoblastic disease; Blood, 7/15/2002. doi: 10.1182/blood-2002-01-0098. http://www.bloodjournal.org/content/100/2/627.long?sso-checked=true

411. R.J. McKallip et al. Cannabidiol-induced apoptosis in human leukemia cells: A novel role of cannabidiol in the regulation of p22phox and Nox4 expression; Molecular Pharmacology, Sep. 2006. doi: 10.1124/mol.106.023937. http://molpharm.aspetjournals.org/content/70/3/897.long

412. C. Lombard, M. Nagarkatti, P.S. Nagarkatti. Targeting cannabinoid receptors to treat leukemia: role of cross-talk between extrinsic and intrinsic pathways in Delta9-tetrahydrocannabinol (THC)-induced apoptosis of Jurkat cells; Leukemia Research, Aug. 2005. doi: 10.1016/j.leukres.2005.01.014. http://www.ncbi.nlm.nih.gov/pubmed/15978942

413. T. Powles et al. Cannabis-induced cytotoxicity in leukemic cell lines: the role of the cannabinoid receptors and the MAPK pathway; Blood, 2/1/2005. doi: 10.1182/blood-2004-03-1182. http://www.bloodjournal.org/content/105/3/1214.long?sso-checked=true

414. D. Vara et al. Anti-tumoral action of cannabinoids on hepatocellular carcinoma: role of AMPK-dependent activation of autophagy; Cell Death & Differentiation, Jul 2011. doi: 10.1038/cdd.2011.32. https://www.ncbi.nlm.nih.gov/pmc/articles/PMC3131949/

415. M. Guzmán, C. Sánchez, I. Galve-Roperh. Control of the cell survival/death decision by cannabinoids; J. Mol. Med. (Berlin, Germany), 2001. PMID: 11269508. http://www.ncbi.nlm.nih.gov/pubmed/11269508

416. M. Guzmán. Effects on cell viability; Handbook of Experimental Pharmacology, 2005. PMID: 16596790.
http://www.ncbi.nlm.nih.gov/pubmed/16596790

417. C.Y. Lee et al. A comparative study on cannabidiol-induced apoptosis in murine thymocytes and EL-4 thymoma cells; Int'l Immunopharmacology, May 2008. doi: 10.1016/j.intimp.2008.01.018.
http://www.ncbi.nlm.nih.gov/pubmed/18387516

418. S. Leelawat, K. Leelawat, S. Narong, O. Matangkasombut. The dual effects of delta(9)-tetrahydrocannabinol on cholangiocarcinoma cells: anti-invasion activity at low concentration and apoptosis induction at high concentration; Cancer Investigation, May 2010. doi: 10.3109/07357900903405934.
http://www.ncbi.nlm.nih.gov/pubmed/19916793

419. V.M. Pushkarev, O.I. Kovzun, M.D. Tronko. Antineoplastic and apoptotic effects of cannabinoids. N-acylethanolamines: protectors or killers?; Experimental Oncology, Mar. 2008. PMID: 18438336.
http://www.ncbi.nlm.nih.gov/pubmed/18438336

420. A. Athanasiou et al. Cannabinoid receptor agonists are mitochondrial inhibitors: a unified hypothesis of how cannabinoids modulate mitochondrial function and induce cell death; Biochem Biophys Res Commun., 12/7/2007. doi: 10.1016/j.bbrc.2007.09.107.
http://www.ncbi.nlm.nih.gov/pubmed/17931597

421. A.A. Izzo, M. Camilleri. Cannabinoids in intestinal inflammation and cancer; Pharmacological Research, Aug. 2009. doi: 10.1016/j.phrs.2009.03.008. http://www.ncbi.nlm.nih.gov/pubmed/19442536

422. N.M. Kogan et al. HU-331, a novel cannabinoid-based anticancer topoisomerase II inhibitor; Molecular Cancer Therapeutics, Jan. 2007. doi: 10.1158/1535-7163.MCT-06-0039.
http://mct.aacrjournals.org/content/6/1/173.long

423. M. Guzmán et al. A pilot clinical study of Delta9-tetrahydrocannabinol in patients with recurrent glioblastoma multiforme; British Journal of Cancer, 7/17/2006. doi: 10.1038/sj.bjc.6603236.
http://www.nature.com/bjc/journal/v95/n2/full/6603236a.html

424. I.W.Y Mak, N. Evaniew, M. Ghert. Lost in translation: animal models and clinical trials in cancer treatment; American Journal of Translational Research, 1/15/2014. PMC3902221.
http://www.ncbi.nlm.nih.gov/pmc/articles/PMC3902221/?report=classic

425. "Report of Partial Findings from the National Toxicology Program Carcinogenesis Studies of Cell Phone Radiofrequency Radiation in Hsd: Sprague Dawley® SD rats (Whole Body Exposures)"; NTP, Draft 5/19/2016. doi: 10.1101/055699.
http://biorxiv.org/content/biorxiv/early/2016/05/26/055699.full.pdf

426. "Cell Phone Radiation Boosts Cancer Rates in Animals; $25 Million NTP Study Finds Brain Tumors"; Microwave News, 5/25/2016.
http://microwavenews.com/news-center/ntp-cancer-results

427. IARC classifies radiofrequency electromagnetic fields as possibly carcinogenic to humans; IARC press release No. 208, 5/31/2011. http://www.iarc.fr/en/media-centre/pr/2011/pdfs/pr208_E.pdf

428. L. Frassetto et al., Diet, evolution and aging--the pathophysiologic effects of the post-agricultural inversion of the potassium-to-sodium and base-to-chloride ratios in the human diet; European Journal of Nutrition, Oct. 2001. PMID: 11842945. http://www.ncbi.nlm.nih.gov/pubmed/11842945

429. D.I. Abrams et al. Milking the Evidence: Diet Does Matter; Journal of Clinical Oncology, 8/1/2014. doi: 0.1200/JCO.2014.56.629. http://jco.ascopubs.org/content/32/22/2290.full.pdf+html

430. F.I. Arnaldez, L.J. Helman. Targeting the insulin growth factor receptor 1; Hematology/Oncology Clinics of North America, June 2012. doi: 10.1016/j.hoc.2012.01.004. http://www.ncbi.nlm.nih.gov/pubmed/22520978

431. Y. Yang, D. Yee. Targeting Insulin and Insulin-Like Growth Factor Signaling in Breast Cancer; Journal of Mammary Gland Biology and Neoplasia, Dec. 2012. doi:10.1007/s10911-012-9268-y. http://link.springer.com/article/10.1007%2Fs10911-012-9268-y

432. S. Mamur at al., Does potassium sorbate induce genotoxic or mutagenic effects in lymphocytes?; Toxicology in Vitro, Apr. 2010. doi: 10.1016/j.tiv.2009.12.021. http://www.sciencedirect.com/science/article/pii/S0887233309003853

433. K. Kitano et al., Mutagenicity and DNA-damaging activity caused by decomposed products of potassium sorbate reacting with ascorbic acid in the presence of Fe salt; Food and Chemical Toxicology, Nov. 2002. doi: 10.1016/S0278-6915(02)00119-9. http://www.sciencedirect.com/science/article/pii/S0278691502001199

434. The Effect of pH on Potassium Sorbate Effectiveness; Hawkins Watts, 9/7/2009. http://www.hawkinswatts.com/documents/The%20Effect%20of%20pH%20on%20Potassium%20Sorbate%20Effectiveness.pdf

435. Alice G. Walton. How Much Sugar Are Americans Eating? [Infographic]; Forbes, 8/30/2012. http://www.forbes.com/sites/alicegwalton/2012/08/30/how-much-sugar-are-americans-eating-infographic/#db241621f718

436. S. Walker-Samuel et al. In vivo imaging of glucose uptake and metabolism in tumors; Nature Medicine, 2013. doi:10.1038/nm.3252. http://www.nature.com/nm/journal/v19/n8/full/nm.3252.html?message-global=remove

437. Dr. Mercola. 5 Things I Wish All Women Knew About Mammograms; healthy holistic living. http://www.healthy-holistic-living.com/5-things-wish-women-knew-mammograms.html

438. A Akpan, R Morgan. Oral candidiasis (Review); Postgraduate Medical Journal, 2002. doi: 10.1136/pmj.78.922.455. http://pmj.bmj.com/content/78/922/455

439. A. Ramirez-Garcia et al. Candida albicans and cancer: Can this yeast induce cancer development or progression?; Critical Reviews in Microbiology, 2016. doi: 10.3109/1040841X.2014.913004. http://www.ncbi.nlm.nih.gov/pubmed/24963692

440. Dr. Carolyn Dean, MD, ND. Yeast and Inflammation; Total Health and Longevity Magazine Sept 2006.
http://www.drcarolyndean.com/articles_yeast_and_inflame.html

441. IARC strengthens its findings on several carcinogenic personal habits and household exposures; IARC press release No. 196, 11/2/2009.
http://www.iarc.fr/en/media-centre/pr/2009/pdfs/pr196_E.pdf

442. P. Quillin. Cancer's Sweet Tooth; Mercola.com, from the April 2000 issue of Nutrition Science News.
http://www.mercola.com/article/sugar/sugar_cancer.htm

443. Alpha 101 Ketones. Alpha Health Products.
http://alphahealth.ca/pages/alpha-101-ketones

444. M.B. Frank et at. Frankincense oil derived from Boswellia carteri induces tumor cell specific cytotoxicity; MBC Complementary & Alternative Medicine, 3/18/2009. doi: 10.1186/1472-6882-9-6.
https://www.ncbi.nlm.nih.gov/pmc/articles/PMC2664784/

445. M.G. Dozmorov et al. Differential effects of selective frankincense (Ru Xiang) essential oil versus non-selective sandalwood (Tan Xiang) essential oil on cultured bladder cancer cells: a microarray and bioinformatics study; Chinese Medicine, 7/2/2014.
    doi: 10.1186/1749-8546-9-18.
    https://www.ncbi.nlm.nih.gov/pmc/articles/PMC4086286/

446. T. Ranjbarnejad et al. Methanolic extract of Boswellia serrata exhibits anti-cancer activities by targeting microsomal prostaglandin E synthase-1 in human colon cancer cells; Prostaglandins & Other Lipid Mediators, Vol. 131, July 2017, Pg. 1-8. doi: 10.1016/j.prostaglandins.2017.05.003.
https://www.ncbi.nlm.nih.gov/pubmed/28549801

447. C. Schmidt et al. Acetyl-lupeolic acid inhibits Akt signaling and induces apoptosis in chemoresistant prostate cancer cells in vitro and in vivo; Oncotarget, 7/8/2017. doi: 10.18632/oncotarget.19101.
https://www.ncbi.nlm.nih.gov/pubmed/28723662

448. M.A. Khan et al. Pharmacological evidences for cytotoxic and antitumor properties of Boswellic acids from Boswellia serrata; Journal of Ethnopharmacology, 9/15/2016, Vol. 191, Pg. 315-323. doi: 10.1016/j.jep.2016.06.053. https://www.ncbi.nlm.nih.gov/pubmed/27346540

449. A.A. Bhat et al. Potential therapeutic targets of Guggulsterone in cancer; Nutrition & Metabolism, Vol. 14, 2017. doi: 10.1186/s12986-017-0180-8.
https://www.ncbi.nlm.nih.gov/pmc/articles/PMC5331628/

450. Nagalase in Blood; European Laboratory of Nutrients, Health Diagnostics and Research Institute. http://www.hdri-usa.com/tests/nagalase/

451. C. Sobolewski et al. The Role of Cyclooxygenase-2 in Cell Proliferation and Cell Death in Human Malignancies; International Journal of Cell Biology, Vol. 2010. doi: 10.1155/2010/215158.
https://www.hindawi.com/journals/ijcb/2010/215158/

452. C. Sobolewski et al. The Role of Cyclooxygenase-2 in Cell Proliferation and Cell Death in Human Malignancies; International Journal of Cell Biology, Vol. 2010, Article ID 215158.
doi: 10.1155/2010/215158.
https://www.hindawi.com/journals/ijcb/2010/215158/

453. Mark F. McCarty. Minimizing the cancer-promotional activity of cox-2 as a central strategy in cancer prevention; Medical Hypotheses, Jan. 2012, Vol. 78, Issue 1, pp 45-57. doi: 10.1016/j.mehy.2011.09.039. http://www.medical-hypotheses.com/article/S0306-9877(11)00492-0/fulltext

454. S. Rinelli et al. Circulating Salicylic Acid and Metabolic and Inflammatory Responses after Fruit Ingestion; Plant Foods for Human Nutrition, Mar. 2012, Vol. 67, Issue 1, pp 100-104.
doi: 10.1007/s11130-012-0282-4.
https://link.springer.com/article/10.1007/s11130-012-0282-4

455. J.R. Paterson et al. Salicylic Acid Content of Spices and Its Implications; J. of Agricultural and Food Chemistry, 3/21/2006.
doi: 10.1021/jf058158w.
http://pubs.acs.org/doi/abs/10.1021/jf058158w?journalCode=jafcau

456. A. Wood et al. A systematic review of salicylates in foods: Estimated daily intake of a Scottish population; Molecular Nutrition & Food Research, 2/23/2011. doi: 10.1002/mnfr.201000408.
http://onlinelibrary.wiley.com/doi/10.1002/mnfr.201000408/abstract

457. U.S. Judge Finds Medical Group Conspired Against Chiropractors; The New York Times, 8/29/1987. http://www.nytimes.com/1987/08/29/us/us-judge-finds-medical-group-conspired-against-chiropractors.html

458. Full text of "Fitzgerald Report To Congress CANCER"; Internet Archive.
https://archive.org/stream/FitzgeraldReportToCongressCANCER/fitzgerald%20report%20to%20congress%20CANCER_djvu.txt

459. 1953 Fitzgerald Report - Suppressed Cancer Treatments; Chris Gupta Share The Wealth, 4/3/2007.
http://www.newmediaexplorer.org/chris/2007/04/03/1953_fitzgerald_report_suppressed_cancer_treatments.htm

460. Vagbhat. Astanga Hridaya Sutra Sthan; Page 344. http://ayur-veda.guru/books/astanga-hridaya-sutrasthan-handbook-pdf.pdf

461. I.F. Robey, L.A. Nesbit. Investigating Mechanisms of Alkalinization for Reducing Primary Breast Tumor Invasion; BioMed Research International Vol. 2013. doi: 10.1155/2013/485196.
https://www.hindawi.com/journals/bmri/2013/485196/

462. I.F. Robey et al. Bicarbonate Increases Tumor pH and Inhibits Spontaneous Metastases; Cancer Research, March 2009, Vol. 69, Issue 6. doi: 10.1158/0008-5472.CAN-07-5575.
http://cancerres.aacrjournals.org/content/69/6/2260.full

463. I.O. Farah et al. Assessing the survival of MRC5 and a549 cell lines upon exposure to pyruvic Acid, sodium citrate and sodium bicarbonate - biomed 2013, Biomedical Sciences Instrumentation, 2013. PMID: 23686189.
https://www.ncbi.nlm.nih.gov/pubmed/?term=23686189

464. Documentary - "Cancer - The Forbidden Cures".
https://www.youtube.com/watch?v=gWLrfNJICeM

465. Gerson Institute; Dr. Max Gerson. https://gerson.org/gerpress/dr-max-gerson/

466. N.S. Rizzo et al. Nutrient Profiles of Vegetarian and Non Vegetarian Dietary Patterns; Journal of the Academy of Nutrition and Dietetics, 8/27/2013. doi: 10.1016/j.jand.2013.06.349.
https://www.ncbi.nlm.nih.gov/pmc/articles/PMC4081456/

467. R.L. Veech. The therapeutic implications of ketone bodies: the effects of ketone bodies in pathological conditions: ketosis, ketogenic diet, redox states, insulin resistance, and mitochondrial metabolism; Prostaglandins Leukotrienes, and Essential Fatty Acids, March 2004. doi: 10.1016/j.plefa.2003.09.007.
https://www.ncbi.nlm.nih.gov/pubmed/14769489

468. Mike Vrentas, ICRF. Budwig Diet Protocol; July 24, 2017.
https://www.cancertutor.com/budwig/

469. A. Dikshi, K. Hales, D.B. Hales. Whole flaxseed diet alters estrogen metabolism to promote 2-methoxtestradiol-induced apoptosis in hen ovarian cancer; The Journal of Nutritional Biochemistry, Apr. 2017. doi: 10.1016/j.jnutbio.2017.01.002.
https://www.ncbi.nlm.nih.gov/pubmed/28178600

470. A.V. Mali et al. Enterolactone Suppresses Proliferation, Migration and Metastasis of MDA-MB-231 Breast Cancer Cells Through Inhibition of uPA Induced Plasmin Activation and MMPs-Mediated ECM Remodeling; Asian Pacific Journal of Cancer Prevention, 4/1/2017. doi: 10.22034/APJCP.2017.18.4.905. http://journal.waocp.org/article_45886.html

471. S. Chikara et al. Enterolactone Induces G1-phase Cell Cycle Arrest in Nonsmall Cell Lung Cancer Cells by Downregulating Cyclins and Cyclin-dependent Kinases; Nutrition and Cancer, May-June 2017. doi: 10.1080/01635581.2017.1296169.
https://www.ncbi.nlm.nih.gov/pmc/articles/PMC5500210/

472. M.V. Varghese et al. Attenuation of arsenic trioxide induced cardiotoxicity through flaxseed oil in experimental rats; Redox Report, 2/17/2017. doi: 10.1080/13510002.2017.1289313.
https://www.ncbi.nlm.nih.gov/pubmed/28209094

473. International Cyanide Management Code For the Gold Mining Industry.
http://www.cyanidecode.org/cyanide-facts/environmental-health-effects

474. History of the Enema and Frequently Asked Questions; Lavage Wellness Center. http://lavagewellness.com/files/LavageWellness_FAQs.pdf

475. Betsy S. Exton, MA, Advanced Certified I-ACT Colon Hydrotherapist.
http://pureonmain.com/betsy-exton/

476. Dean Ornish. Changing Your Lifestyle Can Change Your Genes; Newsweek, 6/16/2008. http://www.newsweek.com/changing-your-lifestyle-can-change-your-genes-91323

477. Dean Ornish et al. Changes in prostate gene expression in men undergoing an intensive nutrition and lifestyle intervention; PNAS, 6/17/2008. doi: 10.1073/pnas.080308010. http://www.pnas.org/content/105/24/8369.full.pdf

478. Jill Sakai. Study reveals gene expression changes with meditation; University of Wisconsin - Madison News, 12/4/2013.
http://news.wisc.edu/study-reveals-gene-expression-changes-with-meditation/

479. H. Strasburger, B. Waldvogel. Sight and blindness in the same person: Gating in the visual system; PsyCh Journal, 10/15/2015. doi: 10.1002/pchj.109. http://onlinelibrary.wiley.com/doi/10.1002/pchj.109/full

480. Chia-Wei Cheng et al. Prolonged Fasting reduces IGF-1/PKA to promote hematopoietic stem cell-based regeneration and reverse immunosuppression; Cell Stem Cell, 6/5/2014. doi: 10.1016/j.stem.2014.04.014. https://www.ncbi.nlm.nih.gov/pmc/articles/PMC4102383/

481. Suzanne Wu. Fasting triggers stem cell regeneration of damaged, old immune system; USC News, 6/5/2014. https://news.usc.edu/63669/fasting-triggers-stem-cell-regeneration-of-damaged-old-immune-system/

482. F.M. Sacks et al. AHA Presidential Advisory: Dietary Fats and Cardiovascular Disease: A Presidential Advisory From the American Heart Association; Circulation, 6/15/2017. doi: 10.1161/CIR.0000000000000510. http://circ.ahajournals.org/content/early/2017/06/15/CIR.0000000000000510

483. Creative Commons. https://creativecommons.org/licenses/by-sa/3.0/

9 781979 637527